MW00775511

PSYCHOTHERAPY AS RELIGION

Psychotherapy as Religion

The Civil Divine in America

WILLIAM M. EPSTEIN

University of Nevada Press ▲▲ Reno & Las Vegas

University of Nevada Press, Reno, Nevada 89557 USA
Copyright © 2006 by University of Nevada Press
Manufactured in the United States of America
Library of Congress Cataloging-in-Publication Data
Epstein, William M., 1944–
Psychotherapy as religion : the civil divine in America /
William M. Epstein.
p. cm.
Includes bibliographical references and index.
ISBN-13: 978-0-87417-678-0 (hardcover : alk. paper)
ISBN-10: 0-87417-678-6 (hardcover : alk. paper)
1. Psychotherapy—Social aspects. 2. Clinical psychotherapy—
Social aspects. I. Title.
RC480.E67 2006
616.89′14—dc22   2006000847
The paper used in this book meets the requirements of American
National Standard for Information Sciences—Permanence of
Paper for Printed Library Materials, ANSI z.48-1984. Binding
materials were selected for strength and durability.

FIRST PRINTING

15   14   13   12   11   10   09   08   07   06
5   4   3   2   1

I do not like thee Dr. Fell,
The reason why I can now tell.

CONTENTS

Psychotherapy in America is immensely popular but consistently ineffective. It persists because it reaffirms basic American values of self-sufficiency and individualism. Rather than a successful clinical practice of psychic, emotional, and mental healing, psychotherapy is a civil religion—a social and political fable. From the perspective of those with material needs for housing, income, family, education, and so forth, psychotherapy is a form of denial.

Psychotherapy has always been ineffective as a solution to personal and social problems. Yet it has perfused the activities and disciplines of the American welfare state—social work, counseling, public administration, and management—frequently justifying their core interventive strategies. Psychotherapy has provided much of the language of modern understanding, ritualizing strongly held, widely shared national values. It creates the corrective myths that enforce the national credo of social efficiency, the notion that any approach to a social problem must be politically feasible, that is, relatively inexpensive and socially compatible. Psychotherapy is best understood as a pseudoscience and a cultural institution rather than as a scientifically credible clinical discipline.

Psychotherapy is an excuse to explore the curiosity of social belief through a cultural institution, but the more general goal is to raise issue with many other social structures, examining the processes that create social authority. Taking the convenience of its long popularity in the Western world and the United States in particular, psychotherapy is a fertile area in which to consider the contemporary dynamics of ideology. No attempt is made to be comprehensive or to provide an exhaustive compendium of research or treatment. Nevertheless, a large amount of the field's most scientifically credible and current research is analyzed in order to underscore its clinical ineffectiveness, a precondition for considering its social meaning. Indeed, there would be little to explore if psychic cure was the routine result of clinical practice. It is the very absence of a true clinical role that occasions the broader exploration of its popularity as social ideology.

Psychotherapy is a ceremony of cultural belief that pantomimes concrete production functions, its scholars mimicking a truly scientific community of researchers. Despite its apparent organization and provenance in medical schools and other disciplines that claim a scientific clinical base, the field is symbolic, a political institution of social preferences, rather than substantive.

In the face of recurring doubts about effectiveness, psychotherapists often fall back on the excuse that they practice an art form; yet they do not look to aesthetics for collegial testimonials from painters, dancers, writers, and singers. Rather, they invoke the findings of standard scientific methodologies in defense of their practice. At least they try to.

In order to explore the social meaning of psychotherapy, the argument proceeds by first prying the fingers of belief off of the credibility of the field's experimental literature. There is an absence of any rational, that is, scientific, evidence that psychotherapy can cure, prevent, or rehabilitate. Deprived of rationality and a recourse to scientific practice, psychotherapy's persistence and meaning become more believable as a wonderment of culture.

Naive choice, made by a nation that does not know any better than to seek help from therapists, may perhaps be a reasonable explanation under the duress of imperfect and incomplete information. However, it does not explain psychotherapy's persistence, since the problems of the field's literature are obvious and widely discussed at least within the technical research community. On the contrary, in spite of its inadequacies the culture sustains psychotherapeutic practice. But why? The answers, drawn from prevailing social preferences and institutions, are necessarily speculative. Yet the field cannot turn back to any credible evidence that it provides effective assistance to individuals with mental and emotional problems as a way to explain its popularity. As that evidence does not exist, something else must be going on.

Psychotherapy is a typical instance of the manner in which social institutions develop as generalized adaptations to social belief streaming through inchoate culture rather than as planned or even reasoned responses to articulated social goals, as monuments to the coherence of a conscious will. Other related social institutions, notably the social services, serve similar functions, heavy on ceremony and light on substance. They are the live melodramas, cautionary tales, and fables of America's social ethos, the ceremonies and rituals of civil religion.

The literature of psychotherapy is immense and could not be read through in four lifetimes. Indeed, each year the field creates another lifetime of literature. Thus a highly selective search strategy is necessary in order to make any statement about even a small portion of the field. The subsequent comments about the effectiveness of psychotherapy rely upon the best evaluative research that appeared during the past decade or so in the most rigorous, influential journals. Studies were considered if they addressed effectiveness, employed a randomized controlled design, and appeared in one of the field's three top journals: the *American Journal of Psychiatry*, the *Archives of General Psychiatry*, and the *Journal of Consulting and Clinical Psychology*. In addition, the three therapies that are specifically discussed in separate chapters—psychodynamic psychotherapy, behavioral therapy, and cognitive-behavioral therapy—are the most frequently employed therapeutic orientations (Norcross, Karg, and Prochaska, 1997).

The social sciences' evaluation skills have overtaken implicit, idiosyncratic tests of program outcomes, porous, unreliable measures, and inadequately controlled experiments. However, credible research methods continue to be routinely defied in psychotherapy research. There has been little progress in reported outcomes or methods since *The Illusion of Psychotherapy* (1995), which covered the field's claims to effective clinical practice before 1990. Psychotherapeutic intervention has not demonstrated any benefit to any patient group under any circumstances. Moreover, the denial of systematic evaluation calls attention to flagging professional will, occupational resistance, and most important, subtle social motives that block accountability.

In any enterprise that invokes science in order to establish its authority, the responsibility rests with the new treatment, invention, or product to prove effectiveness and safety; the burden of proof rests with the engineer, the physician, the drug maker, and the psychotherapist. As a scientific enterprise, psychotherapy clearly carries the burden of its clinical ambitions to certify the achievement of its clinical goals—cure, prevention, and rehabilitation. Just as clearly, the burden has been shifted by cultural influences to the shoulders of the skeptic. The long-standing tolerance for the ambiguities of psychotherapy's outcomes speaks volumes about social attitudes, about the quiet but deep meaning of psychotherapy in the United States as a secular religion—a social ideology and a series of rituals that justify and dramatize embedded culture preferences. Its performance as civil religion supplants its apparent clinical activities. Thus the criticism of psychotherapy is transformed into a criticism of American values and is only coincidentally a comment on its ability to treat emotional and mental illness. In this way too, the insistence on evidence of effectiveness to evaluate psychotherapeutic practice becomes the novelty that needs justification for displacing a comfortable social institution, an acceptable way for Americans to go about being American. But this logic turns science and clinical accountability on its head, replacing knowledge with faith and objective proof with social satisfaction.

A social role that is rationally false can be culturally true. The paradox is perhaps resolved in the Enlightenment hope for social progress: that the rigors of knowing are not antithetical to feeling but rather shape experience; that rationality, however difficult, is a tolerably beneficial ideal. Psychotherapy has not pursued these goals despite the avalanche of its humanistic pretensions and the rehearsed genuineness and practiced spontaneity of its practitioners.

To the contrary, psychotherapy is a Romantic denial of reality that in its most common expression realizes the dominant preferences of contemporary society. Postmodernism won out in psychotherapy without a struggle. Psychotherapeutic practice is benign during benign times and predatory when culture turns a more solemn face to social and personal need.

While the heroic ideals of individuality and extreme personal responsibility dominate psychotherapy, there are many alternative theories of treatment—and nuances even within heroic therapies—and perhaps too, many patients who have enjoyed more communal, accepting, realistic, and less doctrinaire experiences. Still, heroic individualism dominates practice and explains the persistence of psychotherapy as America's civil religion. Psychotherapy promotes creativity as a heroic form rather than as a personal one; it stigmatizes deviance; and most profoundly, it substitutes an implicit dialogue of scolding and guilt for more concrete communal provisions for people in distress. The rarest therapist ever references basic deprivations—material insufficiencies—as a precondition for more philosophical reflections on being; indeed, overcoming great deprivation is part of the heroic myth and a fair target for therapy itself. The rarest therapist ever concedes that the psychological discussion is little more than ontological speculation, a dialectic of personal behavior and moral expectation that is probably unrelated to any behavior change within the limits of the clinic.

The present argument does not discuss drug therapy in its own terms, although the research that is reviewed often includes pharmacotherapy as an experimental condition. Medication represents perhaps the cheapest and least disruptive intervention to change behavior: as a pill, it is the reality of which psychotherapy is only the metaphor. However, drug therapy fails as satisfying social ritual; it is too clinical and antiseptic, without much educational opportunity for social drama or narrative. The complexity of pharmacological interventions for behavioral change requires a separate analysis of the many methodological pitfalls of the pill trials, their side effects, the professional and ethical dilemmas of practice, and the philosophical challenges presented by medical responses to personal deviance, which may be as political and social as they are psychiatric.

Following the introduction, chapters 1 through 4 document the consistent inability of the recent clinical literature of depression, anxiety, eating disorders, the addictions, and other disorders to certify any benefit resulting from psychotherapy. These chapters reinterpret the research as fables, little morality tales of social instruction. Chapter 5 discusses the problems of the measurement instruments and their uncertain achievement of the most fundamental requirement of scientific research: reliable measurement of the phenomena being studied. Chapter 6 elaborates the social role of psycho-therapy and the clinical vehicle—the therapeutic relationship—by which psychotherapy seems to create false evidence. Chapters 7 through 9 interpret the three dominant forms of psychotherapy—psychodynamic psychotherapy, behavioral therapy, and cognitive-behavioral therapy—as civil religion.

The final chapter extends the role of psychotherapy as civil religion to its broader social and political meaning, its consistency with American social welfare policy and the traditional American preference for classical liberalism. American religion, like classical liberalism, is bedeviled by a contradiction, namely the problem of civil virtue emerging from personal greed. Heroic individualism is ironic and contradictory, since heroic action is predicated on sacrifice for the community, not the self-absorption of individuals. America's civil religion—in its ideal of heroic individualism, which gives purpose to psychotherapy—may be promoting the very problems of maladaptation and unhappiness that both the civil religion and psychotherapy profess to handle. The cure may be a cause of the disease.

ACKNOWLEDGMENTS

The only way to make an impression with a book is to write a five pounder and drop it on selected heads, from great heights and repeatedly. The potential damage of this light volume is humble in spite of the encouragement and assistance of many: Denis Boyles, Kristin Brown, Kathleen Bergquist, Carole Case, Trishul Devineni, Tana Dineen, Ralph Dippner, Robert Dippner, Paul Epstein, Ronald Farrell, Howard Karger, Jamie Kelly, Arnold Lazarus, Duncan Lindsey, Brij Mohan, Paul Moloney, Leroy Pelton, Jonathan Reader, Jessica Rohac, Albert Roberts, Jerry Rubin, Linda Santangelo, David Smail, David Stoesz, E. Fuller Torrey, Ysela Tellez, Joanne Thompson. Despite threat of litigation by the jealous, the errors are mine, all mine.

Introduction

If only it were possible for troubled people to find relief through the wisdom of personal disclosure and guided insight. Unfortunately, psychotherapy is not effective and probably cannot be. The histories of psychotherapy, written as though with each succeeding chapter the doors into bliss, understanding, and self-awareness opened a bit wider, are unintentionally grim and determined narratives of denial, mystification, and professional ambition (Dryden, 1996; Bankart, 1997; Jackson, 1999). They flaunt science and accountable clinical practice.

Prominent recent histories of psychotherapy are celebratory. From Freedheim's (1992) anthology of prominent therapists and researchers:

> Psychotherapists have become first and foremost doctors of the psychological interior (p. 5). The need for psychological services continues. In fact, the demand for psychological services has steadily increased over the last 40 years as the public has grown to understand psychological and behavioral problems and to accept the provision of psychotherapeutic care (p. 97). During the last half of the present century, psychotherapy has grown from a narrow medical specialty to a welter of activities to ameliorate, if not to resolve, a number of psychiatric disorders as well as the gamut of problems that are grouped under the heading of "problems in living" (p. 307). The scientific study of psychotherapy by empirical methods has emerged as an enterprise of considerable magnitude and sophistication (p. 308). In its short history, psychotherapy has played an important role in acquiring insight into and providing relief from the complexity of our lives (p. 897).

From Ward (2002): "Psychologists and their knowledge were not just relegated to laboratories or universities but were present in schools, corporations, courtrooms, disaster sciences, marriage retreats, talk shows, as well as in abstentia in self-help books, personality measures, intelligence tests and codes of civility" (p. 221).

From Stone (1997) in concluding his elaborate history of psychiatry: "For the personality disorders or for the many persons whose personalities have been damaged . . . , these people, along with the even greater number of those whose lives have been adversely affected by the early loss of a parent, by ineffective though not cruel parenting, by entrapment in ungratifying marital or other relationships, by the loss of trust and faith in humankind (however this may come about)—all these people will continue to need individual or group psychotherapy" (p. 428).

Perhaps 250,000 therapists treat tens of millions of people each year (Freedheim, 1992, p. 97). Yet the central meaning of psychotherapy extends beyond its direct practice in psychiatry, psychology, social work, the ministry, and education. It pervades the culture; it provides the language by which at least Americans communicate with each other. It is an institution of the nation's values. However, psychotherapy persists because of its cultural role; its clinical role has failed. Psychotherapy only has social meaning; its pervasiveness is explained not by what it does with patients in the clinic but rather by its ideological content—its affirmation of central social values, notably a misguided sense of individualism that is disingenuously heroic and that may be socially destructive.

Wittgenstein (1980) found exactly the right words for modern psychotherapy: "Psychological concepts are just everyday concepts. They are not concepts newly fashioned by science for its own purpose, as are the concepts of physics and chemistry. Psychological concepts are related to those of the exact sciences as the concepts of the science of medicine are to those of old women who spend their time nursing the sick" (p. 12e).

The absence of any scientifically credible grounds on which to accept the effectiveness of psychotherapy poses a challenge.[1] Deprived of a clinical role, why does psychotherapy persist? Is its endurance and success simply a result of conspiratorial silence and ignorance, or is it possible that the field fulfills a nonclinical role?

Psychotherapy and Pseudoscience

The field is enamored of the belief that real psychotherapies accept real clinical science, while fake psychotherapies employ pseudoscience. In fact the entire field is pseudoscientific and best understood as an elaborate mysticism only differentiated from frank religion, even its crackpot fringes, by a seemingly modern orientation and the cant of science.

Lilienfeld, Lynn, and Lohr's (2003) contributors spent considerable energy sorting through psychotherapy to distinguish the authentic from the contrived. In the end they failed. Without credible tests of the effects of its interventions and, to a great extent, because of the persistence of this failure, psychotherapy remains pseudoscientific. The community of its researchers has failed to pursue credible methodologies and credible measures or to appropriately and fully apply current methods. Thus the research is pseudoscientific both because of its tolerance for technical pitfalls and, perhaps more importantly, because the society seems not to demand better. Psychotherapy as pseudoscience has enjoyed a social sanction.

Lilienfeld et al. (2003) clearly identified the characteristics—"subjective and unreliable methods" (p. xiii)—that define pseudoscientific clinical interventions such as thought field therapy, facilitated communication, critical incident stress debriefing, rebirthing, and many others. They lamented the weak claims of these practitioners to successful treatment. "Many of the people making these claims were psychiatrists and clinical psychologists, along with social workers and generic 'psychotherapists' who had taken a weekend course somewhere. . . . Had no one taught them about control groups, memory, child development, the limitations of hypnosis?" (pp. xiii–xiv).

Yet the curious distinction between psychological scientists who presumably abide by science and the many clinicians who ignore the research and practice pseudoscientific therapy does not hold up in practice itself. The failure of the best of the research to adopt scientific procedures drops all of psychotherapy into the realm of the pseudoscientific. The difference is one of style, not substance, as the researchers create belief through disingenuous mimicking of credible science and the clinicians get by with novel clinical enthusiasms. The researchers are high church, practicing the arcane rituals of a distorted science—the mystifications of statistics and scientific method; the practitioners are low church, inducing faith in the immediacy of therapeutic evidence that has still to achieve scientific probity.

All the authors in Lilienfeld et al. (2003) argued that it is possible to identify "mental health claims with and without adequate empirical support," but adequate empirical support does not exist. Better said, what is adequate for the clinician does not constitute credible evidence of effectiveness. At best there are therapies that have not been tested and therapies that have been very inadequately tested. "We believe that the preceding chapters have made clear that the scientific underpinnings of the field of clinical psychology are threatened by the increasing proliferation of unsubstantiated and untested psychotherapeutic, assessment, and diagnostic techniques" (p. 461). They concluded with a call for psychological organizations to impose sanctions for practices that are not empirically supported. However, none of their evidence constitutes "empirically supported treatments." Empirically based practice cannot exist without credible empiricism. The gestures of empiricism, the manners of science, the rituals of rationality are not enough. Some treatments enjoy a consensus of support among researchers—cognitive-behavioral therapy, behavioral therapy, psychodynamic therapy—and some do not. Rather than the issue of rigorous testing, what "we believe" has become central to the field.

The high-church contributors to Lilienfeld et al. (2003), employed in academia to train conventional practitioners and conduct research, were protecting their franchises from the low-church fringes, a posture of reasonability and taste suffering vulgar enthusiasms. Yet again, approved clinical techniques are not separated from the pseudoscientific by credible scientific evidence; conventional practice is protecting itself from novel practice but without credible clinical science. The meaning of the field is derived not from objective evidence of effectiveness but from the preferences of the culture—a sociological marvel rather than a clinical one. Indeed, without a tested clinical role, the persistence of psychotherapy must be explained by nonclinical factors, its activities in forming and sustaining central cultural values.

Psychotherapy has not immunized itself by credible research against the biting criticisms that rationality makes of cultural fraud. Park's (2000) notion of voodoo science, Gardner's (1952) pseudoscientific fads and fallacies, the idea of clinical "know-nothings" (Hunt, 1999), and particularly Frank's (1974) affection for nonspecific effects—a true mysticism of human motivation softened into placebo effects—apply equally to psychotherapy and the frankly crackpot, such as space abductions, flying saucers, psionics and perpetual-motion machines, power lines causing cancer, the transmigration of souls and reincarnation, "natural" and alternative medicines, sleep learning, and many other whimsies. The distinction between the strangely novel and psychotherapy is one of familiarity and social acceptance, not of clinically proven effectiveness. Psychotherapy has been institutionalized by citizen satisfaction, but not because of a clinical utility demonstrated through credible science. Alternative medicine is alternative because of its use of pseudoscience. Psychotherapy is mainstream culture, not mainstream clinical science.

Psychotherapy has not been scrutinized with the same thoroughness as the nineteenth century's enthusiasms of mind and body cures. Perhaps the broad cultural devotion to psychotherapy has limited the criticisms, paying tribute to Gardner's observation that the present time is even more adamantly superstitious than the nineteenth century. In fact, Christian Science practice is a near twin of cognitive-behavioral therapy, and Madame Blavatsky gives Freud a run for his money in the hidden realm of human motivation and wisdom. Science has rarely impeded social mood, personal choice, or individual behavior.

Knowing and believing are not the same. Rationality only exists in the most limited and narrow spheres of the American culture. Psychotherapy is an expression of nonrational urges, a memorial to social ingenuity that creates and affirms belief in socially acceptable forms. Yet despite its pretenses to rationality, psychotherapy ironically serves to convert the rational (science) into the irrational (belief), the clinical into the social, the impulse for change into the strictures of adaptation, and the novel into the conventional. Psychotherapy is a metaphysic and a civil religion rather than a clinical expression of scientific treatment.

Illusion and Myth:
Psychotherapy as a Prototypical American Religion

Psychotherapy's reliance on belief, the power of self-invention through the expectancies of the patient, is so central that illusion has literally become reality in many therapies. The therapist assists the patient to contrive a satisfying series of illusions. "Illusions about oneself and one's world are part of normal development and are necessary for emotional survival . . . the loss of these illusions in the harsh light of reality requires a psychological negotiation" (Teitelbaum, 1999, p. xiii). Yet the forms of illusion are not innocent and unique inventions of creative minds but rather the prescribed devices of socialization. Illusions animate the roles people perform in society. Belief, as it shares common themes, constitutes a society's cohesive values, expressing themselves in shared fables, myths, folklore, and the other forms of communication that justify a society to its members. The pattern of belief affirming moral and ethical choices constitutes a religion, and in the case of psychotherapy, a civil religion propagated to affirm the American society.

The social preferences of psychotherapy, its normative content, have been frequently noticed in the field yet almost invariably as an aside. It is rare for any thoughtful commentator to ignore the degree to which the process of psychotherapy communicates social preferences. But the normative, cultural dependency of psychotherapy is subsumed under the larger issue of clinical treatment: cure, prevention, and rehabilitation. However, without credible evidence of effectiveness, the clinical role evaporates and the social role takes center stage. If illusions promote psychic ease and improve social functioning, then they may confer a direct benefit on the patient. However, illusions may be contrived simply to increase the degree of social cohesion by employing the patient in a morality play of deviance, penance, and rebirth. In this case the society itself rather than the patient becomes the audience for therapy, and clinical outcomes are less important than social acceptance of the values that are affirmed. The illusion for the patient may be the reward for participation. Still, in the end, illusion may be a problematic palliative that puts off a salubrious reckoning with reality.

Metaphors of religion and allusions to psychotherapy's near religious content have been occasionally applied to psychotherapy. Notably Szasz (1974,

1978) but also Frank (1974), Stone (1997), and others have explained the field's activities by falling back on religious parallels. However, none of the parallels actually took the step of identifying psychotherapy as a real religion with the same structural and functional capacities as the more standard types. At most, Frank and Stone identified the supposedly curative effects of talk therapy as being essentially religious, that is, a function of belief. Moreover, psychotherapy is past the cult stage; it is institutionalized and accepted within the normal processes of propagating belief. Put another way, psychotherapeutic wisdom is as standard as Christian theology. Indeed, they may both elaborate the same tradition and underlying impetus.

Szasz reserved some legitimate preserve for psychotherapy, insisting that the field frequently achieves treatment goals. Yet he deplored the inflation of its application to a variety of human conditions that come down to "the perennial interests and institutions of mankind—sex and significance, power and prestige, race, religion, and the family" (1978, p. 206). In this sense religion is employed to deflate some of the scientific pretensions of the field and thus reduce its authority to circumscribe the rights of patients. Szasz saw psychotherapy as a negotiation between the mental patient and those he disturbs, granting great influence to the therapist as arbiter and mediator of social values. However, his insistence on the therapeutic exchange itself depresses the wider significance of psychotherapy as a morality that emphasizes the message to the audience rather the actual outcomes of therapy for the patient. Szasz's religion of psychotherapy is more normative, that is, more value laden than institutionalized. For Szasz, psychotherapy is *like* a religion rather than actually *being* a religion, although a civil one without any necessary god-based content. Yet in the end, Szasz accepted the effectiveness of psychotherapy, its "healing words," despite the absence of credible evidence to support this claim.

Frank (1974) elaborated the priest role in psychotherapy, drawing an exact parallel between the shaman and the therapist. The therapist's ability to induce patient belief explained cure. These expectancies of patient and therapist (and possibly too, the informal, supportive expectancies of the culture) probably define placebo effects. The field has made much of the curative value of belief while avoiding many of its implications. The cultivation of patient belief may not require highly trained and highly paid practitioners but only the common pressures of peer group, social authority, and family. Moreover, placebo effects are probably transitory, as are most of the therapeutic outcomes in the literature. In fact, placebo effects destroy nearly the entire superstructure of psychotherapeutic metaphysics relating to the causes and cures of mental and emotional conditions; the conditions of belief are deeply embedded in culture and are probably not amenable to clinical manipulation. In short, if placebos account for clinical effects, they do so without the provenance, authority, rare skills, or insights of psychotherapy.

Psychotherapy propagates the same values that Bloom (1992) placed at the core of the American religion, notably individualism and a gnomic form of belief. In fact, psychotherapy is itself progeny of those values rather than a scientifically revealed truth that confers an obvious benefit on humankind like the virtues of the automobile, antibiotics, or reinforced concrete. However, psychotherapy is an extreme, heroic form of individualism and relies on a stunning belief in perception's triumph over reality. Indeed, an impoverished culture would not have the wealth to block the intrusions of economic necessity nor the comfort and ease to indulge heroic fantasies.

Psychotherapy fits easily into the traditions of radical self-reliance characteristic of dominant American religions while mirroring the enthusiasms of many American sects, notably Christian Science. Indeed, psychotherapy is also akin to the native superstitions of alternative cures and spiritualism in the manner of Madame Blavatsky. Its style, however, is distinct. In keeping with the symbolism of current authority, psychotherapy fashions itself as scientific, thoughtful, prudent, and humane. Characteristically, the American credo defines responsibility as essentially individual rather than social; truth is certified by personal experience that confers mystical certainty; chosenness or salvation proceeds from these unique values and this knowledge. Indeed, psychological chosenness as the sense of heroic personal destiny and the potential of the individual for creativity and great achievement mirrors the patriotic belief in American exceptionalism—a "manifest destiny" reiterated through the past few centuries in politics as well as the arts and reinforced with the emergence of the United States as the world's sole superpower. In a nutshell, psychotherapy is not at all independent of culture. It should come as no surprise that a central institution of American socialization reflects central American values. The field's intellectual autonomy—its scientific objectivity and neutrality—is imaginary, even fanciful.

Thus psychotherapy includes all the structural characteristics of standard religion except a specific god, although it still derives authority from gnomic, that is, mystical and untestable sources. It has a dogma that explains reality and even creation (developmental stages), a sense of proper behavior (adult autonomy and personal responsibility) and improper behavior (deviance, mental illness, self-defeating behavior), centers for the study of its religious phenomena (university-based training programs, public and private funding institutions), a clergy (therapists), and, perhaps most important, values and beliefs that mirror general social preferences. Psychotherapy has conducted a very successful missionary outreach, enjoying a huge number of communicants and deep cultural acceptance. There is little exaggeration in pointing to its profound penetration of common discourse, the immense degree to which America is the psychological society.

However, the professional claims of psychotherapy rest on evidence that it can predictably handle its defining conditions, mental illness and emotional disorders, not simply on its communicants' feeling better after chatting about themselves for a few hours. If placebo effects largely set the limits on psychotherapy's effectiveness, then the field is reduced to the common banalities and truisms of human discourse: it is nice to be nice. As distinct from an entertainment measured directly by customer satisfaction, psychotherapy as a professional, scientific intervention is held to credible demonstrations of predictable and efficient (in the sense of both social and clinical value) abilities to resolve the problems of mental and emotional distress.

Psychotherapy is one of the many institutions that patrol the boundaries of America's embedded beliefs. Indeed, without a demonstrable clinical role, that is all that therapy does. In fact, the broad social tolerance for the weak and distorted clinical proofs of psychotherapy—the political satisfaction with therapy as a programmatic strategy for handling personal and social problems and the social satisfaction with therapy as a personal intervention—testifies to the embedded, accepted, sanctioned role of psychotherapy as a civil religion, an institutionalized series of social norms and social habits that are expressed in the rituals and ceremonies of American culture to sustain its social structures.

The Critiques of Psychotherapy:
A Scholarship of the Tentative and Beholden

The enormous literature of psychotherapy, routinely insisting on important progress against personal and social problems, is only dotted with occasional disclaimers. However, even the critical work is rarely trenchant or comprehensive; it customarily handles only a particular technique, a single school of intervention, or an isolated ethical issue of practice. Indeed, only recently did Freudian psychoanalysis come into disrepute, while many neo-Freudians still enjoy large practices and considerable prestige as psychic healers. Even the most thoroughgoing criticisms of the field hold out for some form of psychotherapy. Moreover, the criticisms almost invariably emerge from within the field and largely accept the notion that the clinical role is psychotherapy's principle function. Only passing reference is made to the possibility that psychotherapy is sustained by nonclinical considerations, that it acts as a moral guide or a religion. Still, its sociological meaning is customarily added on to its clinical meaning. The overwhelming proportion of the vast psychotherapeutic literature offers itself in testimony to the effectiveness of psychotherapy in handling emotional, mental, and psychic problems.

Yet none of the testimony is credible, and few if any of the criticisms reflect the near universal failure of any form of psychotherapy to cure, prevent, or rehabilitate. The curiosity of a deeply popular, institutionalized social activity, devoid of an ability to fulfill its ostensible goals, draws attention to its symbolism—its significance beyond clinical functions.

After nearly a century of popularity, Freudian theory and practice were finally debunked by profound criticisms that were curiously isolated from psychotherapy itself. Popper (1962) insisted that Freud's psychoanalytic theory immunized itself from empirical testing through hermetic predictions. As one example of hermetic logic, the unconscious plays a central role in Freud's theory of motivation but it cannot be explored directly, only through its putative effects. Consequently, behavior can always be attributed to hidden, untestable motives, while motives that do not eventuate in behavior can be attributed to repression into the unconscious. Thus no evidence disconfirms Freudian theory of the unconscious, which in a scientific sense then becomes meaningless.

Grunbaum (1984, 1993) disputed Popper, insisting that Freudian theory did in fact lead to meaningful assertions amenable to testing but that the psychotherapeutic community had failed in its duty to apply randomized controlled trials, which were required to test the effectiveness of any form of psychotherapy.

The encyclopedic MacMillan (1991), with added flourishes by Crews (1993), and the work of Dufresne (2000, 2003), Masson (1988), and Jurjevich (1974) have unmasked the pretensions of the Freudian legacy. They have extended the criticism of Freudian theory as untestable and untested to every corner of practice: its immorality, its assault on individualism and autonomy, its "corrosion of civilized values" (Jurjevitch, 1974, p. 128), its pseudoscientific procedures, the falsity of its assumptions, and even, but only occasionally, its clinical failure. Indeed, Macmillan's massive tome only devotes six pages to the outcome research, the issue of whether "psychoanalysis is effective as a therapy" (pp. 555–561). Yet curiously, much of the criticism of Freudian psychoanalysis, notably including that of Macmillan, concedes its effectiveness at least in part and takes it to task on other grounds. Moreover, only a few of Freud's critics extend their comments to other therapies (for example, Masson has extended his comments on Freudian analysis to family therapy, gestalt therapy, feminist therapy, and a number of other marginal practices). Yet even the critics frequently rely on case studies—evidence from the couch—rather than objective and systematic data.

The broader criticisms of contemporary psychotherapy have been similarly cautious, incomplete, and tenuous. The critics' book titles usually promise more than their arguments deliver. Indeed, they are often the work of psychotherapy's loyalists, arguing for their own schools; rarely do they deeply question the field's abilities. Dawes (1994) shrewdly promised an iconoclastic analysis in naming his book *House of Cards* but then went on to insist that "psychotherapy works," although he argued that advanced degrees and highly credentialed practitioners are not necessary for successful treatment (p. 73). He built an argument for differential treatment—particular interventions for particular problems—on the extant literature of the field but acknowledged that "success in therapy is far from assured, even though it works overall in a statistical sense" (ibid.). Still, he largely accepted the scientific credibility of the literature.

The basis for Dawes's optimism derived from his analysis of outcomes (Landman and Dawes, 1982), which he claimed sustains Smith and Glass's classic defense of psychotherapy (Smith and Glass, 1977; Smith, Glass, and Miller, 1980). In fact, it does the reverse, highlighting the protectiveness and introversion of even the field's self-proclaimed critics.

Landman and Dawes (1982) reanalyzed a sample of the controlled studies that Smith et al. (1980) included in their analysis. Landman and Dawes found that psychotherapy research consistently supports the effectiveness of treatment, conferring a net improvement of 14 percentage points on treated patients over placebo control patients. In an earlier and complete reanalysis of Smith et al.'s (1980) controlled studies, Prioleau, Murdock, and Brody (1983) reported a net improvement of only 6 percentage points. Epstein (1984a, 1984b) estimated the net improvement within the logic of Smith et al. to be 10 percentage points, although still unadjusted by estimates of obvious expectancy effects and measurement biases. Lambert, Weber, and Sykes (1993) estimated that placebo effects amounted to about 16 percentage-point improvement above the mean of untreated control groups (about .42 effect size) and suggested, perhaps with the driest humor, that randomized controls were unnecessary; experimental outcomes should simply be discounted by the estimate of placebo effects.

In the end then, Dawes (1994) fails as a critic and even as a protector of psychotherapy's effectiveness. The amount of reported benefits of psychotherapy over placebo controls—whether 6 or even as much as 14 percentage points—is still very small, especially since the estimates are inflated by the likely biases of even the best research. Indeed, reasonable adjustments for probable biases, substantially reducing the reported effectiveness of treatment, begin to suggest that psychotherapy may be not just ineffective but routinely harmful. To make much of these small, unadjusted effects is to apply the rosiest eye to interpretations of questionable data.

In fact, Smith et al. (1980), who initiated the popularity of metanalysis, employed many dubious practices in selecting studies for inclusion and then analyzing them. They pointedly included very weak research rather than living up to their own commitment to the canons of science. Only a small minority of the included research was relatively rigorous. Most of the studies employed analogue patients rather than those with actual clinical problems; most lacked true controls and even more lacked placebo controls; measurement was suspect, reactive, and often unreliable. Moreover, they employed a series of statistical summaries that greatly understate the true variability of outcomes.[2] To justify casting a wide net of inclusion, they undercut their stated dedication to rigorous clinical science, ridiculing randomized controlled trials as "'textbook' standards; these methodological rules, learned as dicta in graduate school and regarded as the touchstone of publishable articles in prestigious journals, were applied arbitrarily; for example, note again Rachman's high-handed dismissal on methodological grounds of study after study of psychotherapy outcome" (p. 38). Thus their professed commitment to include only "controlled studies of effectiveness" came to also encompass research that employed uncontrolled pre-post comparisons and nonrandomized comparison groups. Smith et al. (1980) was a gloss on the effectiveness of psychotherapy, a booster's enthusiasm but hardly credible analysis.

Other critics take to task only a small portion of the field or a single school of treatment, reserving praise for their own clinical orientations. Stuart (1973) touted behavioral treatments at the expense of psychodynamic forms. Pope (1997), Loftus and Ketcham (1994), and Dineen (1996) argued forcefully against the factual validity of patient self-reports, pointing to the tragic possibilities of patients' creating memories of events that never took place. Yet they accepted the general effectiveness of treatment.

Zilbergeld's (1983) wonderfully rich discussion of therapy and its failures still insisted that practice is effective—perhaps cognitive therapy for depression and behavioral therapy for a variety of phobias. Similarly, Szasz (1974, 1978), Dryden and Feltham (1992), Gross (1978), and Eysenck (1965) criticized a portion of the field but retained a general loyalty to the therapeutic process. Even Masson (1988) can be read not so much as an indictment of psychotherapy for being ineffective but rather as a political commentary on the costs of its success: it is effective in an inhumane way that undercuts personal expression, freedom, and individual growth. Psychotherapy is not adequately revolutionary for his tastes.

It is curious that except for the rarest critic such as Eisner (2000), the arguments are hermeneutic—analyses of texts and counterproofs that accept the logic of case examples—rather than scientific. However, even Eisner (2002) frequently admires research that is in fact seriously flawed while relying upon only partial and often dated samples of the outcome literature. Even the severest critics, such as they are, rarely assess the scientific merits of the clinical research and therefore ignore the central criterion of the field's rational claims to authority as clinical science. The separate schools of therapy are endlessly contentious but usually only embellish their a priori points of theory (for example, the value of behaviorism) with partisan readings of the evidence. The behaviorists condemn the psychodynamic orientation for failing either to provide testable propositions or to actually test outcomes; the cognitive therapists criticize the behaviorists for reductionism; and the cognitive school is denigrated by the other schools for a shallow eclecticism. Still, all the criticisms may be simultaneously correct, especially in light of the absence of any scientifically credible evidence that any of them have ever successfully treated any mental or emotional problem.

Whatever the putative merits of the ideal practice of therapy, the customary reality is far different and substantially impaired. Masson (1988) and Gross (1978) point to numerous ethical lapses by therapists. Yet even here the evidence is episodic and personal, relying largely on unsystematic case reports.

The Requisite Science: Randomized Controlled Trials

The truth of the scientific method for clinical research, randomized controlled trials, is probably wired into the cosmos like space and time: when only one of several equivalent groups receives an experimentally induced condition, that condition must be the cause of whatever differences eventuate between it and the other groups—the controls. Thus when one group of patients receives psychotherapy and control groups that are equivalent in every other way do not receive psychotherapy, any differences in outcomes— benefits or deterioration—must be caused by the psychotherapy. The absence of superior outcomes in the experimental group means that psychotherapy was not effective.

This axiom of experimental research needs to be further adapted to the special circumstances of psychotherapy. First, because of the possibility that patients respond to their own expectancies for recovery as well as to those of their therapists rather than to the features of the therapy itself, a placebo control is required. A placebo provides all the conditions of therapy, notably belief in receiving treatment but also equivalent treatment settings and equivalent experiences with ancillary personnel, except for the essential psychotherapeutic interventions themselves. A nonplacebo, nontreatment control group also needs to be incorporated into the research design in order to estimate the degree to which maturation, spontaneous recovery, the seasonality of the mental or emotional problem, and other factors external to the treatment itself account for the outcomes. The differences between the outcomes of the experimental group and the placebo provide an estimate of the true effects of the experimental treatment; the differences between the placebo and the nontreatment control provide an estimate of the placebo effect.

Second, in addition to control conditions, multiple blinding is necessary in order to avoid serious bias; neither the patient nor the evaluator should be aware of the patient's assignment to either the experimental group or the control group. Blinding eliminates at least two sources of biased response—the patient and the evaluator, both of whom may exaggerate the actual outcomes of treatment for a variety of personal and professional reasons.

Third, research patients need to be randomly selected from the underlying pool of those suffering from the problem under study in order to assure that the results of the investigation are representative and can therefore be applied broadly to those with the problem. Fourth, research patients need to be randomly assigned to the different conditions of the research in order to assure that groups are equivalent. Fifth, the measures employed throughout the research, especially those that assess the conditions of patient selection and the outcomes of psychotherapy, need to be reliable and accurate. In addition to these fundamentals of credible scientific research, additional protections and cautions—large samples, uncontaminated reports, low attrition and censoring, treatment fidelity, and so forth—need to be instituted to assure the credibility of the research.

The goal of scientific methodology is to eliminate every explanation for the outcomes except the experimental condition. Thus without a placebo control, the outcomes might be attributed to the natural remission of the disease itself, as in the case of depression, which is customarily cyclical. Most depressed patients will eventually become less depressed even without treatment. When measures are biased, the outcomes can be attributed to the researchers' enthusiasm or to professional self-protection. Without random selection, outcomes might not apply to all those with the condition being treated; without randomized assignment, outcomes could be reasonably attributed to demographic differences between the groups in age and morbidity, for example, rather than to the experimental intervention.

It is both clear and broadly accepted by the field (at least formally) that the burden of proof—the obligation to test outcomes fairly—rests with the researcher. As is the case with pharmaceuticals, surgical procedures, and medical interventions, psychotherapy carries the equivalent responsibility to offer credible tests of its effectiveness in allaying the prudent doubts of the informed skeptic. Skepticism is constituted by the relevance of alternative potential explanations for outcomes; scientific methods are adapted to clinical psychotherapy to provide credible responses to skepticism. The skeptical starting point is the assumption that therapists and evaluators are biased, that patients are encouraged to report positive outcomes, and that factors other than therapy account for changes in emotional and mental conditions—in short, that many pitfalls of research contrive positive reports of success.

Psychotherapy's imperfect research, in spite of the self-congratulations of its practitioners, does not refute the skeptical position. Alternative explanations of successful outcomes are invariably more credible than the attempts to establish the potency of therapy itself. The fact remains that against rigorous standards of clinical science, psychotherapy has rarely, if ever, gone through a definitive test of its effectiveness. At best its outcomes are indeterminate; psychotherapy is most likely ineffective; it may even be routinely harmful.

The research is beset by a host of crippling problems. Research patients are most often in acute states of their problems. They are rarely if ever randomly selected from a defined population of emotional or mental need. Most often they are self-selected, responding to public advertisements or following through on clinical referrals. Random assignment to experimental and control conditions, when it occurs, is frequently compromised, notably by high attrition rates but also by a variety of biases that work into the assignment process. The measurement instruments themselves are frequently not reliable, having gone through initial testing in highly dubious circumstances. More often, outcomes rely on patient self-report, which is notoriously flexible. Expectancies are not controlled for. Evaluators are customarily not neutral, as claimed by the research, but are beholden to the research institution or are themselves therapists and graduate students with career interests in the success of the treatments they are evaluating.

Moreover, research is customarily conducted in university settings under the most amenable conditions of treatment—motivated patients, presumably the most skilled clinicians, and tight scrutiny of practice. In fact, the university auspices might be the least neutral situation in which to conduct research as well as the least representative of the customary community settings where most therapy is delivered.

The history of psychotherapy research is a boggling procession of one weak form of research replacing another as newer techniques of research gain popularity without substantially improving credibility. Currently popular "stepped care models," "patient-focused research," "best practice," and "evidence-based practice," all in the tradition of "appropriate treatment," reflect postmodern enthusiasm for heuristics and hermeneutics to supplant "obsolete" science (Heineman, 1981). The changes do not mark scientific progress but rather express subtle professional and ideological, even religious, shifts propelled by changing social imperatives.[3] The apparent progress in statistical sophistication is nullified by ever changing but rebarbative methodological pitfalls.

Summaries of outcomes—systematic attempts to draw generalizations from the vast clinical literature of psychotherapy—are no better than the scientific quality of the underlying, primary research. The current fashion of metanalysis simply hides the imperfections and doubtful authority of the primary research behind summary statistics and the quiet hope that the convergence of findings will dispel skepticism. Yet the culture is extraordinarily homogeneous: biases for positive outcomes that occur in hospitals and universities in Cleveland also exist with similar force in New York, San Francisco, and Atlanta.

A Few Final Introductory Remarks

The fact that a body of research is simply the most sophisticated to date and an improvement over previous efforts does not compel its acceptance as credible evidence. Indeed, psychotherapy research as tribal lore and ritual mocks experimental psychology. Credibility implies good information, not the best available. The demands of cultural authority have preempted credible research in favor of social cohesion, providing the comfort that things as they are are correct, beneficial, and fair. By suborning scientific authority to affirm its institutions, the culture also undercuts any comfort that a scientific practice of social policy has been achieved or even that it is sincerely pursued. Still, the ritual of science—a teddy bear in the terrifying dark—may be enough.

Scripted by society, played out by its institutions, and always with the citizen as audience, the field of psychotherapy is hardly culpable for its misleading work; it cannot take responsibility for itself. Its participants—the therapist, the schools, the journals, the publishers, and so forth—are vehicles of social preference. They are professional roles, social actors, humanity as situationally created expressions of larger forces. Psychotherapy is a dynamic of social meaning, not individual or conscious responsibility.

The irony, of course, is that the essential message of psychotherapy is that the patient take responsibility for him- or herself. But this only has theatrical meaning as civic instruction and moral education, lacking the true force of individual culpability in the same sense that institutionalized preferences relieve the therapist and researcher from the obligation for objective truth. In this way social roles tend to preempt individual responsibility.

Psychotherapy rejects structural explanations for social outcomes and thus rejects social welfare strategies of greater sharing. It is not a passive mirror of American society but an active cultural actor in assessing blame and justifying the procedural remedies of formal legal equality, yet rarely with the material provisions of substantive steps toward greater social, political, or economic equality. Psychotherapy interprets mental and emotional dysfunctions as personal choices and thus character flaws, accepting the social dogma that the individual is heroically self-determinative. Thus clinical practice willfully ignores the powerful and possibly irresistible influence of social institutions—families, communities, schools, labor markets, and so forth—in shaping the individual. The individual bears heroic responsibility for the individual's behavior.

Still, the romance of psychotherapy as credible science deprives its literature of any rational authority. The field persists as a popular cultural institution elaborating the cherished habits of the American people. Psychotherapy is one of the culture's socializing institutions, performing a largely symbolic role in promoting the American religion of an impossible and perhaps even cruel individualism. It proselytizes the ideology of a highly homogenized and centralized society that is even adopted by its lower-status and poorer members out of nationalism, patriotism, and the fear of further stigma for their obvious failures. In its social guise as religion, psychotherapy is a penalty and a rebuke, justifying the rejection of generosity as a moral hazard.

A social role cannot be tested scientifically. No society can be randomized to a variety of experimental and control conditions to see whether particular roles have enumerated effects. Rather, the analysis of role is necessarily weak. It proceeds by eliminating untenable alternatives and accepting those that appear to be consistent with the evidence, such as it is. In this case the possibility of psychotherapy's functioning largely as a civil religion becomes germane as it becomes clear that it lacks any true clinical usefulness. Thus the failure of psychotherapy as clinical treatment necessarily precedes consideration of its role as civil religion.

1: Depression

More than 16% of adult Americans acknowledge that they have suffered from serious depression during their lifetimes and about 7% report serious depression within a single year (Kessler, Berglund, and Demler, 2003). Yet while major depression appears to be a disabling condition, there is little evidence that any psychotherapeutic treatment for it has been effective. Nonetheless, the enormous clinical literature claims routine success in treating adults, adolescents, and a variety of targeted groups.

The contemporary debate about treating major depression centers around whether the three basic forms of psychotherapy—cognitive-behavioral therapy, behavioral therapy, and psychodynamic interpersonal therapy—are superior to drug treatment and placebos. Yet the interventions are consistent in one very important regard; they all involve clinical interventions with the patient as the object of treatment. None implicate the social environment as the principal source of depression. Therefore, none seek a social remedy. There are profound political implications for the emergence of the clinical rather than the political arena as the cultural choice for handling the problem. Indeed, the continuing insistence of the clinical literature on its ability to handle depression, especially through short treatment lasting but a few months, detracts policy attention away from the possibility of social and economic remedies for debilitating psychological reactions.

The best of the clinical literature, that is, its most scientific forms, employs randomized controlled trials, with the findings collected and summarized in a variety of metanalyses. Some areas of treatment, discussed in subsequent chapters, have not been able to achieve even this degree of formal conformity with scientific practice. The studies of studies, together with their base of primary research, constitute the general assessments of the state of the art of clinical treatment of depression. The principal reviews (Casacalenda, Perry, and Looper, 2002; Hamilton and Dobson, 2002, updating Dobson, 1989; Gaffan, Tsaousis, and Kemp-Wheeler, 1995; Robinson, Berman, and Neimeyer, 1990; and a few others) have concluded on the evidence of the best of the experimental literature that psychotherapy is a powerful and predictable cure for depression. They suggest that managed care has exercised a benign influence in reducing the amount of treatment, since short-term interventions, rarely longer than twelve weeks, are as effective as longer-term treatments. As a result treatment costs have declined, together with the disruption of patients' lives.

Cognitive-behavioral treatment seems occasionally to outpace psychodynamic interpersonal therapy, more often behavioral interventions, and sometimes even medication. Still, the metanalyses tout all four as superior to no treatment at all, that is, wait-list and placebo controls. Logically, less disabled patients do better in treatment than severely depressed patients. Even accounting for a number of practitioner and researcher loyalties to particular interventions ("researcher allegiance"), the reported benefits of psychotherapy for depression remain substantial.

Yet the metanalyses are captives of their sources; their conclusions are only as accurate and credible as the research they cite. Unfortunately the best of the research is too methodologically flawed to sustain any conclusion except indeterminacy and ineffectiveness, and always with the undercurrent of possible harm.

Despite reputations for scientific rigor, the apparently sophisticated authors, their hospitals, and their universities routinely ignore methodological pitfalls on the way to findings of effective treatment. The research itself constitutes a cultural manifesto more than scientific evidence for progress against a serious disability.

A critical analysis of the best of the clinical studies reduces their candidacy for scientific authority to social ideology that expresses deeply held cultural values rather than objective truths about repairing human dysfunction and unhappiness. The subculture of professionals that purveys psychotherapy for depression conducts factional negotiations over belief, recruiting science to serve occupational interests. Through faulty research that contrives convenient support for psychotherapy, the clinician and the researcher reveal a blind faith and partisan loyalty that overwhelm a prudent skepticism and the other tenets of science. Psychotherapy for depression is best understood as testimony for social belief rather than as clinical science.

Adults

Psychotherapy's effectiveness in treating depression is not sustained by scrutiny of the most credible research in the field's literature: serious methodological flaws undermine the authority of each and every study; researchers exaggerate their findings and ignore the weaknesses of their research; indeterminacy, ineffectiveness, and perhaps even harm are the only credible effects of psychotherapy for depression. Indeed, in comparison with Casacalenda et al.'s (2002) problematic review, every other metanalysis and summary builds more Panglossian findings on even less credible evidence.

Rather than psychotherapeutic interventions, the improvement that is measured in patients can more plausibly be attributed to the seasonality of depression, the demand characteristics of the research situation itself that is frequently transmitted through "the therapeutic alliance" between patient and therapist, as well as the researcher's allegiance to positive outcomes, measurement distortion, inaccurate patient self-reports, differential attrition, and other factors. These pitfalls of research blemish the experimental literature of psychotherapy like meteorite craters on Mars and the Moon. They seem to be characteristics of the field's research, essential to sustain its social role.

Casacalenda et al. (2002), one of the most selective reviews of psychotherapy's effects on depression, identified only six experiments that employed "randomized controlled double blind trials for well-defined major depressive disorder in which medications, psychotherapy, and control conditions were directly compared and for which remission percentages were reported" (p. 1354). They concluded that psychotherapy was as effective as medication for nonpsychotic patients and that both were about twice as effective as control conditions: 46% remission of symptoms for the two interventions versus 24% for control patients. However, each of the six studies is seriously marred as a scientific statement. Each is a narrative for our times that seduces broad belief, a marketing device for psychotherapists, a dramatic testimonial that observes the rituals of science while negating its defining rigor and skepticism.

The earliest of the six, Herceg-Baron et al. (1979), suffered an attrition rate of 56% within the seventeen weeks of their experiment and concluded with suggestions for maintaining patients throughout the study. Reported elsewhere (DiMascio et al., 1979; Weissman et al., 1979), the clinical outcomes of their four experimental conditions—interpersonal psychotherapy alone, medication alone, a combination of the two, and a "nonscheduled treatment control" (supportive therapy on demand), each provided for the short term of sixteen weeks—are vitiated by the enormous attrition as well as by other problems of measurement. Indeed, differential attrition in all groups by itself may explain any outcome.

The authors found that all of the treatments were effective, that is, significantly superior to the control, but that the combination of short-term psychotherapy and medication was superior to either one alone, usually taking effect after only eight weeks of treatment. Clinical outcomes were measured by the Hamilton Rating Scale for Depression and the Raskin Depression Scale, both of which are highly imperfect assessment tools. It is notable that improvements measured by the Hamilton scale were dramatic for the combined group and large for medication and psychotherapy alone but that the mean improvements were clinically marginal except for the combined treatment. The Raskin improvements were small except, again, for the combined treatment.

However, attrition was very large and differential, with more than 50% of patients failing to complete sixteen weeks of all but the combined treatment, in which only 67% completed sixteen weeks. Moreover, the resulting sample of treated patients was also small, ranging from 17 in the psychotherapy group to only 23 in the medication group.

> All of the patients were seen for clinical assessment after one, four, eight, twelve, and sixteen weeks, or at the termination of treatment, by a clinical evaluator (a psychiatrist or a psychologist) who was independent of and blind to the patient's treatment. Patients were instructed not to discuss with the evaluator the type of treatment they were receiving. The treating psychiatrist also evaluated the patient. . . . [A]greement between clinical evaluator and psychiatrist . . . was excellent. (Weissman et al., 1979, p. 556)

This, however, does not mean that raters were either blind to the group assignments of the patients nor independent. To the contrary, despite instructions to hide their assignments, the patients probably offered clues. After all, the five assessment points provided many patients with a variety of opportunities for disclosure. Further, the agreement between raters employed by the same department in the same research institution, in this case Yale University's medical school, probably reflects the symmetry of their motives, preferences, and commitments more than any capacity to assess neutrally and objectively the outcomes of their chosen craft. The obligation is on the researcher's shoulders to deflect potential criticisms of bias by employing credible methods, but the authors did not make the effort to enlist truly independent raters. To the contrary, their decision to rely on an obviously beholden group of evaluators raises doubts about the independence of the research itself.

In the end, it is provocative that such imperfect research should be cozened by such prestigious and culturally central organizations: Yale University hosted the experiment, the federal government funded it through the National Institute of Mental Health and the Alcohol, Drug Abuse, and Mental Health Administration, and the findings were published in the *American Journal of Psychiatry* and the *Archives of General Psychiatry,* two of the world's most influential and respected periodicals, presumably because of their commitment to the canons of scientific research. The institutional acceptance of faux science begins to suggest that social meaning rather than objective authority was the point of the butchered experiment, a triumph of autobiography over clinical science and imagination over history.

The second of the six, The National Institute of Mental Health's Treatment of Depression Collaborative Research Program (TDCRP), is reported principally in Elkin et al. (1989) but also in additional papers (Imber et al., 1990; Sotsky et al., 1991). It is extensively cited throughout the literature as evidence for the efficacy of psychotherapy. TDCRP assigned a total of 250 patients at three sites to four conditions: cognitive-behavioral therapy, interpersonal therapy, medication, and a drug placebo plus minimal support. Therapy lasted for sixteen weeks.

The researchers concluded that "all treatment conditions . . . evidenced significant change from pretreatment to posttreatment. . . . The results for the two psychotherapies fell between those for [medication] and [drug placebo plus minimal support] (p. 980)." Yet the drug placebo with minimal support therapy is commonly and appropriately employed as a control for true treatments in Weissman et al. (1979). Thus the therapies rarely improved on the effectiveness of the placebo. In a few regards, the placebo group did better than the treated groups; outcomes were measured as personal changes, sleep disturbances, appetite changes, and so forth. Moreover, a host of methodological problems, notably including large and probably differential attrition of 38% as well as practice effects in measurement, further undermined the research.

Rather than explaining the comparability of outcomes among the groups as mysteriously resulting from undefined "core processes" of therapeutic value, the researchers might have more modestly and honestly accepted their drug placebo minimal-support condition as a true placebo control, with the consequence that all of their interventions were largely ineffective. This seems reasonable since sixteen weeks, and frequently less, of uncertain therapy is an improbable strategy for resolving serious mental and emotional conditions. Even though a subsequent replication failed to confirm the TDCRP findings (McLean and Taylor, 1992), Elkin et al.'s (1989) hopefulness and disingenuous research continues to be offered routinely in support of psychotherapy for depression.

A. I. Scott and Freeman (1992), the third of the six, compared four conditions: medication, cognitive-behavioral therapy, social-work counseling and casework, and routine care provided by a general practitioner. The authors concluded that at the end of sixteen weeks of care "the severity of depressive symptoms declined markedly in all treatment groups, and any differences in clinical efficacy between [general practitioner care and the other treatments] were not commensurate with the differences in the length and cost of treatment" (p. 887). At the end of treatment, only the social-work intervention provided significantly better outcomes than general-practitioner care, although the patients in the social-work group were substantially older and less ill than patients in the other group. To its credit, the study counted attrition as treatment failure. However, patients were not blind to the raters; follow-up data were not collected; and the procedures of both the cognitive-behavioral therapy and the social-work treatment were not manualized, with the result that the actual content of treatment in these two groups remains uncertain.

Most important, however, there was no true nontreatment control. The study conveniently relied upon the conclusions of the literature that all of its chosen treatments were effective. This is a problematic assumption (discussed below), emerging from similarly deficient studies that usually compared, but imperfectly, wait-list nontreatment conditions to therapeutic interventions. True placebo controls enormously reduce the reported efficacy of psychotherapy. Furthermore, general-practitioner care provided little psychotherapeutic content even considering the substantial number of referrals that were made to specialized mental-health services. Indeed, general-practitioner care may be a placebo for psychotherapy, in which case the similarity of outcomes, if not an artifact of repeated measurement itself, is a poor testimonial to the efficacy of psychotherapy. It is plausible, in fact likely, that a substantial number of depressed patients would have recovered with no treatment at all; spontaneous remission—self-cure—is a critical tenet of scientific skepticism, especially in clinical research. Thus A. I. Scott and Freeman's (1992) experiment is invalidated by the absence of a true nontreatment control; the likelihood of natural recovery; the important differences between groups in age, sex, and the severity of depression; the lack of blinding; and the inappropriate assumption that all of their conditions were effective. Moreover, the absence of follow-up also prevents an assessment of the duration of effects, including the degree to which some patients may have deteriorated as a result of treatment. A. I. Scott and Freeman (1992) stands as evidence that compromised research leads to agreeable findings that falsely become the credentialized tenets of later designs. This is the process of legend and myth but screened through the lore of science.

Mynor-Wallis, Gath, Lloyd-Thomas, and Thomlison (1995), the fourth study, did employ a placebo control for medication and problem-solving treatment (perhaps analogous to cognitive-behavioral therapy) for depressed patients in primary care. They found that only 3 1/2 hours of problem solving provided a significant improvement over the placebo control: 60% of patients given problem solving had recovered, compared with only 27% of placebo patients. It is intriguing that the placebo condition seems to be the same one employed by TDCRP—drug placebo plus standard clinical management, that is, "supportive therapy"—but the TDCRP results were very different, with comparable success for all of the treatment conditions. It seems plausible that the different research assumptions about drug placebo plus standard clinical management were transmitted as subtle demand characteristics in creating the different findings. TDCRP considered the condition a treatment and created measurement incentives to report efficacy; in contrast, Mynor-Wallis et al. (1995) and Weissman et al. (1979) considered the condition to be a placebo and thus created the incentives to minimize its success. Yet Mynor-Wallis et al. (1995) did not conduct a follow-up assessment, which would seem to be necessary to estimate the value of the recovery past the treatment situation itself. Indeed, reports of recovery may diminish as patients are freed from any obligation or gratitude to the therapist or clinic.

Mynor-Wallis et al. (1995) also claimed that the assessments of outcomes "were made by one of two experienced research interviewers who were blind to the type of treatment" (p. 441). However, this seems unlikely, as A. I. Scott and Freeman (1992) recognized, especially after raters may conduct as many as three interviews with the same patients, who probably provide clues to their assignment. But most important, the instruments themselves, even when applied by neutral judges, are inadequate and unreliable (as discussed in chapter 6). They often rely upon patient self-report, which is greatly affected by a variety of research conditions that influence the patient's response. It is a standing and near universal indictment of psychotherapeutic research that it fails to enlist evaluators who are independent of the research situation or of the occupational protectiveness of therapists.

Furthermore, 26 of 91 patients failed to complete 6 sessions of treatment over the 12 sessions of treatment; this 29% attrition rate is increased by an additional six patients who apparently refused to be interviewed ("data missing"). Thus the effective attrition rate climbs to 34%, far higher than the 20% that the authors initially suggested was tolerable. They apparently did not include the lost patients as treatment failures, which probably would have wiped out their reported gains. Yet their results are reported for patients who completed a minimum of only 4 sessions of treatment. Such a large number of superficially treated patients reinforces the possibility that the study's outcomes are artifacts of distorted measurement procedures rather than true effects of the experimental interventions.

The fifth experiment endorses specialized care for current major depression. Shulberg et al. (1996) claimed that patients receiving medication or interpersonal psychotherapy were better off eight months after the beginning of treatment than primary-care patients. Yet again, attrition rates were stunning: only about 50% of the medication group and the psychotherapy group completed acute treatment, while fewer than 30% of the medication group and only 42% of the psychotherapy group completed continuation care. While some patients left treatment by themselves, others were "dropped when judged by their clinicians to be nonresponders" (p. 916). Only 10 of 92 patients dropped out of primary care. If noncompleters are considered failures (and their initial Hamilton rating scores are carried through the analysis), then the positive findings evaporate. As it is, outcomes measured as the severity of depression among the groups, while statistically significant, are not large. Differences between psychotherapy and usual physician care are actually tiny. Moreover, even these very credulous authors raise a question about initial selection bias, since many acutely depressed patients refused to participate in their experiment.

Thus Shulberg et al. (1996) proved nothing at all except that supposedly sophisticated funding sources, including the National Institute of Mental Health and a roster of the most prominent American research foundations, were more anxious to endorse a cultural form than to practice science. Funding sources reviewing Shulberg et al.'s initial research protocols should have voiced concern about sampling, measurement, and analysis, raising cautions that the research was premature and badly designed. This did not occur, intruding the possibility that motives of social compatibility rather than treatment success justified the research. Moreover, by publishing the findings in their present form, the *Archives of General Psychiatry* becomes complicit in propagating this fiction of clinical efficacy.

The last of Casacalenda et al. (2002) six studies purports to prove the superiority of both cognitive-behavioral therapy and medication to a placebo control (clinical management and placebo medication) as treatments for major depression with atypical features. Jarrett, Schaffer, McIntire, Witt-Browder, Kraft et al. (1999) randomized 108 patients to the three groups for ten weeks of treatment. Twice as many patients in the treated groups as in the placebo group benefited, although a more stringent definition of success wiped out the differences. Jarrett et al.'s control was the same as TDCRP's control, but here placebo medication and clinical management produced little benefit. Attrition was low in the treated groups but 23 of 36 patients dropped out of the placebo group; presumably many sought alternative care; perhaps only the most persistent and the most debilitated stayed. No follow-up was reported, and again ratings were claimed to be blind. The authors raise questions about the representativeness of the treated sample, since many prospective participants refused to participate, resulting in a typical patient who "was a white female approaching midlife with a moderate level of depression" (p. 436). It is intriguing that 53% of the placebo patients as opposed to 93% of the live-medication patients reported side effects, hinting at the power of research conditions over patient behavior and self-report and thus the seriousness of the demand characteristics in any research situation.

In the end, Casacalenda et al.'s (2002) metanalysis is more disturbing than convincing. Not one of their six studies—the best of the best of the literature—can sustain its conclusions against rudimentary scientific skepticism. Casacalenda et al. acknowledge that the studies did not conduct follow-up evaluations and that the research trial was not typical of customary care. But their conclusions are not bounded by the multiplicity of basic methodological imperfections in the primary research, notably sampling, attrition, and measurement problems.

The best of the other metanalyses sustain the basic line of psychotherapy's effectiveness for depression, yet on more tenuous grounds. They focus on the best of the literature, usually large randomized clinical trials, although they loosen their inclusion criteria to pick up far more than six studies. Yet they customarily increase the spin of the underlying primary research.

In their "comprehensive review of controlled outcome research," Robinson et al. (1990) analyzed 58 studies, reaching conclusions that sustain Smith, Glass, and Miller (1980). At the beginning of treatment, the average patient in both the psychotherapy groups and the controls are at the 50% point. However, at the end of treatment, patients receiving psychotherapy were better off than 77% of controls; the therapeutic effects persisted at follow-up with 25% of treated patients better off than controls. Robinson et al. (1990) obligingly reported that comparisons with wait-list controls produced evidence of enormous effectiveness (80% of treated patients better off than controls). However, when treated patients are compared with placebo controls, they are better off than only 61% of controls, a difference that is not statistically significant. Placebos that control for the effects of being in a treatment situation (the "nonspecific effects") are the appropriate comparison, not wait-listed patients who may falsely report continued symptoms to stay eligible for treatment. In any event, the difference between the two kinds of controls is perhaps an estimate of the extent to which the treatment situation itself accounts for reports of improvement. In this case, about two-thirds of the reported improvement (about 20 out of 30 percentage points) seems due to patient expectations rather than psychotherapy itself.

Yet Robinson et al. (1990) chose to ignore the placebo studies on the excuse that wait-list controls are "the more frequently occurring type of control" (p. 34). This justification for method on the basis of popularity rather than rigor also reflects the ease of putting together wait-lists as well as their agreeable tendency to sustain the effectiveness of treatment. Yet attrition on wait-lists is usually large, with stayers perhaps being more adamant about their illness or even sicker than those who drop off. Not surprisingly, compared with wait-lists, Robinson et al.'s (1990) findings are joyful antidotes for professional depression over comparisons with placebo controls. Robinson et al. celebrate that "Cognitive, Behavioral, and Cognitive-Behavioral" therapies are all wildly successful. Their distortions were published by the *Psychological Bulletin,* another of the world's leading journals.

Apart from the frank biases of the metanalyses, the greatest vulnerability of Robinson et al.'s (1990) happy conclusions lies with the primary research that they summarize. Even when the clinical research appears to conform to the broadest dictates of scientific rigor, it is fatally impaired by methodological pitfalls that stand in the way of accepting any conclusion except perhaps the ineffectiveness of psychotherapy for depression.

Differing from the First Sheffield Experiment by varying the duration of psychotherapy, the Second Sheffield Experiment, conducted during the early 1990s in England, is one of the most cited sources of evidence for psychotherapy's effectiveness. It evaluated the two most common forms of psychotherapy—cognitive-behavioral therapy and psychodynamic interpersonal therapy—provided in a short dose of 16 sessions and an even briefer dose of 8 sessions. Shapiro et al. (1994) reported that "there was little evidence that [cognitive-behavioral therapy] was generally more effective or acted more rapidly than [psychodynamic interpersonal therapy], or vice-versa, or that one treatment was more effective than the other with relatively more severe or less severe clients" (p. 526). However, both treatments seemed to be very effective, with the outcomes sustained at three-month follow-up. Indeed, on the Present State Examination, patients moved on average from their pre-treatment scores of 50% to the 99th percentile; on the Beck Depression Score patients moved from 50% to the 96th percentile. The raw score improvements were just as dramatic.

"However, there is scant evidence of added benefit from 16 weekly treatment sessions, compared with 8" (Shapiro et al., 1994, p. 527). This "negatively accelerated dose effect," that is, the diminishing returns of psychotherapy, was further analyzed by pooling patient data from the Second Sheffield Experiment and the TDCRP (Barkham et al., 1996). The reanalysis by and large refuted the initial findings: "the negative acceleration was not evident . . . the change in particular symptoms looked approximately linear," with patients benefiting from eight additional weeks of psychotherapy. Nevertheless, the Sheffield patients' perceptions of therapy sessions suggested that the degree of positive reports, perhaps largely measures of patient satisfaction that the authors hopefully relate to therapeutic outcomes, improved less with time (S. Reynolds et al., 1996).

Pointedly, the Second Sheffield Experiment failed to employ any nontreatment control, simply assuming that the efficacy of psychotherapy had been previously established. Further, the pooled findings ignored the improvements in TDCRP's placebo, often equivalent to those in the treated psychotherapy groups. Thus, rather than as a result of therapy, the seasonality of depression—self-cure, spontaneous remission—may have accounted for the measured improvements as depression naturally ebbed. Moreover, the repeated measurement procedures, the faulty measures themselves, the questionable neutrality of the raters, and the subtle demand characteristics of both experiments may well have induced patients to exaggerate their improvements. Aside from the patients' appreciation for the therapists' sympathetic attentions to their sorrows, patients may also have been returning gratitude for the free care.

Attrition was a smaller problem in the Second Sheffield Experiment than in TDCRP. However, Sheffield only recruited patients who were "professionals, managers, and white-collar workers" and was initially even selective about whom it accepted for treatment among this group (Shapiro et al., 1994, p. 524). From an initial referral of 540 applicants for treatment, 257 completed intake interviews, 150 patients were randomized to treatment, 138 entered treatment, and 117 completed treatment—a relatively low attrition rate in these sorts of clinical experiments of only about 22% between randomization and completion. Those who completed treatment were somewhat older and better educated than those who did not.

Referral (especially self-referral), recruitment, and solicitation of depressed people as research patients seriously limits the applicability of the findings to the general population of depressed people or even to the population of depressed people who enter treatment. Since depressed people characteristically feel "hopeless, helpless, and worthless . . . the disorder may preclude seeking treatment, because many patients with depression feel they are not worthy of feeling better" (Insel and Charney, 2003, p. 3168). In this way, depression studies face the difficulty of demonstrating that they are not simply screening the depressed for the most amenable, those who have the psychic strength to seek cure. The likelihood of many self-selected patients in depression research and psychotherapeutic experiments in general increases the desirability of employing placebo controls as well as taking other design precautions against undue researcher influence over patients with a possible proclivity to enhance reports of their recovery.

The Second Sheffield Experiment assumed on the basis of previous research that the forms of therapy it compared were effective. Proven effectiveness creates a standard of treatment that becomes the control for any new therapy. In this way, the standard treatment replaces a nontreatment control, and research only carries the future obligation to explore the relative ability of different therapies to resolve depression. Unfortunately, contemporary clinical practice has settled the issue of psychotherapy's effectiveness in treating depression on grounds of convenience rather than scientific rationality.

Dobson (1989) identified 28 studies that were comparable in employing the Beck Depression Inventory to assess the outcomes of cognitive-behavioral therapy. However, only 5 of the 28 studies employed wait-list controls and only three included placebos. As noted, one of the three placebo studies, TDCRP, concluded that there was no difference in outcomes between the placebos and psychotherapy; another only employed cognitive-behavioral treatment along with a drug placebo for medication but did not include a placebo for psychotherapy.

The third study, Beutler, Scogin, Kirkish, Schretlen, Corbishley et al. (1987), seemed to corroborate TDCRP, finding that none of the treatments were superior to the placebo at any point in the twenty weeks of therapy or three months after the termination of treatment. Yet Beutler, Scogin, Kirkish, Schretlen, Corbishley et al. suffered enormous attrition: 75 patients were initially included, 56 were assigned to the four conditions, and only 29 patients completed treatment, an overall average attrition rate of 61%. The experiment also had excluded 4 of the 75 initial patients because they were "placebo responders," that is, those whose depression subsided after two weeks of a "placebo washout" period. Thus only an average of about seven patients in each group completed treatment, sample sizes so small that they constitute case studies rather than samples.

Gaffan et al.'s (1995) metanalysis of the next cohort of outcome research sustained the basic effectiveness of cognitive-behavioral therapy but reduced Dobson's (1989) estimate by about 50% on the grounds of researcher "allegiance," that is, the preference a researcher has for a particular intervention. Curiously, Gaffan et al. (1995) shied away from labeling the effect a bias, tactfully writing only about the extent to which researcher allegiance "predicted" the extent of reported effectiveness. Of course, commitment may be a rational choice; or it may be the wellspring of belief and bias; or *homo credulus* and *homo economus* may live in peace with each other. The whole issue could, of course, be avoided by neutral evaluation and reliable measures. But this has not occurred, and those with the greatest material stakes in outcomes are typically allowed if not actually encouraged to evaluate their own practice.

Subsequently, Hamilton and Dobson (2002) cited Clark, Beck, and Alford's (1999) analysis to conclude that "a wealth of empirical data derived from randomized controlled treatment outcome studies support the relative efficacy of [cognitive-behavioral therapy] of depression" (p. 875). However, Clark, et al. (1999), among the inventors of cognitive-behavioral therapy, failed to identify any credible research that employed placebo controls. Additionally, research subsequent to Dobson (1989) that employed placebo controls (Jarrett et al., 1999, and Mynor-Wallis et al., 1995, discussed above) contained numerous pitfalls that undercut their positive findings.

Other major research is perhaps even more flawed than the Second Sheffield Experiment and TDCRP. Citing Dobson (1989) as proof that "cognitive-behavioral therapy has been found to be an effective treatment for clinical depression," Propst, Ostrom, Watkins, Dean, and Washburn (1992) still prudently employed two controls, wait-list and "pastoral counseling treatment-as-usual," in testing the relative effectiveness of two types of cognitive therapy, the customary form and one with religious content, for treating depressed religious patients. Of these patients, 64% identified themselves as "evangelical or fundamentalist" and only 24% as "mainline Protestants." Both religious and nonreligious therapists delivered about 19 one-hour sessions over a period of three months to each patient. Of the 68 patients who were selected for the study, 11 persisted through the wait-list and 48 completed one of the three therapy conditions. Results were mixed. First, only the cognitive-therapy group exposed to religious content improved significantly at the end of treatment, and only on one score. Second, on one measure of depression the pastoral-counseling group and the religious-content cognitive-therapy group achieved clinically important changes by the end of therapy; however, employing a second measure of depression, only the religious-content group achieved clinically important changes. Patients in each of the three therapy conditions remained "substantially less depressed at both the 3-month and 2-year follow-ups than at the pretest" (Propst et al., 1992, p. 100). Importantly, patients who completed treatment, compared with those who did not, scored significantly "higher on intrinsic religiosity, committed religiosity, orthodoxy, [and] reported religious experience" (p. 97) and were perhaps more prone to exaggerate their recovery, possibly out of an intrinsic sense of ecclesiastical duty to appear more cheerful after so much therapeutic reliance on the Bible. The authors made no methodological provision (such as a control of nonreligious patients) to test whether religious people with such a bent for inerrancy and unquestioning belief were reporting an imagined religious experience rather than an actual psychological improvement.

However, treatment groups and the wait-list control were tiny; the evaluators were graduate students in counseling psychology, as were the therapists, and had little clinical experience. Most intriguing, the pastoral counseling treatment was more like a placebo for the religious content group than a true treatment group. The pastoral counseling manual "used in our study specified that each session should include approximately 75% of the time spent in nondirective listening and 25% of the time spent in discussing bible verses or religious themes that might relate to the patient's concerns" (Propst et al., 1992, p. 96). This sort of pastoral counseling seems similar to time-structured interest groups and contains little if any therapeutic core, or better said, only nonspecific elements. The fact that the cognitive-behavioral conditions did little better than pastor counseling is hardly an endorsement. The occasional differences from the wait-list patients are most likely due to the problems of wait-list reliability more than to any true therapeutic effect. Indeed, to the extent to which the wait-list is a nontreatment control and pastoral counseling is a placebo, Propst et al. (1992) suggest the ineffectiveness of psychotherapy but rather a large placebo effect, perhaps abetted by the natural seasonality of depression. In any event, the likely absence of measurement neutrality as well as the tiny group sizes vitiate any hard conclusion and, notably, any serious claim for the effectiveness of psychotherapy.

Again, for all its many flaws, Propst et al. (1992) is among the most credible outcome research in the field. The other leading sources for the authority to employ psychotherapy for depressed adults are crippled by similar flaws (Jarrett, Kraft, Doyle, Foster, Eaves et al., 2001; Thase et al., 1997; Barber and Muenz, 1996; Whisman et al., 1991).

Skepticism

As troubling as the weak research is the fact that the field consistently minimizes the occasional notes of skepticism that are noted in the literature (regarding researcher allegiance, patient alliance, and patient factors, for example). The patient's alliance with the therapists in both the Second Sheffield Experiment and TDCRP has been tortuously reinterpreted as a requirement of therapy (Zuroff et al., 2000; Stiles et al., 1998) in spite of scant proof of its beneficial effects (Blatt et al., 1996). The field consistently ignores the possibility that strong emotional bonds and broad common understandings between therapist and patient may signal an unhealthy discipleship, a desire for transformation and surrender that supplants patient autonomy and growth with a cultish denial of individuality and a craving for the therapist's affirmation. Addiction to psychotherapy may be one of its routine harms.

Suggesting that therapeutic outcomes resulted from factors outside of therapy, Barber and Meunz (1996) found that certain patient characteristics predicted their outcomes in a variety of TDCRP's conditions: married patients did better with cognitive-behavioral therapy, single patients with interpersonal psychotherapy. It is more than simply provocative that the actual content of psychotherapy has been so rarely related to actual patient outcomes (Stiles and Shapiro, 1994), or that the quality of the therapeutic relationship has only modest influence on outcomes (Blatt et al., 1996), or that the active factors in cognitive-behavioral therapy, for one, defy experimental verification (Jacobson et al., 1996). Still, Barber and Meunz (1996) went on to bravely endorse differential treatments for patients with different demographic characteristics while ignoring the enormous attrition that marred TDCRP and the further likelihood that it was not at all random but highly selective. Indeed, the psychotherapeutic community's deference to its highly imperfect clinical experiments by itself testifies to the power of research allegiance, hinting at the field's inability or unwillingness to test practice fairly or to confront the possibility of its routine ineffectiveness and harm.

Although they do not establish treatment effectiveness, a number of the stronger experiments such as Jarrett et al. (1999) invite serious consideration of their positive findings, but only as starting points for truly rigorous and systematic investigation. But then again, given the generally weak condition of research in the field, the few studies with even marginally defensible methodologies that produce positive findings may reflect a group of patients unusually amenable to therapy, undiscovered but severely differential attrition, or an undisclosed quirk in the randomization procedures. To paraphrase a prominent sociologist's comment on faith's dominating data, it is simply foolhardy to ever expect psychotherapists, the group with the greatest stake in beneficial outcomes, to evaluate their own effectiveness (Rossi, 1994, p. 464). But then again, the malleability of imperfect research may be the social motive that funds just such a system.

The absence of credible research means that the effectiveness of psychotherapy for adult depression has not been established. The studies that compare different treatments with each other are premature and presumptive. The overwhelming majority of all research in psychotherapy employs standard treatments in the place of controls but without having established the effectiveness of those treatments against placebo controls. Yet the absence of placebo controls, debilitating in itself, is still not a unique failure of the research. Even taken on their own, none of the initial certifying experiments—that is, the previous research that did incorporate wait-list or placebo controls—are credible. The descent of authority from weak studies whose tenets and findings eventuate in even weaker experimental designs has pro-

duced psychotherapy's specious clinical literature. The effectiveness of psychotherapy for depression has been accepted through a cultural process but not
rationally through credible science. The authority of psychotherapy is grad-
uated from skepticism to belief but without the credentials of achievement,
a social promotion rather than a scientific advance.

   In the end the primary research concerning adult depression, and therefore the summary statements of psychotherapy's effectiveness for depression,
are about as reliably positive as advertised testimonials for breakfast cereal but
equally suspect and self-serving. After all, cereal and psychotherapy both
occupy competitive market niches. The research failures are obvious, not
obscure, suggesting that a broad consensus quietly sanctions the deception.
If the primary research is the testimonial of missionaries, then the summaries
are the sermons for an immense congregation of believers—the society itself
even more than those who seek treatment.

Adolescents

The literature on treating adolescent depression with psychotherapy is far less
extensive than that for adults but just about as pretentious, misleading, and
weak. Mufson, Weissman, Moreau, and Garfinkel (1999) reported that interpersonal psychotherapy for depressed adolescents was much more acceptable
and effective than a clinical monitoring control. Interpersonal psychotherapy
consisted of twelve weekly sessions and some additional phone contact during the first four weeks. Therapy addressed six areas of development common
to adolescents: "separation from parents, exploration of authority in relationship to parents, development of dyadic interpersonal relationships [that is,
dating], initial experience with the death of relative or friend, and peer pressure" as well as problems concerning single-parent families (p. 574). In contrast, clinical management was available for thirty minutes per month unless
the patient initiated additional, usually emergency requests. Those who
delivered the clinical management condition "were given a brief treatment
manual instructing them to refrain from advice giving or skills training, and
to use the sessions to review depressive symptoms, school attendance, assess
suicidality, and just listen supportively" (p. 574). The psychotherapy group
suffered only 12% attrition compared to 54% in the clinical monitoring control. Most importantly, the therapy group evidenced far fewer depressive
symptoms after twelve weeks of treatment than did the control.

   The experimental findings, however, fall apart on the research's imperfections. First, the clinical support control was designed as an "ethical wait-list
condition" rather than as a placebo. It therefore failed to control for the

placebo effects of the clinical setting and simple attention, since control patients were acutely aware that they were not receiving care, which may have affected their self-reports as well as the way they presented themselves for evaluation. The neglect of wait-list status may even have exacerbated their symptoms, arguing once again for the necessity of true placebo controls. Indeed, denying patients care in a situation that may actually provoke their symptoms or at least encourage their misreporting hardly seems ethical.

Second, all of the patients were initially screened by the lead author applying the Hamilton scale, which is dependent upon the evaluator's judgment of symptoms, thus suggesting the possibility of a bias toward inflated estimates of depression. Subsequently, evaluations of progress were conducted by research staff, with the possibility of inflated estimates of improvement. The blunt statement that evaluators were blind to the status of the patients seems forced. If the experiment was truly committed to independent, neutral evaluation it would have employed evaluators uncommitted to therapy and organizationally unattached to the treating clinic, in this case part of the Columbia University medical complex. Third, it is noteworthy that at the end of treatment, experimental patients did not report on the Beck Depression Inventory (which is independent of the evaluator's judgment, relying entirely on patient self-report) any improvement in depressive symptoms compared with those of the control patients. The improvements in depressive symptoms were recorded by evaluators applying the Hamilton Rating Scale for Depression. Fourth, "most patients were self-referred or referred by parents or mental health professionals from school-based clinics," which leaves the question of how representative they were of the population of depressed adolescents (p. 574). Finally, the authors failed to conduct a follow-up, nor did they bother to check the reliability of the scaled scores of the adolescents' conditions and behaviors either during or subsequent to treatment from either parents, teachers, or the partner in their "dyadic interpersonal relationships."

Mufson et al. (1999) fits nicely into the intransigent research tradition of psychotherapy, offering little understanding of adolescent depression and even less evidence of interpersonal psychotherapy's effectiveness. On some measures, experimental patients did better than controls, although too many of the wait-list controls dropped out of treatment to allow a valid comparison. Moreover, treated patients did not report the improvement; the decline in depressive symptoms was estimated by the experimental staff—those with an obvious professional stake in successful treatment. The society comfortably abides practitioners evaluating their own practice and the implicit waiver of science to inconvenient truths.

Birmaher et al. (2000) and Brent, Holder, and Kolko (1997) exemplify psychotherapy's tortuous science in creating myths of psychic cure. Their experiment compared three therapies for depressed adolescents: cognitive-behavioral therapy, systematic behavioral family therapy, and nondirective supportive therapy. At the end of treatment, only about 17% of cognitive-behavioral therapy patients reported major depressive disease, compared with about 32% of patients who received systematic behavioral family therapy and 42% who received nondirective supportive therapy. Cognitive-behavioral therapy patients also showed gains over the other two groups in severity of depression, remission, and a number of other measures (Brent et al., 1997). However, at two years following treatment the outcomes were equivalent; patients in all three groups showed improvement from their initial problems (Birmaher et al., 2000). Yet nondirective supportive therapy is similar to placebo conditions in TDCRP as well as other studies. Thus all three treatments were equally ineffective; remission and recurrence rates followed the natural course of adolescent depression suggested throughout their paper.

Birmaher et al. (2000) acknowledged that cognitive therapy "did not confer any long-term advantage over family or supportive therapy with regard to rates of remission, recovery, recurrence, or level of function" (p. 33). However, they went on to press the clinical effectiveness of all three interventions, since "most of the participants (84%) recovered from their index episode of depression, mostly within 1 year from baseline (p. 33) . . . along with substantial improvement in functional status" (p. 34). Still, "there was a lag in between the clinical and functional improvement, with most subjects showing functional improvement during the follow-up phase of the study" (p. 34).

A less complimentary explanation replacing the insistence by the authors and their field that the gains are attributable to psychotherapy seems more plausible simply on the basis of the information offered by Birmaher et al. (2000). It is intriguing that after eleven months, those who dropped out of therapy were just as well off as those who completed therapy. Indeed, the authors reported that "naturalistic studies have shown that in clinically referred samples, the median duration for a pediatric major depressive episode is approximately 8 months, with a recovery rate up to 90% over 1 to 2 years from the onset of the depressive incident and a rate of recurrence of 40% to 70% over a period of 2 to 5 years" (p. 29). This is very close to what Birmaher et al. (2000) discovered in the patients who received therapy.

These naturalistic, that is, uncontrolled studies were very suggestive, since they actually employed controls to the extent that one of their experimental conditions (as in the TDCRP) was a placebo rather than a form of psychotherapy. Conversely, if the questionable condition—usually some form of nonspecific support—does indeed offer nonspecific therapeutic elements, then the benefits of psychotherapy, to the extent that they exist, puncture the field's pretensions. In this case, the benefits of therapy cannot be attributed to the rare skills of the therapist but rather to caring, warmth, and patience, which may be even more common among the general population than among frequently robotic and indifferent professionals. Many studies do indeed contain true, unacknowledged controls, especially when their treatments have not been credibly tested against placebos in prior research or when the prior research does not credibly establish their superiority to placebo treatment. Nondirective support therapy was designed intentionally for this experiment "to control for the nonspecific aspects of treatment" (Kolko, Brent, and Baugher, 2000, p. 606). It is questionable whether these elements—the passage of time, the amount of therapist contact, and empathy—require professionals to be administered, and therefore whether nonspecific support should be considered a treatment or a placebo. In fact, nondirective support therapy looks just like the placebo control in the Vanderbilt studies (Strupp and Hadley, 1979) rather than being a true form of psychotherapy that justifies the advanced training of licensed clinicians. The Vanderbilt studies found no difference in the ability of nontherapists and trained therapists to treat troubled college students.

Kolko et al. (2000) further analyzed the Brent et al. (1997) experiment to identify specific elements of the various treatments that related to different outcomes. Enormous problems in defining the elements of treatment, assuring that they were delivered as intended, and then measuring the outcomes prevented any hard conclusions that distinguished between what patients might have been induced to report out of loyalty to their treatments, the treatment situation, and their therapists on the one hand and their actual experiences and outcomes on the other. Still, the authors identified few differential effects of treatment and even fewer that were consistent between the end of treatment and the two-year follow-up. "Neither cognitive nor family measures were found to moderate the acute effects of treatment," and therefore they concluded that treatment is robust. However, the lack of specificity and difference between the treatments again endorses the notion that nondirective supportive therapy is a placebo for psychotherapy or alternatively that psychotherapy itself offers little more than the strategized patience to await the natural remission of depressive symptoms, contact with an accepting human being, and personal warmth. Yet these are the everyday elements of human decency and conventional wisdom, not the rarefied skills that justify the specialized, highly trained professional psychic healer on grounds of predictable clinical effectiveness.

With adolescents as with adults, experimental conditions are labeled place-bos or active treatments at the convenience of the researcher and within clin-ical situations that may well pass along to patients the demand characteris-tics of the researcher's hypothesis through porous methods and imperfect assessment instruments. Birmaher et al.'s (2000) similar recovery rates after one year for patients who completed treatment and those who did not may be explained by the seasonality of depression—its natural course—and by changes in the adolescents' situations as they moved out of their parents' house, went to college or work, established agreeable adult relationships, and so forth.

Moreover, Birmaher et al.'s (2000) repeated use of the Beck Depression Inventory to measure outcomes may account for the initial superiority of cognitive treatment. Participants in cognitive treatment may have appreci-ated the time spent alone with a high-status caring adult; those in treatment with their family may have resented the confrontation with parents; and those in nondirective therapy may have interpreted nondirection as neglect. In short, the Beck scale, trusting self-report, may be more reactive to the treatment situation than to the conditions of depression.

The field refuses to place a moratorium on expensive research pending the development of rigorous designs that employ reliable instruments. Birmaher et al. (2000), loyalists to their field, acknowledged some of the limitations of their research but never the fact that those flaws undercut proof of effective-ness. Instead they pushed on to recommend ever greater doses of psycho-therapy for persistently depressed adolescents. The provision of structural alternatives—nurturing, low anxiety, supportive alternatives to families, atten-tive schools, engaging communities, and the like—rarely if ever crosses the lips of the psychotherapeutic literature or even enters the experimental research as a true control for psychotherapy. The myth of treatment is inex-pensive; improving basic social institutions is immensely more costly.

Rudd et al. (1996) tested an enhanced outpatient intervention against cus-tomary care for suicidal young adults in the military. "The experimental treat-ment was structured on a partial or day hospital format in which patients spent approximately 9 hours each day at the treatment facility for a 2-week period" (p. 182). Therapy involved three types of groups: experiential-affective discussions, psychoeducational classes, and extended problem solving. In contrast, the customary treatment group received a variety of services, includ-ing many of the same kinds of outpatient therapeutic content, averaging seven days of inpatient care.

Rudd et al. (1996) reported no differences between the groups at either one, six, or twelve months after treatment, while insisting that improvement for both groups was similar and was large. At both six and twelve months after treatment, equal percentages of both groups, sometimes reaching 90% depending on the measure, achieved clinically significant change. "Both groups evidenced quick remission of reported symptoms and significant improvement across all areas or domains assessed, including suicidal ideation and behavior, symptomatology, and general problem solving" (p. 188). The authors even went on to boast that their sample "offers a number of strengths relative to previous research," namely, representative young adults who are disproportionately affected by suicide.

Any nontreatment control for acutely suicidal patients is unconscionable. Yet the other flaws of the study are so severe as to question why the research was conducted, written up, or accepted for publication. First, the experimental intervention seemed to be very similar to the standard treatment control, so much so as to undercut the wisdom of a full-blown trial. Second, attrition was huge and, as the authors acknowledged, seemingly selective, with the most severely depressed dropping out. By the six-month follow-up about 50% of both groups had dropped out, and by twelve months more than two-thirds had disappeared from the research. Still, long-term attrition is more appropriately measured against those who were initially randomized to the two groups rather than against those who completed treatment. In this case the base for attrition in the experimental group rises to 181 from 143, with a proportionate increase in the actual attrition rates: at one year, about 75% in both groups. At two years, attrition reached about 95% percent in both groups, and the authors finally allowed modesty to silence their conclusions. The authors still proudly asserted that their experimental group retained more of the poor problem solvers than the control retained.

In fact, the enormous attrition blocks any conclusion at all. It is suggestive of the social motives in the field rather than its clinical commitments that the authors were permitted to present any finding except the confession of weak research and unwarranted conclusions. Yet with so little ability to distinguish between the interventions, it is difficult to justify the effort and expense that went into the research to begin with or to pin much on an analysis that found no difference in outcomes. The general finding that the treatments are equivalent is actually harmful if it convinces the military health system to provide less of the standard treatment in the expectation of financial savings from inpatient expenses. It is a wonder that Rudd et al. (1996) sits among the better experiments in the field and even more provocative that it appears in one of the world's most influential journals.

Weersing and Weisz (2002) measured the outcomes of psychotherapy for depressed youths who received treatment in community mental-health centers and then compared them to the outcomes reported in the literature for similar youths who received cognitive-behavioral therapy. More of the youths in the community-care samples than in the experimental benchmarking studies were minorities and were therefore probably poorer. The outcomes of the "research standard of care" were markedly different than the outcomes of community care for depressed youth until about one year after treatment, when the differences evaporated. While acknowledging that "it is unclear whether the eventual improvement in the [community] sample should be attributed to the effects of [community] therapy or rather to natural remission of depressive symptoms," the same skepticism was not applied to the benchmark. Indeed, the authors might well have asked whether the greater initial benchmark improvements were due to natural remission and biased measurement techniques (along with the other serious faults of the research).

Weersing and Weisz (2002) obviously did not apply symmetrical doubt in the rush to endorse Brent et al. (1997) findings that push the superiority of cognitive-behavioral treatments over psychodynamic treatment for depressed youth while offering a series of suggestions to improve community care. The actual differences among the therapies have been persistently questioned (Luborsky, Singer, and Luborsky, 1975). Yet to the extent to which the community youth may have suffered the situational depressions of poverty, it is notable that Weersing and Weisz (2002), in the manner of the psychotherapeutic literature itself, ignored extrapsychic—social and economic—solutions for adolescent depression. Nor did they provide the advocacy of truth by acknowledging through responsible research that psychotherapy has failed to help depressed youth transcend their deficient families, communities, or schools. The research refuses to state or even experiment with the possibility that socially normative situations are prerequisites for beneficial mental and emotional adjustment.

Largely ignoring the equivalence of outcomes at one year after treatment, Weersing and Weisz (2002) concluded that the differences between community-clinic treatment and experimental outcomes measure the superiority of cognitive-behavioral treatment over community care, which they claimed is frequently psychodynamic. Weersing and Weisz relied upon the community therapists to describe their own therapeutic approaches, but without manuals and evaluations of videotaped sessions the study cannot assure treatment fidelity. Indeed, the community treatment may have included many elements of cognitive-behavioral therapy.

Yet the benchmark may estimate only an optimal level of care that is impossible to achieve outside of a research situation. Research settings usually provide greater scrutiny of service and probably employ more gifted, motivated,

and responsible therapists. Thus, as marginal as the reported benefits of optimal care may actually be after adjusting for the enthusiasms and allegiances
of the researchers, the routine effects of psychotherapy outside of research situations are probably even less successful, possibly including a sizable amount
of frank patient deterioration and practitioner abuse. Indeed, if the benefits
of community care are accounted for largely by natural remission, it looks
as though optimal care provides only short-lived and small benefits, if any
at all. A difference between community care and benchmark care may not
exist. Plausibly, Weersing and Weisz (2002), in the manner of the literature,
simply contrived a number of artifacts through a factional study that reflected
the ambitions of the psychotherapeutic community rather than its ability
to handle adolescent depression and the needs of unhappy children with
problems.

Prevention

Various studies have attempted to prevent relapse among patients treated for
depression. Rare experiments have actually attempted to prevent its initial
occurrence among high-risk groups. The research is as flawed as the basic
treatment studies.

Fava, Rafanelli, Grandi, Conti, and Belluardo (1998) provided cognitive-
behavioral therapy as a follow-up strategy subsequent to drug treatment to
prevent relapse. The study targeted patients with histories of recurrent depression but who responded well to initial treatment. Relapse prevention treatment consisted of ten thirty-minute cognitive-behavioral therapy sessions
every two weeks for experimental patients and clinical management, that is,
supportive therapy for controls. Both groups were completely weaned from
their drugs during the twenty weeks of the study. Because 80% of control
patients but only 25% of experimental patients relapsed during the two years
after prevention treatment, the authors concluded that their experiment "provides important clinical insights regarding the treatment of recurrent, unipolar, major depressive disorder" (p. 818). However, all of the treatments were
provided by only one psychiatrist. Additionally, patients were assessed at eight
points during the two-year follow-up by "the same clinical psychologist who
had performed the previous evaluations and who was unaware of treatment
assignment" (ibid.).

However, it is farcical to maintain that blinding was preserved or that the
single treating psychiatrist failed to transmit his displeasure at relapse to the
patients. Further, no effort was made to obtain the full treatment histories of
patients during the two-year follow-up in order to dispel the possibility that

many sought mental health treatment elsewhere. It is even more suspect that such a light dose of cognitive-behavioral therapy—five hours spread over twenty weeks—would constitute, even in the hands of its most zealous advocates, a curative minimum, notably for people with recurrent and severe depression.

While suffering far greater attrition, the literature customarily reports eight hours as the shortest extent of cognitive therapy. The imperfect literature also rarely reports such dramatic effects. Since the shorter cognitive treatments are associated with the better outcomes, perhaps it is worth asking whether the optimal outcome may be reached with no intervention at all. With less humor, it is worth considering that the research took almost no precautions against researcher expectancies, opening itself up to the charge that the improbable findings are not credible.

In a similar study but handling patients with residual symptoms, Paykel, Scott, and Teasdale (1999) reported only a small difference (16%) in relapse sixty-eight weeks after treatment between patients receiving cognitive therapy and the controls, who received only supportive therapy. Cognitive therapy consisted of sixteen sessions over the first twenty weeks plus two booster sessions. However, all patients received clinical management and drugs. Thus the cognitive-therapy patients received more hours of clinical contact and not simply different kinds of therapy. Attrition was 20% for the 158 patients who were randomized to the two study groups. However, the study had initially recruited 230 patients "who appeared to meet criteria" for inclusion. Paykel et al. (1999) were silent on the loss of the 72 patients who never reached the point of randomization. Presumably they represented a serious attrition that circumscribed the study's representativeness. A difference of only 16% (especially with large differences in the amount of care received by the research groups) muddies interpretation of the findings and is hardly remarkable except to further sustain suspicion toward the power of cognitive-behavioral therapy that Fava et al. (1998) reported.

In another similar study but without drug treatment, Jarrett et al. (2001) reported a 21% difference between the cognitive-therapy group and the supportive-therapy control two years after treatment. Patients who had responded favorably to 20 sessions of cognitive therapy were randomized to an additional 10 sessions of cognitive therapy provided over the subsequent eight months or to a control. Yet the control, receiving nothing but evaluation, failed as a placebo for the cognitive-behavioral therapy, while attrition and measurement problems also undercut the findings.

Clarke et al. (2001) tested the value of psychotherapy for adolescents whose parents were treated for depression in a very large health-maintenance organization. The experimental psychotherapy condition provided "15 one-hour sessions for groups of 6 to 10 adolescents"; the usual-care control was free to utilize any of the HMO's services. Corroborating their earlier experiment, Clarke et al. (2001) concluded that preventive psychotherapy for these youths was very successful, that "the adjusted risk for development of depression in the control group was more than 5 times that of the prevention group" (p. 1133).

Yet the differences between the experimental and control groups were inconsistent across measures and never very large. Two of the principal outcome measures favored the experimental group at completion of treatment and for the twenty-four-month follow-up period; one did not. Most benefits fell off considerably over time. Suicidal tendencies were greater for the control than the experimental group, although the amount is not specified. Major depressive episodes were greater for the control (28.8%) than the experimental group (9.3%). Of the initial 49 youths in the control group, 12 developed a mood disorder (mean time to onset of 14.0 months) within 24 months, while 9 of the 45 youths who received psychotherapy did so (mean time to onset of 6.3 months). Moreover, youths receiving psychotherapy "reported an average of 33 fewer depressed days in the year after intake than did control subjects (11 versus 44).

However, these modest findings might be accounted for by biased reporting. The youths in psychotherapy may well have learned, through the vehicle of group support and an affection for their therapists, to suppress the report of their suicidal thinking, the number of days they actually felt depressed, and even their mood disorders. The opposite motivation among the controls— perhaps to exaggerate depressive symptoms in pursuit of treatment—may have falsely increased their reported differences with the experimental patients. Whether attributed to Kelly's "patient-hiding" (2000), Orne's (1962) demand characteristics, or Rosenthal and Rubin's (1978) expectancy bias, the study did not take steps to assure that therapy itself rather than the reports of subjects accounted for the positive results, such as they were.

Moreover, the final randomized sample of 94 was a highly screened, tiny fraction of the group of 2,995 families of depressed parents who were initially "judged appropriate for the study." Only 65 of the 94 randomized youths provided information at the twenty-four-month follow-up. Apart from the questionable representativeness of the research sample, the enormous amount of lost information at follow-up by itself undercuts claims for treatment effectiveness. Finally, the corroboration between different studies that encourages the field to reach for greater clinical authority is probably due to symmetrical biases in similarly flawed research more than to true scientific replication.

Depression Associated with Other Disorders or Conditions

A large multiyear, multisite clinical trial to test the ability of cognitive-behavioral therapy to enhance recovery from coronary heart disease produced provocative results (Writing Committee, 2003). The trial strikingly involved almost 2,481 patients instead of the small samples characteristic of the literature. Patients who had suffered heart attacks and were depressed or reported low social support or both were randomized to a psychotherapeutic treatment group that received individual and group cognitive-behavioral therapy or to a customary treatment control that received care from their physicians. Treated patients averaged eleven therapy sessions. Follow-up evaluations occurred six months after randomization and then annually for four years.

There was no substantial difference in any measure of coronary disease improvement at any time during the four-year follow-up. The gains for depressed patients in the treatment group compared with those for the control patients were very modest. The improvements in depression and social supports in both groups can easily be attributed to improvements in health and spontaneous remission. The substantial number who subsequently died from their heart attacks were not available for follow-up interviews.

About six months after treatment began, depressed patients in the treatment group showed a very small gain over controls of 3.1 points on the Beck Depression Inventory and 1.8 points on the Hamilton Rating Scale for Depression. The Beck Depression Inventory gains had evaporated by the time of the thirty-month follow-up. The gains for patients with perceived low social support over controls were even smaller and had disappeared by the forty-two-month follow-up. While the Writing Committee (2003) cited Robinson et al. (1990) and Dobson (1989) to justify the effectiveness of cognitive-behavioral therapy, the actual results of their experiment failed to replicate the size of improvements reported in both reviews.

Still, even the Writing Committee's small gains are open to interpretation as biases of the therapeutic situation—reporting less severity and fewer symptoms in order to repay the concern of therapists—rather than as the effects of psychotherapy. The very small gains of experimental patients over controls and even the modest improvements of both groups over their initial levels of depression reported by the Writing Committee (2003) encourage skepticism toward the effectiveness of cognitive-behavioral therapy and reprise the likelihood that a variety of biases and methodological pitfalls account for reported successes. The Writing Committee tends also to dampen enthusiasm for mind cures of physical ailments—the possibilities that deep thinkers can walk through walls and that depression dissipates as people are enjoined to harbor only happy thoughts.

Other studies that tested the value of psychotherapy in handling depression coincidental with medical, social, or mental conditions were far more impaired that the heart disease study. Markowitz et al. (1995) provided short-term interpersonal psychotherapy or supportive therapy to depressed HIV-positive patients. Both therapies demonstrated large gains, but interpersonal psychotherapy achieved significant larger improvements. Gallagher-Thompson and Steffen (1994) claimed to have successfully treated depressed family caregivers. Brown et al. (1996) succeeded with depressed and anxious patients; C. F. Reynolds et al. (1999) with the bereaved elderly; Lenze, Dew, and Mazumdar (2002) with late-life depression; O'Hara, Stuart, Gorman, and Wenzel (2000) against postpartum depression; and Hardy et al. (1995) with depressed patients who also suffered from avoidant, obsessive-compulsive, or dependent personality disorder.

In contrast to the Writing Committee (2003), these studies share a number of common threads: therapists apparently committed to one condition of psychotherapeutic intervention in the study (usually cognitive-behavioral intervention or interpersonal psychotherapy), small samples, recruitment procedures that undercut their representativeness, questionable measures, uncertain measurement procedures, substantial attrition, limited follow-up, and exaggerated interpretations of findings. The studies were published in leading journals. These deficits characterize the psychotherapeutic literature itself and are the reasons why its knowledge is contrived rather than scientific and consequently why psychotherapy is a pseudoscience rather than a true clinical science. Psychotherapy is alternative to medicine because its research methods remain alternative to science.

In the End

When adults, adolescents, and others resolve their depression during psychotherapy, it is probably coincidental to their treatment, not a result of it. The influential summary reviews simply transform the debilitating methodological problems of the basic clinical research into virtues by ignoring them with breathtaking indifference. Recall Smith et al.'s (1980) dismissal of rigor as too fastidious. More recently, Robinson et al. (1990) acknowledged that comparisons with wait-list controls sustained the efficacy of psychotherapy, while comparisons with placebo controls did not. They then proceeded to throw out the placebo comparisons and accept the wait-list comparisons on grounds of popularity. Moreover, their evidence of "research allegiance" to one form of intervention or another, still large after adjustments for long-established loyalties, by itself reduced the efficacy of four out of six types of comparisons.

The most revealing failures of psychotherapy for depression emerge from the weakness of the primary studies rather than from the technical imperfections and obliviousness of the reviews in putting together the results of disparate research. The researchers act more through their true belief in therapy, their critical scientific eyes blinded to the pitfalls of their own research and that of others but sensitive to the vast cultural congregation of cobelievers. They consistently make a premature peace with distorted evidence, offering lame state-of-the-art excuses that their imperfect research is still better than nothing at all and good enough to prove the effectiveness of psychotherapy for depression. The field seems to react against criticism with an extraordinary defensiveness in the manner of two psychologists condemning some of their critics who

> attribute these positive ratings to other factors such as social desirability, demand characteristics and the like. . . . Such criticisms are impossible to refute with certainty in this or any other research on such topics. . . . Such criticisms often can be placed in the 'universal general deficit' category. There are some technically legitimate criticisms that can always be leveled at any research with essentially no fear of disproof. Harcum (1992) called such a reviewing ploy the Carp and Quibble Tactic. (Harcum and Rosen, 1993, pp. 164–165)

Surely the research on treatment for depression has become more sophisticated, both methodologically and statistically. However, it remains porous science—protoscience at best but usually pseudoscience—too leaky to credibly sustain any conclusion in spite of ever more intricate methodological embellishments. It has not provided protection against researcher bias. Notably, clinicians typically evaluate their own practice, an invitation to bias. There does not appear to be any instance—perhaps the Writing Committee (2003) is an exception—in which the evaluation of any form of psychotherapy has been turned over to neutral investigators who stand apart from factional preferences and, more important, from a belief in the efficacy of intervention itself. Researchers' allegiance to psychotherapy, the efficacy of relatively short-term, superficial talk cures, is stronger than their allegiance to any particular intervention.

The primary research on psychotherapy for depression is also bounded by problems that question its applicability to depression generally. The research does not study representative samples of depressed people but only depressed people who seek care or are referred to care. Not one study drew its patients randomly from the underlying population of the depressed. In this way, the findings of the research, such as they are, only speak to the more active, self-aware, motivated, and assertive among the depressed, characteristics that by definition suggest a more amenable group of patients. But because research patients seek treatment on their own or respond to advertisements or agree to referrals, the suspicion lingers that psychotherapy may be largely coincidental with the reduction of their symptoms rather than the reason for the reduction.

Beginning with a group of patients who are probably unrepresentative of the larger number of depressed patients, the primary research then goes on to inflate its findings through additional methodological pitfalls, demand characteristics, and likely biases. Skepticism is endorsed by a persistent observation: psychotherapy patients enjoy little if any advantage over placebo patients; larger benefits for psychotherapy are reported through weaker research. The strongest research reported no benefit for psychotherapy (Writing Committee, 2003).

Without credible evidence that psychotherapy can treat depression, the relationship between patient and therapist takes on the tragedy of a folie à deux, a mutual self-deception providing the would-be healer with status and income that sustains an allegiance to the field and the patient with a compelling but false hope that introspection is a valuable remedy for melancholy. The impulse to look outside of psychotherapy in order to explain it is given force by the persistent inability to relate the qualities of the therapeutic relationship to actual patient outcomes. Patients, and notably those who stay the course, are often protective of their psychotherapists, perhaps believing that they become ennobled by a putative journey of self-discovery and the thought that there is something ineffable to grasp.

Curiously for a process of self-discovery that boasts independence as an outcome, many patients reject out of hand the possibility that the remission of their symptoms is a result of their own will or the seasonality of their sadness and self-doubt or the conditions of their social milieu. Many patients feel the need to export their recoveries to an external force, preferring to believe in psychotherapy as religion and the affirming therapists as spiritual vicars who have conferred a specialness on them. They seek affirmation through discipleship and cherish the process as an epiphany of conversion.

But the pursuit of autonomy and emotional maturity, asserted at the core of psychotherapy, conflicts with the practice of psychotherapy, especially when depression reflects depressing environmental conditions. The language of psychology's humanism includes its euphuistic scientisms, a series of incantations that transform the superstitious dependence of the credulous into a social symbol of individual responsibility. For some it even induces an addiction to the soothing reassurances of therapists complicit in the fiction of emotional progression to Zen master heights of individual wisdom and power—the Oneness of the Twoness of Life and Death—or to Scientology's "clear." Demanding unquestioning belief, the cult of psychotherapy scorns challenges to its pseudoscientific proofs of effectiveness, denigrating nonbelievers as heretics and skeptics as quibblers.

The longstanding social adoration of psychotherapy turns its back on the absence of scientific evidence that psychotherapy is an effective treatment for depression. However, treatment is not the point of its popularity. In spite of their regrettable failures of practice and intellect, clinical psychotherapy and its inseparable scholarship may both be useful as expressions of social ideology—a paradox of treatment resolved by political choice. The strong and large relationship between income, education, and the prevalence of depression (Kessler et al., 2003) occurs in a society that cherishes intrapsychic approaches to social problems not for the beauty of their clinical prowess but because they thwart more material, costly provisions and promote the nation's heroic individualism.

2: Anxiety

The same cunning and compromise with scientific rigor that obscure the ineffectiveness of psychotherapy for depression also hide the failure of individual psychotherapy to treat anxiety and related problems. In the process of its repetitive and ponderous failures, it has put together impressive fables for a credulous and needy public. Witches, elves, goblins, trolls, hobbits, werewolves, and vampires—only children and lunatics believe in their literal presence. But only the ignorant and oblivious discount them as child's tales. Psychotherapy, like other social rituals, is of a piece with the pageantry of the fantastic. They are all insubstantial truths but formative in their metaphorical importance.

The society accepts with only the merest and most belabored proofs the ability of psychotherapy to handle emotional and mental problems. Lacking rational evidence of effectiveness, psychotherapy persists as metaphor, ritualizing the culture's values in a popular, accessible format. The meaning of psychotherapy lies outside the clinic, in the creation of authority to ratify mass belief, a bulwark of social cohesion against disorder. The clinic is a stage for the melodrama of morality. Yet belief in modern society is induced through the culture's touchstones of its traditions. The shaman as scientist affirms the clinician through a language of stunning obscurity that pervades the dialectics of mental disease, deviance, and treatment in practice, scholarship, and publication. It is not so much that science confers authority as that authority demands scientific conformity with social imperatives.

The undercurrents that actually create the forces of culture are only dimly perceived; they may be unknowable, a tragedy of semievolved consciousness. Nevertheless, their expressions are tangible: psychotherapy for phobia, for one, is contained in a series of experimental papers and critically assessed against scientific criteria. The actual momentum of psychotherapy's social force and its expressive importance emerge as the tangible evidence of effectiveness crumbles under scrutiny. The possibility of critical analysis has never been hidden or even obscure; it is part of the canon of higher education. The field's patent fecklessness is incidental to social belief in the same way that historical inquiry does not bust itself to prove that Samson had his hair cut, that the Red Sea waters parted as plumbed walls, that Red Riding Hood was propositioned by the wolf, that Mother Hubbard lived in public housing not a shoe, that George Washington threw a pfennig not a dollar across the Delaware, and that Moses and the ancient Hebrews chiseled the Ten Com-mandments. Psychotherapy is the legend of which stuff is made—social belief, not scientific truth.

Anxiety, Phobia, and Panic

In one of the better designed and conducted experiments, Heimberg et al. (1998) compared cognitive-behavioral group therapy and drug therapy in treat-ing social phobia. Each treatment was carefully matched with an appropriate placebo: a placebo pill for the drugs and educational-supportive group ther-apy for the psychotherapy group. The cognitive-behavioral group therapy—twelve 2.5 hour sessions to groups of between 5 and 7 patients—consisted of a sequence of four cognitive restructuring steps that are standard for cognitive-behavioral therapy patients: identification of automatic thoughts, identifica-tion of the logical errors in the automatic thoughts, formulation of reasonable alternatives, and formulation of measurable goals. The therapy also included exposure to feared situations, practice with cognitive skills and handling reac-tions to feared situations, behavioral tasks, and homework in practicing cog-nitive restructuring.

Educational-supportive group therapy presumably offered about the same number of sessions and hours but simply discussed topics related to social phobia rather than offering processes of psychological change, nor did it "instruct patients to confront feared situations" (p. 1135). One hundred and thirty-three patients recruited at two different clinics were randomly assigned to each of the four groups. Attrition was modest, with only 26 patients (19.5%) reported as dropping out of their groups early, although only 65% of patients completed drug therapy and only 58% completed psychotherapy; many would cite 42% as the true rate of attrition. One "independent assessor" per-formed the patient ratings.

After twelve weeks of treatment, the authors claimed that drug treatment and psychotherapy were both successful and the literature, repeatedly citing their research, apparently believes them:

> Compared with pill placebo and attention-placebo conditions, both [treatments] were associated with higher rates of response after 12 weeks. . . . The 2 treatments produced equivalent outcomes. Seventy-seven percent of patients receiving [drugs] and 75% of patients under-going cognitive behavioral group therapy who completed treatment . . . were classified as responders, significantly more than [control-group patients]. (Heimberg et al., 1998, p. 1139)

While drug treatment obtained quicker and better responses among a greater percentage of patients, both treatments were presented as conferring large benefits on patients. Unfortunately, the actual data of the study as well as its many pitfalls will not sustain these conclusions. First, only one assessor apparently evaluated all patients. While Heimberg et al. were proud of their design, which tested allegiance to either drug or cognitive therapy, their design ignored the possible effects of allegiance to treatment generally. While perhaps independent in an existential sense—free to pursue happiness and occupational passion—the assessor was obviously not independent of the research nor its clinical stakes. The signature of a paycheck has a clarity in defining allegiance quite apart from the heroic musings of the payee. It is unlikely that the sole assessor was unaware either of treatment assignment in many patients who received psychotherapy or of even telltale clinical evidence of the drugs (phenelzine in this case).

But even granting for the moment the integrity of the measures and the measurement process, the measured benefits themselves were customarily small and very uneven. Indeed, they were frequently so small as to belie any clinical significance. While 6 of the 8 measures made by the assessor were statistically significant and favored the treatments, only 4 of the 10 outcomes rated by patients were statistically significant, favoring the treatments. Patients were also provided 4-minute tests of their ability to handle feared situations. Two of the three measures were statistically significant and favored the treated groups.

Heimberg et al. (1998) presented the magnitude of benefits through effect sizes, citing specific measures on which the treatments appear to be moderately effective. Yet in no case did they reach Smith, Glass, and Miller's (1980) overall effect size of .85. Moreover, effect sizes only convey the relative improvement of patients over controls; they do not indicate the actual size of improvement. In fact the 21 measures that Heimberg et al. (1998) report are customarily small, frequently not statistically significant, and at times underscore the gains of the placebo groups. Moreover, not one of the 12 effect sizes for cognitive-behavioral therapy reached .50; seven were below .25. Again, effect size says nothing about clinical significance. Contrary to Heimberg et al. and notably related to research that suffers a multitude of threats to its rigor, until effect sizes surpass .50 (where about 40% of treated patients are better off than controls), they are probably not worth attention.

It is more than a little curious that in both the analysis of all enrolled patients and the analysis of only those who completed treatment, the pill placebo group consistently outpaced the educational-supportive therapy control. Moreover, on a number of outcomes in all categories of assessment (by the independent assessor, through self-rating, and by the behavior test), the pill placebo group was better off than the cognitive-behavioral treatment patients. While the differences were small, between 5% and 10%, and the study was leaky, these findings raise questions about the possibly pernicious dynamics of therapy itself. The pill placebo group received only a pill and presumably clinical monitoring. Yet almost 40% of pill placebo patients were rated as responders after twelve weeks. Thus the measured benefits of the pill placebo patients were due either to placebo effects or to natural remission. Educational-supportive therapy apparently suppressed either or both of these effects, all the more remarkable since the provided support logically should have increased the placebo effects. Yet this point is speculative in light of the large number of patients who did not complete treatment and the resulting very small samples of patients who did complete it.

While Heimberg et al. (1998) is notable for its carefully designed placebo controls, its other flaws—characteristic of anxiety, phobia, and panic studies generally—undercut any conclusion of positive outcomes, at least for the psychotherapeutic interventions: recruitment and self-selection, measurement, variable outcomes at the end of therapy, and especially the issue of follow-up, that is, whether the benefits of therapy are sustained.

Liebowitz et al. (1999) addressed the issue of sustained benefits in a follow-up study of those who had responded well in Heimberg et al. (1998) to either drug therapy or cognitive-behavioral group therapy. Liebowitz et al. provided maintenance therapy for six months after initial treatment then terminated all treatment and monitored patients for another six months. Maintenance therapy consisted of monthly cognitive-behavioral group therapy sessions of 2.5 hours each and weekly homework assignments or continued drug treatment. Of the 21 psychotherapy patients and 20 drug-treatment patients eligible for this study (that is, those who responded to earlier treatment), 7 of the former and 6 of the latter refused to continue. Thus of the 133 initial patients randomized for treatment in Heimberg et al., only 24, that is 21%— an attrition of 79%—continued into follow-up maintenance.

Liebowitz et al. (1999) reported that only 3 of the 14 drug-treatment patients relapsed during maintenance, 1 dropped out, and another 3 relapsed during the nontreatment period; in the psychotherapy group, 1 patient relapsed and 1 dropped out during maintenance. While outcomes were comparable between the two treatment conditions, they are also comparable to the outcomes of the two initial placebo conditions. Of the 67 patients initially randomized to treatment, only 18 had continued to respond six months after treatment, a proportion that is slightly lower than the approximately 22 of

66 patients who had responded to placebo conditions by the end of active treatment.

Curiously, the researchers abandoned controls during the follow-up without a nontreatment control during maintenance therapy or comparisons between the treatment responders and the placebo responders at any follow-up point. Thus the causes of the outcomes are ambiguous, whether improvements, limited as they were, resulted from psychotherapy or simply from the motivation of responders, the seasonality of their social phobia, or placebo effects.

Yet the study's serious problems did not inhibit the authors' rosy, differentiated conclusions: psychotherapeutically "treated patients may have less chance of relapse; however [drug] treated non-relapsers maintained greater gains" (Liebowitz et al., 1999, p. 95). The authors identified the small sample sizes as a limitation of the study but only in reducing the precision of measurement, ignoring the many problems of bias created by tiny samples and what they acknowledged to be "somewhat arbitrary" criteria for improvement. Yet on their way to boast of the study's methodological strengths, notably the presence and length of maintenance phases, they failed to acknowledge the enormous number of problems that undercut any conclusion at all. The benefits of the interventions, notably cognitive-behavioral group treatment, were unimpressive and, considering the problems of measurement and controls, probably nonexistent.

The actual size of the gains made by treated groups over controls was small and suspiciously inconsistent. Indeed, so many problems mar both the treatment study and the follow-up study that the authors might have more profitably sacrificed them as offerings to skepticism and restraint. But no such modesty softened their conclusions nor provoked the prestigious journals in which they appeared to insist upon a more cautious write-up of the experiments.

In light of the many problems of design that were foreseeable—attrition, low completion rates, measurement problems, and the issue of controls for the follow-up—a prudent experimenter might have refused to embark on such a scientifically quixotic venture. But the research is neither prudent nor scientifically rigorous, largely because the society demands the fictions of clinical success and the community of psychotherapeutic researchers is politically responsive. The studies by Heimberg et al. (1998) and Liebowitz et al. (1999) are not moments for celebration but rather for wonderment that such imperfect experiments should call attention to anything but their deficiencies and the motives of the audience that credulously accepts them as true science.

Serious ethical problems also emerge from jerking around troubled patients when no tenable finding is possible. Moreover, informed consent is not an informed protection when the researchers and their institutional review boards refuse to comment on the quality of the research design but only on the possible harms of treatment itself. The criticism becomes deeply troubling after one realizes that Heimberg et al. (1998) and Liebowitz et al. (1999) represent the very best of the clinical research, far more sophisticated and aware than the great majority of what passes for authority and rigor in the clinical literature of psychotherapy.

Both Heimberg et al. and Leibowitz et al. consistently presented their data selectively, in a manner that enhanced the appearance of effective treatment. They offered additional data and complied with requests rapidly and fully. Nevertheless, the published presentations are both deceptive and capricious. Putting the best foot forward, a principle of polite society but certainly not of science, means it is never stubbed against either the skepticism of the field, its journals, or a public pursuing realistic cure for serious mental and emotional problems. To the contrary, the faulty and misleading research is given the same permission for fabulism as a Disney production and with the same purpose of fabricating fables of social conduct, morality plays, dramatizations of deep cultural values, and evidence of small steps toward idealized goals. In each case, the self-positing ego triumphs over social responsibility. The subtlety of the scientific pretensions of the psychotherapeutic literature rests with the authors' medical degrees, fancy doctorates, and cosmetic use of statistics, scales, and controls. Yet its sublime meaning rises through its contrivances as ideology, careerist boosterism, and the meekness of those who have seen the god of culture and bowed to its imperatives—not science, not truth, not service to the distressed, not the bafflement of intelligence confronting the conundrums of culture. All the rococo contrivances of cleverness have been whittled into statues of the grotesque.

The Heimberg project is Aesopean in quality and meaning, an entertainment for the culture, appreciated and rewarded. The other research aspires to public service with the same esurient ambition for prominence and expertise. Provocatively, Butler, Fennell, Robson, and Gelder (1991) concluded that cognitive-behavioral therapy is superior to behavioral (relaxation) therapy in handling generalized anxiety disorder, while both are superior to the wait-list control. Although the customary problems of measurement impaired the research and its samples were relatively small, the findings were large and consistent across a variety of measures—some reported by patients and others recorded by the perennial "independent assessor"—and persisted at six-month follow-up with very low rates of attrition. Wait-list patients maintained the levels of their symptoms across twelve weeks.

In contrast, it is intriguing that among J. Beck, Stanley, Baldwin, Deagle, and Averill's (1994) control group of patients who received only minimal contact (enquiry and empathetic listening, once weekly by phone)—similar clinically to Butler et al.'s (1991) wait-list patients—fully 36% were assessed to be "responders," that is, their clinical improvements were substantial enough to constitute cure. The large changes in J. Beck et al.'s control, compared with the persistence of symptoms in Butler et al.'s wait-list patients, begs for explanation. If in fact wait-list patients falsify their symptoms to stay eligible for treatment and if reported outcomes of the minimal-contact control indicate an underlying seasonality of emotional problems and self-cure, then Butler et al.'s (1991) impressive gains for psychotherapy, especially cognitive-behavioral treatment, evaporate. Yet the minimal-contact control did not seem to be a placebo, since the patients were not told and therefore could not have believed that they were in therapy. Thus the stark differences between the outcomes of the controls in the two studies beckon ever more forcefully to the volatility of the research and the possibility that findings may be more frequently induced than simply recorded. In fact, the impressive Butler et al. findings may simply be projections of the researchers' preference for cognitive therapy over relaxation therapy and psychotherapy in general over no treatment at all. The research is given added irony by Butler et al.'s (1991) confession that "there is no consensus on criterion measures of generalized anxiety disorder" (p. 69), which still fails to slow the march toward enhanced findings.

Therapy itself transmits an expectation of recovery to patients. Therefore in order to create an adequate control that approximates the environment of therapy but without its defining curative elements, minimal-contact conditions might profitably verbalize an expectation by the interviewer that the patient will improve. Even better, by recognizing that the effectiveness of psychotherapy has not been established, patients might be given instructions that all group assignments are therapeutic, thus creating a true placebo.

Telch, Schmidt, Jaimez, Jacquin, and Harrington (1995) insisted that cognitive-behavioral therapy improved the lives of panic-disorder patients. However the statistically significant improvements were small, inconsistent, and clinically marginal. A 12% effect size improvement over a community comparison group reported in a different study is very small, even while it obscures the actual size of the improvement. Moreover, attrition and censoring were high; the loss of data for a number of analyses and comparisons approached

50% at six-month follow-up; all of the measures relied on patient self-report; differences between the wait-list control and the treated sample, although not statistically significant, were often sizable.

Barrowclough et al. (2001) insisted that cognitive-behavioral therapy "was an effective treatment for anxiety problems in older adults and that the benefits observed at the end of therapy were maintained over the 12-month follow-up" (p. 761). However, cognitive-behavioral therapy was superior on only two self-reported measures to supportive counseling, a form of therapy that they employed as a control. Supportive counseling relies on the therapist's empathy, respect, and practiced genuineness to achieve patient changes. The research employed neither a nontreatment control nor a placebo condition. Attrition reached 41% in the cognitive-behavioral group, going far to explain its occasional superiority to the supportive counseling group, which only suffered 18% attrition. The samples were tiny. Similarly inflated claims for emotion-focused psychotherapy in treating panic disorder (Shear, Houck, Greeno, and Masters, 2001) and for brief dynamic psychotherapy in reducing relapse rates (Wiborg and Dahl, 1996) are similarly punctured by the deficiencies of the experiments: small samples, high attrition, questionably relevant differences between treated groups, the absence of meaningful controls, measurement bias, rater bias, and so forth.

Treating Youths for Anxiety and Phobia

It is déjà vu all over again. Adolescents with anxiety and phobia do not fare any better talking to their psychotherapists than do adolescents who are depressed. Barrett, Dadds, and Rapee (1996) discovered large and persistent benefits for cognitive-behavioral therapy—even greater when paired with family management—in treating youths with anxiety disorder. However, with anxiety disorder in particular, their wait-list control was singularly inappropriate; apart from the possibility of inducing false reports of symptoms, the wait-listing may actually exacerbate anxiety.

In any event, the size of their success seems proportionate to the softness of their measures. Principal measures of success came from "clinicians who were unaware of the child's treatment condition," which is implausible since in repeated and extensive interviews, it becomes quite obvious that patients are on a wait-list when they tip to not seeing a therapist, or that children are being treated by themselves when their parents either confess to seeing a therapist or disclose that only their child sees a therapist. Moreover, the use of clinicians to judge clinical outcomes defies any canon of objectivity—only the use of therapists to rate their own patients would be worse. Indeed, to rely upon the implicit judgments of those with a professional interest in the outcomes is to actually thumb a research nose at science. Their other measures were derived from the self-reports of the youths and their parents.

It is startling that every outcome measure consistently improved across each point of assessment: pretreatment, post-treatment, six-month follow-up, and twelve-month follow-up. This level of regular progress is nearly unique in the literature and points to the experiment's other problems in addition to its soft measures and self-serving measurement procedures. Samples were small; the reliability of the initial diagnoses was modest; attrition at follow-up reached 17% and there was no attempt to count dropouts as failures; there were large and significant differences between one of the treated groups and the wait-list patients at pretest; patient recruitment as well as the outcomes of the wait-list patients after treatment were not reported.

Even more serious, by relying upon an inappropriate wait-list Barrett et al. (1996) ignored the likelihood that positive outcomes, rather than being a result of treatment, arose naturally from a self-selected group of adults sufficiently motivated to seek treatment for their children and to subject themselves to scrutiny of their parenting. Thus the research fails to handle the extent to which anxiety naturally dissipated over time among amenable patients or the possibility that the results were simply artifacts of the experiment as patients fulfilled the expectations of their therapists in describing their conditions. Indeed, it seems to be definitional that patients who suffer anxiety disorder would seek to please their therapists. After all, confessing failure to an authority figure, mentor, or beloved confessor would in itself increase their anxiety. On their part, Barrett et al. did not risk any twinge of anxiety by applying scientific skepticism to their experiment.

Kendall et al. (1997) compared an average of 18 sessions of cognitive-behavioral therapy with a wait-list control. They claimed their treatment for anxious youths demonstrated so many gains that it should be considered "generally efficacious." Therefore, future tests need not include nontreatment controls but only comparisons against "an alternative therapy such as family treatment, group treatment," or eventually drug treatments (p. 378).

But not so fast, as their conclusions again far outpaced the value of their data. It is commendable that the research employed a range of measures from a variety of raters: clinicians, parents, teachers, direct observations of the youths' behavior during interviews, and the youths' self-reports. Most of the measures favored the treated children and were sustained one year afterward. However, the teachers found no gains. The authors attempted to explain this away on grounds that "a substantial number of children with anxiety disorders are not seen by teachers as troublesome in the classroom" (Kendall et al., 1997, p. 378). This may be the conventional wisdom, but it is offered without any substantiating reference to research. Moreover, only a few of the behavioral observations were significant; but again, the authors discounted their importance, since "in another study the behavioral codes did not discriminate between youths diagnosed with anxiety disorders and those who did not meet the criteria for a diagnosis" (ibid.). Then why did the authors include these measures in the study? Were they fishing for corroboration?

An even greater threat to their happy conclusions was the fact that the wait-list control was more compromised in this research than it was in other studies. The authors' sensitivity to the problems of wait-list controls, however, did not prevent their misuse in analysis. "A 16-week (4 month) waiting-list was deemed too long for clinically referred cases. Such a long wait period may increase attrition (and differential attrition), with many parents seeking alternate treatment for their children during the wait period and, thereby, reducing the representativeness of the resulting sample" (Kendall et al., 1997, p. 369).

Therefore, out of concern for the patients' suffering, the research only maintained the wait-list for eight weeks but by doing so reduced the comparability of their wait-list control. Thus the principal findings are derived from faulty comparisons between treated patients at sixteen weeks (termination) and one year follow-up and wait-list patients at eight weeks. Attempting to resolve the control problem, the authors assumed that the first portion of treatment simply sets up the second portion, enactive exposure, which contains the therapeutic gold of cognitive-behavioral treatment. Therefore, their second analysis compared treated patients at termination with wait-list patients after they subsequently received the initial eight weeks of treatment. But the patients were not handled at the same time by the therapists, who, obviously aware of patient assignment as either control or treated, may have adjusted their interactions, transmitting different expectations.

More serious, the wait-list experienced enormous attrition: 9 of 34 patients had dropped off before their treatment phase, presumably because they sought treatment. It is likely that the departure of these more energetic parents of anxious children left the more seriously disturbed on the wait-list, thus exaggerating their differences from treated patients at any point in the analysis. Six more dropped out during the treatment phase, for a total debilitating attrition of 44%. Nine of the 60 treated patients dropped out, possibly the more debilitated, who did not or could not respond. Thus the findings of the research need to be discounted due to the likelihood of substantial differences between the study groups—an overly anxious group of control patients and a less anxious group of treated patients—that by themselves may well have accounted for the reported treatment benefits.

Many of the findings were statistically significant, but the actual size of the gains, largely drawn from the self-reports of the youths and their parents, were quite modest and even smaller in light of the subsequent improvements of the wait-list patients during the initial nontherapeutic eight weeks of their therapy. Moreover, in an attempt to measure clinical significance, the authors reported that perhaps 20% more of the treated than the nontreated patients returned to nonclinical levels of anxiety; this modest benefit was based on parent and teacher reports but apparently was not sustained by the youths' reports, which were not presented in the published research. Thus the positive gains, small and inconsistent to begin with, were undercut by the deficiencies of the controls and large, probably differential attrition.

In addition, the authors seemed oblivious to the likelihood that the self-reports of the treated patients and their parents indicated gratitude for the affections of their therapists more than actual improvement. Indeed, Kendall et al. (1997) found no relationship between either the quality of the therapist's relationship with the children or the quality of parental involvement in treatment (as measured by the therapists) and the reported outcomes. These relationships are expected, and their absence raises the question whether there is, indeed, any relationship between psychotherapy and reported outcomes. The possibility that the demand characteristics of the research situation transmitted the desires of engaging therapists for confirming reports from their patients, anxiously seeking approval, constantly intrudes itself. Yet none of the frank imperfections of the research were adequate to caution the authors that cognitive-behavioral treatment might not have been adequately tested. Indeed, a placebo would have seemed to be obligatory in light of the problems of wait-lists and the unproven effectiveness of cognitive-behavioral therapy for youth with anxiety disorder. Still, neither clinicians nor their funding source—again, the National Institute of Mental Health—nor their institutional review boards accepted prudent methodological safeguards against concocted evidence of clinical effectiveness.

The imperfect research is accepted as definitive by subsequent studies that are grateful for the encouragement to ignore design problems. Indeed, the consecutiveness of weak proofs seems to be periodically renewed as a sacrament of allegiance, a ritual of solidarity in a professional interest group that is ever more needful of exaggerated tributes to its clinical power. Dropping out even wait-list controls from their design, Cobham, Dadds, and Spence (1998) are able to report that treatment for youths with anxiety disorder was enormously successful—over 80% in a number of their groups that received cognitive-behavioral treatment. Cognizant of Kendall et al. (1997) and imitating many of their problems, Öst, Svensson, Hellström, and Lindwall (2001) reported large self-reported gains for *one* session of exposure therapy for motivated youths with specific and relatively mild phobias who were maintained at one-year follow-up; indeed, there may even be some truth to Öst et al., except that they failed to follow-up their wait-list for one year, during which they might have discovered that a goodly amount of exposure therapy for fear of spiders, snails, birds, and ants occurred naturally.

Post-Traumatic Stress Disorder (PTSD)

Traumatic stress, usually caused by violence such as war combat, rape, and serious assault, presumably creates traumatic memories that, through panic and anxiety, seriously disrupt customary social and psychological behaviors—sleep, thought, memory, social interactions, and so forth. Various behavioral interventions have been tried to dispel the traumatic memories. Eye-movement desensitization and reprocessing (EMDR) is one of the more controversial.

During EMDR the patient holds in mind "an image of the trauma, a negative self-cognition, negative emotions, and related physical sensations about the trauma" and then moves the eyes "quickly and laterally back and forth for about 15 to 20 seconds, following the therapist's fingers," reporting back changes in thoughts and emotions (S. A. Wilson, Becker, and Tinker, 1995, p. 928). "This recursive procedure continues until desensitization of troubling material is complete and positive self-cognitions have replaced the previous negative self-cognition" (ibid.). EMDR is presumably effective in just a few sessions, while more standard exposure therapies such as systematic desensitization and flooding usually require more than ten sessions.

In designing their experiment, S. A. Wilson et al. seemed aware of the methodological weaknesses of previous research: "there was no objective or standardized post traumatic stress disorder diagnosis, the research design did not control for nonspecific treatment (placebo) effects or therapist demand characteristics, the novelty and complexity of the EMDR treatment was not controlled for, and the sample size was small" (pp. 928–929). Their own design randomized 80 patients to two conditions: EMDR treatment and a "delayed treatment" control, that is, a wait-list. They found that on every measure EMDR was superior to the control at post-treatment and at 90-day follow-up. The wait-list patients, when treated, mirrored the gains of the initial EMDR group.

Yet awareness of the invalidating pitfalls of previous research was not sufficient to stir S. A. Wilson et al. to safeguard their own experiment. They did
not incorporate a placebo, and they acknowledged that "behavioral measures
of outcomes were not used." Thus all their measures, notably including reports
of anxiety and panic that are central to diagnosing the disorder, depended on
patient self-report. Randomization by itself does not provide adequate justification for a complex trial. In fact, it seems wasteful to conduct any research
on post-traumatic stress disorder at this late date without first resolving the
problem of measurement reliability and then assuring that demand characteristics are properly eliminated.

Feske and Goldstein (1997) contradicted S. A. Wilson et al. (1995) in an
experiment with more appropriate controls. Feske and Goldstein assigned
patients to EMDR, a placebo group similar in every way except that it did not
receive eye movement, and a wait-list. While EMDR patients mirrored the
gains over wait-list patients reported in S. A. Wilson et al., they were only
slightly improved over the placebo. Notably, all differences evaporated at
three-month follow-up. Unfortunately, Feske and Goldstein's groups all num-
bered fewer than twenty participants, and again, the measures were based on
patient self-report. Thus the distinctions between the two studies may be
explained as much by initial attitudes of the researchers toward EMDR as by
the true conditions of their patients.

The same concerns about EMDR were voiced by Devilly (2001a,b) but not
well answered by Lipke (2001), who relied on issues of professional loyalty
rather that the quality of the research itself. It is notable that in order to sustain the effectiveness of EMDR, Lipke (2001) simply recorded patient gains
subsequent to treatment, with little appreciation for the vagaries of self-
report within research environments that promote the effectiveness of the
tested treatments. Because effectiveness depends on the experimental group's
gains over placebos, behavioral treatments, even the most customary, that
frequently employ uncontrolled single-subject designs have fared poorly,
producing little credible evidence of their benefit (Corrigan, 2001).

Foa, Rothbaum, Riggs, and Murdock (1991) compared four interventions
to treat rape victims for post-traumatic stress disorder: stress inoculation training, prolonged exposure, supportive counseling, and wait-list. The authors
consider the first two to be cognitive-behavioral therapies rather than behavioral therapies similar to systematic desensitization or flooding. Treatments
were provided in nine 1.5-hour sessions spread over about four months.

Initially, Foa et al. reported that "all conditions produced improvement on
all measures immediately post-treatment and at follow-up" (p. 715). They
then went on to torture their findings for evidence that treatment was supe-

rior to the wait-list, reporting that the superiority of the cognitive-behavioral treatments "was evidenced only on post traumatic stress disorder symptoms" but not on any of the other measures of psychopathology (p. 721). Yet they failed to bracket their small point by commenting on the tiny number of subjects (45 spread across the four conditions), the weak self-reported data, or the large pretreatment differences among groups. However, the inability to demonstrate improvement over the nontreatment control compels a conclusion of frank ineffectiveness. Without any notable gain of one condition over any other but gains in all conditions over time, it is a point of wonderment that Foa et al. refused to confront the folk wisdom that time heals all wounds or the possibility that the treatments were absurd and ineffective intrusions into the lives of victims of violence. It hardly seems a point of feminist advocacy to promote an ineffective treatment rather than to acknowledge the continuing difficulties of seriously abused women.

Marks, Lovell, Noshirvani, Livanou, and Thraher (1998) repeated many of the customary methodological errors in driving to a conclusion the idea that therapy is effective against post-traumatic stress disorder. The reactive measures, small samples, treatment allegiances, recruitment patterns, absence of true controls, and attrition should have dampened their enthusiasm that "prolonged exposure, and cognitive restructuring . . . were each superior to relaxation" (p. 317). Instead, they pressed on to a mystical explanation for the equally curative abilities of different therapies: "An emotion can be reduced by action on certain strands in its skein of responses. Attenuating one strand can then weaken others" (p. 324). They might have contemplated the alternative possibility that the findings were contrivances of the research situation rather than bragging that sample sizes under 20 in each group are large.

A Few More Comments

It is an act of faith among the easily led that psychotherapy resolves panic, anxiety, phobia, PTSD, and related problems. Yet the uninitiated are barred from research in the field. There is not one discoverable study of the effects of psychotherapy conducted by someone who is not a therapist or enrolled professionally in the community of clinicians. Indeed, entry into the nests of therapy research are protected more sedulously than eagles' chicks. This is a true marvel, as dissidents have routine access to government but apparently not to government funds in its psychotherapeutic territories.

The trip through the faulty studies of psychotherapy's clinical outcomes bumps along to an exasperated question: "Is psychotherapy effective?" Yes indeed it is, but as an entertainment of social education rather than as clinical science. The consensus of practitioners, the most obvious stakeholders in the game, is allowed to substitute for credible proof of clinical effectiveness. The field is not moved by a demanding public to conduct credible tests of its effectiveness. Instead, a cherished social institution is enjoined to clutch science to its mothering breast while it is relieved of the obligation to provide authentic proof. The clinical literature has achieved democratic popularity without rational acclaim.

It is as though psychotherapy were in the motion-picture business, with a market test hovering over its head. It seems detached from accountability to clinical criteria for cure, prevention, or rehabilitation. It endures because enough tickets are bought to sustain the industry. It is acceptable to critics as popular culture, even high culture, in its cognitive and emotive (psychodynamic) forms that flatter the successful and affirm the wisdom and justice of the society's ethos. Its truths are guided into the realm of full-screen epics by biblical shepherds in lab coats babbling about statistics and mystical mental dynamics, epiphanies of the divine.

Psychotherapists separate themselves from the frankly crackpot by the distance of social class, not substance; by emotional intelligence, not insight; by social acceptability, not content. Their little lies are not terrible; they are the quotidian deceits of social meaning and culture. They are the way that people get on with life and carve out a bit of self-respect and social position. Unfortunately, the perfidies of psychotherapy play out ideologically in consistent support of a social policy of inexpensive, unambitious social-welfare programs that impose an enormous amount of personal responsibility on those least able to bear it. But just as psychotherapy did not create itself from a series of tests and proofs of what works, so it is that people do not form themselves in spite of their heroic beliefs in self-creation and personal responsibility.

Psychotherapy is compatible with a society deeply attached to an ethos of self-invention, a fiction that dispels the terror of confronting humanity's miserably evolved self-consciousness, deep ignorance, and vast inability to control its urges or its environment. The benefits of self-deception, perhaps political stability and cultural coherence, are probably paid for by the persistence of social problems—actual social progress, necessitating attention to social problems, being undercut by an ideology of social progress that denies them.

3: The Addictions

The extent of the social and personal problems caused by the addictions draws sharp attention to the extraordinarily consistent failure in treating them. Certainly there are some patients whose recovery occurs during and after psychotherapy. Yet cure is rare, often associated with the age of thirty and explained by the addict's personal motivation and social circumstances, suggesting that in the few instances of success, psychotherapy may be more an irrelevant ceremony of cure than its actual cause. While a number of strategies seem to offer hope of reducing the damage of addiction—"harm reduction" programs and methadone—neither one incorporates psychotherapy or cures the dependency; both accept the addiction; both work with a selected group of patients.

Yet without offering much chance of remission, psychotherapy for addicts serves perhaps a more theological function of condemnation, blame, and perhaps stigma even when the therapist is as value free and without judgment as the textbooks prescribe. The demand that patients take responsibility for themselves, pressed with the futility and passion of skid-row preaching, underscores the intransigence of the patients without providing a solution for the addiction itself. Just like the mission to the forlorn, participation in psychotherapy is the socially approved devotional obeisance demanded of the impenitent and improvident before they receive some small, concrete benefit: rice Christians who sit through a sermon being allowed into the mess hall, and rice addicts who endure psychotherapy as a condition of hospitalization or housing or other basic services. However, the benefit is not small when participation in psychotherapy is a condition for probation or parole.

Psychotherapy for the addictions is customarily paired with some sort of social sanction; it is rarely voluntary; yet it remains persistently ineffective. However, the continuing popularity of psychotherapy may be suggested by its placement of responsibility on addicts—their failure to take responsibility for themselves—rather than in a medical condition over which they have as little control as over a virus infection or the flow of their blood. Quite to the point, psychotherapy's role is consistent with the mood of America expressed with some force in eliminating the eligibility of addicts for Supplemental Security Income in the 1996 welfare-reform legislation. That act (the Personal Responsibility and Work Opportunity Reconciliation Act of 1996) separated addicts from the seriously mentally ill, no longer accepting the drug and alcohol dependent as medically disabled but rather denouncing them as rebarbative, self-indulgent, hedonistic, and irresponsible. The failure of psychotherapy in treating the addictions is compensated by the ideological benefits of readily available bad examples to underscore the virtues of American self-sufficiency. Still, psychotherapists are far too well trained, deeply conscious of social motives, and insightful about themselves to be simple, unwitting accomplices in this social melodrama of righteousness.

Drugs

Winters, Fals-Stewart, O'Farrell, Birchler, and Kelley (2002) compared behavioral couples therapy with individual-based treatment in treating alcohol and drug abuse among a sample of married or cohabiting female subjects.[1] Behavioral [sic] couples therapy and Individual-based treatment both provided cognitive-behavioral therapy "in developing coping-skills behaviors conducive to abstinence" (p. 347); the females in the Behavioral couples therapy condition participated in one-hour individual sessions and ninety-minute group sessions without their "intimate partners" and in one-hour sessions with their partners. Individual-based treatment did not provide any conjoint therapy, only one-hour individual sessions and ninety-minute group sessions without intimate partners. Both treatment conditions covered twenty-four weeks, with participants scheduled for 56 treatment sessions. In short, "the only difference between the Behavioral couples therapy and Individual-based treatment conditions was that during the twelve-week primary treatment phase, the Behavioral couples therapy cases received 1 couples therapy session and 1 individual session each week, whereas the female patients in the Individual-based treatment condition received 2 individual sessions each week," with both conditions receiving one weekly group-therapy session (ibid.). Behavioral couples therapy was delivered by master's level therapists; Individual-based treatment was delivered by state-certified substance abuse counselors trained by a psychologist in cognitive-behavioral therapy. Treatments were manualized, and fidelity was checked by rating videotaped sessions. The 75 research subjects were randomly assigned to the two different conditions and were followed for one year after treatment.

The sample was obtained from "277 married and cohabiting women entering treatment for substance abuse" (p. 346). Of the 277, 31 declined to participate and another 171 were excluded because the partners were abusing drugs or alcohol. Of the 75 patients who participated in the experiment, 26 entered through the coercion of either the courts or the welfare department under threat of incarceration or loss of benefits. On average, women in both groups were about thirty-three years of age, had completed more than twelve years of schooling, had been living with their partners for about six years, and had about two children. They had substantial histories of substance abuse.

Dependence was measured prior to treatment, at the end of treatment, and every subsequent three months for one year after treatment. Urine tests and breath tests but not hair tests were given to the women at each point of data collection after pretreatment. In addition, a variety of other outcome measures related to the social impact and severity of addiction were collected from subjects through semistructured interviews. Abuse was measured by self-reported percentage of days abstinent (PDA). Not surprisingly, patient reports agreed well with urine and breath tests . . . so long as patient reports were paired with the more objective tests.

While there were no significant differences between the outcomes of the two treatment conditions twelve months after treatment, both groups achieved large and clinically significant gains compared with their pretreatment levels of abuse. Behavioral couples therapy reported a pretreatment mean PDA of 42.3% and a twelve-month PDA of 74.2%, an improvement of about 30 percentage points. Individual-based treatment participants moved from 45.2% PDA to 65.4%, a gain of about 20 percentage points. About 60% of the behavioral couples therapy subjects and 40% of the individual-based treatment subjects reported continuous abstinence one year after treatment. In addition, both groups reported impressive drops in the indicators of the severity of their addictions. Unfortunately these results are neither applicable to the general population of drug addicts, even female drug addicts, nor credible estimates of the outcomes of the experiment. First, the subjects were among the most amenable and highly motivated for treatment; although about one-third were forced to seek treatment, two-thirds of the subjects sought treatment voluntarily. The women had also reached the magic age of thirty, at which deviance of all sorts becomes increasingly burdensome. They were mothers in fairly stable families that were threatened by their addiction. Their partners were not addicts and presumably were encouraging their sobriety.

Second, while the experiment randomized subjects to two treatment conditions, it still lacked essential controls. There was neither a nontreatment condition nor a placebo treatment condition, and thus the motivation of the clients and the expectations for recovery apart from treatment remained alternative explanations for whatever improvements may have occurred.

Yet the measurement problem is more debilitating. The measures of substance abuse and thus the extent of recovery are uncertain. The patients' self-report of their pretreatment substance abuse was not checked with any objective test, rather relying on recall for one year prior to treatment. As one of the authors admits, substance abuse immediately prior to treatment may be greater than in the whole one-year period. Indeed, in order to obtain treatment patients may inflate the actual severity of their addictions. The true extent of pretreatment abuse was probably considerably less that the study's reported levels, and thus the likely extent of recovery was also proportionately less. Furthermore, urine tests were scheduled at all follow-up points, with the strong likelihood that some patients obscured their abuse. The failure to employ hair analyses at any time is puzzling, since hair tests reliably cover three months (the period for follow-ups), while the kidneys usually purge opiate traces in about seventy-two hours. Thus the study's estimates of "days of continuous abstinence after treatment" are speculative.

In addition, the self-reports of addiction severity—referring to substance abuse, employment, and family and social functioning—may be more reactive to the patients' relationships with their therapists, the courts, and the welfare department than they are indicative of their actual social circumstances. In fact, self-reported treatment success may itself be a form a denial.

In the end, then, the creaming of patients, the absence of relevant controls, and the porous, unreliable quality of the measurements undercut the study's claims that its interventions were effective in achieving substantial remission for substance-abusing patients. To a far greater extent than is acknowledged in the field, motivated, older addicts with strong stakes in relationships threatened by their addictions are the most likely to achieve sobriety even without treatment. But taking into consideration the measurement problems of the experiment, even these highly conducive motivations failed to achieve a substantial amount of recovery.

Woody, McLellan, Luborsky, and O'Brien (1995) is typical of the strange juxtaposition in the addiction research of weak methods and questionable outcomes with inflated claims for treatment efficacy. Woody et al. (1995) compared the relative effectiveness of supportive-expressive therapy (a form of psychodynamic treatment), and drug counseling in treating opiate-dependent patients with psychiatric symptoms who were taking methadone. The intention was rehabilitation—reducing drug dependency—and improving the patients' psychiatric problems. Each treatment was delivered once a week for six months. Supportive-expressive therapy helps patients "identify the core relationship patterns and work through relationship themes . . . [especially those] that are involved in drug dependence, the role of drugs in relation to problem feelings and behaviors, and how problems may be solved without recourse to drugs" (p. 1303). In contrast, drug counseling emphasizes current problems, support for change, compliance with clinic rules, and referrals. The study was a replication of two earlier studies; it intended to resolve their contradictory results by improving their designs.

Woody et al. (1995) reported that the supportive-expressive therapy was more successful than drug counseling in reducing methadone dependence although the reductions were small and, as they acknowledge, perhaps not clinically important. Drug use declined along with addiction severity in both groups; however, only the supportive-expressive therapy patients sustained the gains at six-month follow-up. Nonetheless, Woody et al. concluded that "we have demonstrated that a substantial portion of psychiatrically symptomatic patients in community-based methadone programs are interested in professional psychotherapy, that it can be delivered in these settings, and that the use of psychotherapists [as distinct from nondoctorate counselors] can add to the gains achieved by additional drug counseling, in much the same manner as in" their successful earlier study (p. 1307).

Yet the actual numbers belie their optimism. First, participants were volunteers and thus among the most motivated patients; therefore, the results, such as they are, are probably not representative of similar clinical patients who did not volunteer. Even so, about 45% of both groups tested positive each week for opiate use during the twenty-four weeks of treatment; about 22% of the supportive-expressive therapy patients and 36% of the drug-counseling patients tested positive for cocaine use during treatment. About 30% of both groups tested positive for at least one additional drug during the same time, in addition to substantial alcohol use. The amount of drug use is even more startling, since the patients were already taking methadone and presumably had made a commitment to abstinence.

The authors claimed that Addiction Severity Index scores and psychiatric symptoms improved for supportive-expressive therapy patients during the six months after treatment but deteriorated for the counseling patients. However, the Addiction Severity Index information is all self-reported and amenable to an enormous amount of falsification, notably in the absence of random urine tests, and the authors do not report the amount of improvement, only the fact that it was statistically significant. The effect size estimate of the superiority of the supportive-expressive group was tiny at one-month follow-up (0.07) and only 0.26 at six months, implying that supportive-expressive patients had moved up about 10% over drug-counseling patients, a difference so small that it is probably clinically meaningless. More to the point, the study did not employ a nontreatment or placebo control, obstructing any estimate of the natural amount of remission in motivated, that is, volunteer patients. Moreover, the small improvements that were reported by the patients may simply have been artifacts of the relationship with their therapists or perhaps their reactions to the styles of the different interventions. It is also commonly understood that the uncorroborated reports of drug addicts greatly underestimate their actual use. In the end, then, Woody et al. (1995) simply failed to face the continuing weaknesses of their replication or to acknowledge that both interventions appeared to be ineffective in reducing the drug dependencies of psychiatrically debilitated addicts on methadone.

Moreover, the entire experiment was conducted in chaotic situations that undermined both treatment integrity as well as simple faith that procedures were followed:

> We had to drop one of the clinics where we originally began work because it was unable to supply the required number of patients and was using such low doses of methadone . . . that outcome data would probably have been seriously confounded. Other problems encountered were the general difficulty in obtaining medical and psychiatric services and the difficulty in hiring psychotherapists who felt comfortable at the sites. Two of the clinics were located in areas that made female therapists uncomfortable; thus only one of the five therapists was female. Still another problem was the instability of program staff. Two of the clinics had staff turnover exceeding 100% during the course of the study, and the clinical director of one program changed more than three times. (Woody et al., 1995, p. 1308)

Chaos is actually the principal finding of interest: the society has refused to establish reasonable treatment programs for debilitated people. Drug treatment is obviously not the role that sustains the community clinics, offering programs that do not supply minimally competent medical care or basic safety for the staff, let alone the patients. Rather the methadone clinics, even for seriously mentally ill patients, are places of medical and service neglect, moral indifference, and yet, social importance. They provide Night of the Living Dead consequences for hedonists who turn to drugs.

From the outset, the design of the study was incapable of providing credible data to answer its central questions. Yet the researchers plowed on to unreliable findings and implausible conclusions, oblivious all the while to the broader meaning of their research. Still, Woody et al. (1995) were more restrained than much of even the very best research. Thus Iguchi, Belding, Morral, Lamb, and Husband (1997), employing behavioral techniques, vouchers for conforming behaviors, produced only very modest gains among methadone patients. Their insistence that it was wise to "reinforce behaviors other than abstinence" was made ridiculous by a follow-up of only six weeks and a treatment gain of only about twenty percentage points in the number of clean urine samples among presumably the most motivated patients, that is, addicts with extraordinarily high drug use seeking methadone treatment.

Indeed, the improvement was so small and sustained for such a short time that without a substantial follow-up period, nothing should be claimed except that a few patients seemed to adapt to the hopes of therapists for a short period of time. Moreover, Iguchi et al. jeopardized even these small gains with their observation that "participants were aware that other interventions existed in addition to the one to which they had been assigned; this knowledge may have had a negative effect on participant motivation and satisfaction with treatment. For example, [some] participants may have felt 'cheated' that they were required to remain drug-free to obtain vouchers" (p. 426).

It is notable that Kirby, Marlowe, and Festinger (1998) failed to replicate even these small benefits for vouchers. Moreover, their second experiment, testing the value of different voucher schedules, produced few and small significant findings. Indeed, the tiny sample sizes in the latter experiment, eleven and twelve, together with substantial demographic differences between the two groups, weakens even these unimpressive findings.

Neither group of researchers confronted the possibility that their interventions were patently ineffective. Indeed, Kirby et al. (1998) seemed astonished that their cognitive-behavioral intervention was so ineffective—reporting that only 17% of one group and 11% of the other completed treatment—but made no effort at all to scrutinize the imperfections of the studies, such as Iguchi et al. (1997), that may have concocted their positive results.

Similarly, Higgins, Wong, Badger, Haug Ogden, and Dantona (2000) reported such small benefits, even while statistically significant, for their schedule of contingent reinforcements that their small samples, commitment to behavioral methods, and methodological defects overwhelmed any claim to success.

Carroll et al.'s (2001) conclusion that these sorts of behavioral techniques play a "substantial role" in treatment is not sustained by the very small measured benefits: less than two-week improvement over twelve weeks in treatment retention and 14 as opposed to 19 opioid-free urine samples. They did not bother with follow-up assessments. Petry and Martin (2002) continued these patterns—small, questionable findings reinterpreted as important progress against addiction despite serious research pitfalls—into community programs.

As is customary, the benefits of behavioral techniques defy any notion of clinical significance, with addicts customarily maintaining their addictions through treatment even while the researchers search assiduously for a small gain in the intensity of use. Moreover, the decision to employ behavioral methods, together with the refusal to acknowledge their consistent weakness, endorses their metaphoric value more than their clinical prowess. Apparently thought and emotion are less important considerations with addicts, who are subtly analogized with Skinner's pigeons through the use of mindless reinforcement schedules.

McKay et al. (1997) tortured their data to discover a few small and variable significant findings that were invalidated by self-reported measures, a highly selective sample, the older age of participants, short-term follow-up, and the lack of rater blinding. The judicious conclusion is that their relapse prevention program had little if any effect and that the group of successfully treated patients they began with continued their addictions at extraordinary levels before, during, and after treatment.

Contrary to their findings and conclusions, Maude-Griffin et al. (1998) failed to establish the benefits of cognitive-behavioral therapy in treating urban crack-cocaine abusers. The 12 percentage-point gain of cognitive-behavioral treatment over twelve-step treatment needs to be disparaged by the fact that only 17 of 134 patients "attended at least 75% of both the group and individual sessions" (p. 834). Moreover, large differences existed between the two groups of patients in abstract reasoning and religious beliefs. Indeed, the small reported differences might easily be attributed to the poorer abilities of the twelve-step patients. The small amount of delivered therapy even suggests that the outcomes, if legitimate, had little to do with therapy itself but were either artifacts of the research or simply differential characteristics of the patients themselves.

On the one hand, Stephens, Roffman, and Simpson (1994) stated that their experimental comparison of cognitive-behavioral treatment and social support

> appears to be the first controlled treatment-outcome study focused specifically on adult marijuana use. Substantial reductions in the amount of marijuana use and related problems were found in both treatment conditions throughout the twelve-month posttreatment follow-up. . . . However, there were few significant differences in outcomes between the two treatment conditions. . . . [Yet] sustained abstinence was the exception, with only 14% of subjects reporting no marijuana use throughout the follow-up period. (p. 98)

On the other hand, all of their measures were self-reported from patients or their designated collateral, while the "relapse curve was steep in the first several months posttreatment" (ibid.). In fact, only about 15% of both groups were abstinent one year after treatment. The rates of relapse were so high and the measures seemingly so biased toward underestimates of marijuana use—hair analysis was not employed—that either condition probably constitutes empty therapy, that is, a placebo control for future research and not the standard treatment control of the literature.

Instead of accepting the conclusion of ineffectiveness, Stephens et al., who are apparently committed to cognitive-behavioral therapy, preferred to conclude that "in the absence of clear treatment differences and a no-treatment control group, it is not possible to attribute outcomes to the treatments with certainty" (p. 98). Though they concluded that "the substantial reductions . . . were at least partially a product of the interventions" (ibid.), they might have alternatively considered that the reductions were at least partially the product of soft measures, amenable to a host of confirmational biases. A motivated group of patients had voluntarily sought to reduce their marijuana dependence, but at one-year follow-up few were abstinent and the amount of gains was small, particularly when discounted by both patient falsification at the beginning of treatment and by their coy disremembering at the end. Instead of defending cognitive-behavioral techniques on specious grounds, the authors might have reevaluated their devotion to psychotherapy for marijuana addiction.

Young Addicts

Addicted youngsters do not fare any better in therapy than adults—if anything, worse. Latimer, Newcomb, and Winters (2000) reached the conclusion that pretreatment psychosocial protective factors—the degree of social support of various kinds—rather than the severity of alcohol and drug abuse predict successful outcomes of treatment for adolescent addicts. Unfortunately, their analyses were hampered by the unreliability of their data as well as by the likelihood that very few adolescents improved in treatment and that the improvement that did occur was probably not associated with treatment but with independent family and peer influences.

The study compared the outcomes of 225 adolescents entering either a 30-day inpatient treatment center or a thirty-day outpatient treatment program for alcohol and drug addiction, both offering extensive aftercare. Both programs, including their aftercare, were modeled on the Alcoholics Anonymous twelve-step approach. Success was measured as the difference between their pretreatment and follow-up use of alcohol, marijuana, and other illicit drugs. Yet in spite of urinanalyses, their data depended heavily on uncorroborated self-reports, since the tests were scheduled and were only accurate for use during the previous seventy-two hours. Furthermore, no tests for alcohol use were possible. Consequently, at one-year follow-up patients took a scheduled urine test but were asked to recall their substance use for the previous six months.

This was a prescription for misreporting, especially in the absence of hair tests. The authors' pride in the high reliability of self-report and urine tests under these conditions was pointedly oblivious to their porous testing procedures, especially with youths who did not feed their addictions daily but were capable of abstaining for 3 days in order to obscure their dependency.

Furthermore, attrition was enormous, at 36%: 225 patients at intake but only 144 at one-year follow-up. Yet contrary to the prudent custom of counting patients who drop out of drug treatment as failures, Latimer et al. (2000) simply ignored them, conducting their analyses on available patients. Indeed, they made no comment on attrition. In this way the large gains by one-year follow-up can be accounted for by attrition and misreporting. For example, the authors reported that 33% of the patients had abstained from illicit drugs during one year before treatment but 63% had abstained for the previous six months one year after treatment. However, if the patients who dropped out are counted as continuing users, then the number of one-year abstainers drops to 44% of the total. Moreover, the pretreatment estimates by the youths could obviously not be corroborated by urine tests. It is quite conceivable that drug use actually increased. Except for the data, every aspect of their very sophisticated pathway analyses was superb.

Moreover, the authors' central findings were not methodologically tied to treatment, since the experiment did not include randomized assignment nor, importantly, any true nontreatment control—even a community sample. Thus whatever changes took place among a voluntary group of adolescent patients may well have been incidental to treatment and simply an instance of the authors' suspicion that the youths' psychosocial environment—parents, communities, and peers—was the main factor in their subsequent use of drugs and alcohol, an unremarkable consideration pushed aside by the passion for clinical treatment.

The influence of parents, communities, and peers might well have been explored with profit for social policy if the authors had been open to interventions besides therapy, notably Alcoholics Anonymous. Alcoholics Anonymous has never credibly demonstrated success with any type of addiction. Its popularity is built on an obsessive conviction that the individual freely chooses addiction or sobriety. Indeed, Alcoholics Anonymous, with its commitment to a Higher Power, actually combines the God-based religion of the church with the secular religion of psychotherapy. Both insist that individuals take responsibility for themselves in denial of a social obligation for psychosocial support, that is, substantial, enduring, and concrete investments in repairing deficits of family, community, schools, and so forth.

Waldron, Slesnick, Brody, Turner, and Peterson (2001) provided better evidence of patient falsification in reporting their drug use than of modest reductions in marijuana intake as a result of four different treatments. The authors concluded that each of their tested interventions—cognitive-behavioral therapy, family therapy, a combination of the two, and group drug therapy—reduced adolescent dependence on marijuana: small reductions in the days of use but greater increases in the percentage of each group that used marijuana at minimal levels. Yet the probability of inflated pretreatment rates of use wiped out the reported gains in days of use. Furthermore, the fact that "positive urine screens were found for 84% at pretreatment, 81% at 4 months and 76% at 7 months" (even more troubling because point-in-time urine screens are low estimates of use during any period longer than three weeks) mocks the other findings (Waldron et al., 2001, p. 809). Rather than the oracular insight that "potential interpretations of the findings can be offered in relation to the theoretical mechanisms of change of each intervention," the authors might more judiciously have recognized that their basic data, drawn from the self-reports of their patients, was inaccurate. Yet they went to great lengths to state that the self-reports were somehow validated by the urine screens that established the "convergent validity" of the self-reports (p. 811). In fact, it seems likely that the four interventions had little impact at all, especially since the analysis did not carry forward the large number of dropouts as failures.

Alcohol

As with illicit drugs, so with alcohol. The studies are uniformly marred by methodological pitfalls that facilitate unwarranted conclusions, usually inflating the curative powers of the researchers' favored psychotherapeutic interventions. Miller, Benefield, and Tonigan (1993) achieved spectacular results with heavy drinkers—an overall reduction of 57% in drinking after a two-session intervention—but alas, none of the data are credible. The two styles of intervention consisted of either a confrontational or a "client-centered" presentation of the results of a medical examination and social review "for drinkers who wanted to find out whether alcohol was harming them in any way" (p. 456). The interventions were provided in two sessions: a two-hour evaluative session and then, one week later, a feedback session. Both groups were compared with wait-list patients at intake and six weeks after the evaluative session. At the time wait-list patients were given treatment, then all groups were compared one year later.

To begin with, the authors did not discount the 57% reduction in drinking among the treated patients by the reduction among wait-list patients. In this event, the improvements would fall by about 35 percentage points to only about 22%. Even this modest gain, still impressive for only a two-session intervention, needs further discounting. The principal measures of outcomes—weekly consumption and days drinking—were self-reported and corroborated by collaterals identified by the drinkers. Peak intoxication, reported as "blood alcohol level," was simply a computer-generated estimate based on the other two measures. However, reliabilities between the drinkers and their collaterals, while statistically significant, were only moderately related (frequently only about .5). It is also curious that the treated patients who began on the wait-list deteriorated on all outcome measures at the one-year follow-up, while the pattern for non-wait-list patients was mixed.

Further, the gains of the two interventions were associated with interviewers who were disposed toward one or the other. That is, none of the interviewers were neutral, but all were negative toward nonintervention. Thus likely expectancy biases of the researchers were uncorrected, unadjusted, and unacknowledged. Attrition and the loss of data, particularly among collaterals, were serious, exceeding 50% at twelve-month follow-up.

Finally, while the authors stated in their first sentence that their goal was to address the "lack of motivation for change" among alcoholics, they tested their interventions on a group of patients who were among the most motivated (p. 455). The sample was composed of educated, middle-aged drinkers, frequently with families, who did not suffer extremely severe addictions or associated isolation and loss. About three quarters were currently working. For all patients, "this was the first time they had sought help or consultation of any kind with regard to their drinking," and they had quickly volunteered to participate in the study on the basis of a single unrepeated advertised solicitation for people concerned about the effects of their drinking (p. 457). Indeed, with so many assaults on the integrity of research, it is surprising that Miller et al. (1993) were only able to produce a 22% improvement. Why bother doing such weak research? Why accept it for publication? Perhaps again, social efficiency—the putative luster of achieving great gains against alcoholism with only two uncomplicated, inexpensive sessions of treatment—was a more compelling motive than accurate program evaluation.

McKay et al. (1997) reported no difference in outcomes between inpatient and outpatient care whether patients were allowed to pick their own treatment or were randomized. Their data also suggested that treatment was uniformly ineffective in reducing drinking. Yet the groups differed greatly in age, ethnicity, drug use, employment, use of welfare, and other measures that undercut any interpretation of the data. These differences complicate any interpretation of the data, raising the issue of why the experiment persisted after group assignment.

Longabaugh, Wirtz, and Beattie (1995) provided data for the startling effectiveness of each of their three therapies for alcoholism: brief broad-spectrum therapy, extended relationship-enhancement therapy, and extended cognitive-behavioral therapy. Twenty sessions of each were planned, but patients only attended an average of ten sessions. Moreover, 35% of patients in two of the treatments and 16% of patients in the other one never attended any session at all; no patient in two of the three therapies attended more than seven sessions. The authors only presented patient self-reports, although they claimed corroboration with unpublished reports from collaterals. While the patients seemed to be living in stable conditions, many had been arrested and many had failed in previous hospitalizations for alcoholism. Moreover, their alcoholism seemed very severe, reportedly averaging about ten standard drinks per day for one month prior to treatment.

In the three months before treatment, patients reported that they were abstinent for between 26% and 38% of the days. Fifteen months after treatment, patients in all three groups reported that they were abstinent for more than 80% of the days in the previous three months (in one case almost 90%). Thus in spite of receiving a small number of the intended treatments, the overwhelming proportion of patients were largely sober. No other treatment has reported such enormous success through a similarly designed study.

Still, the research did not include a nontreatment or placebo control. Yet the findings are so large and sustained for so long, and the patients at baseline seem so debilitated, that the magnitude of the findings cannot be explained away simply as the result of extraordinarily motivated patients. Nevertheless, these findings have not been independently replicated in an appropriately controlled study. Yet if they are not true treatment effects, then they are the product of confluent factors: unusually powerful expectancy biases and demand characteristics of the research situation, highly motivated patients, and their reporting distortions, among others. Indeed, all of these possibilities, together with large placebo effects, might begin to substitute for treatment as an explanation of the outcomes. Nonetheless, they beg for replication. Moreover, skepticism is sustained by the refusal of sophisticated researchers to employ adequate controls and by the fact that many patients who received little therapy became abstinent. Thus if the treatment effects are not genuine, then the study is an important cautionary tale, signaling the importance of objective, corroborated measures and placebo controls. The authors' credulity regarding their findings also spurs a reluctance to herald their three interventions as advances in alcohol treatment.

In sharp contrast, O'Malley et al. (1996) reported data that suggest thoroughgoing failure, although predictably they struggled to retrieve some benefit derived from the interventions in their discussion. They compared four different treatment conditions for alcoholism: coping skills or supportive therapy, each provided with drug treatment or placebo. By the sixth month after treatment, both the rates of drinking and the rates of heavy drinking had returned to pretreatment levels. Indeed, in a few cases they actually increased *during treatment* as well as at the six-month follow-up.

The methodology followed by O'Malley et al. is as questionable as that of Longabaugh et al. (1995), filled with the customary measurement weaknesses and failures to protect against researcher biases. Yet O'Malley et al. incorporated some controls (although there was no nontreatment control for the psychotherapy conditions), while the findings were diametrically opposite to those of Longabaugh et al. To make a very broad comparison, if supportive therapy in O'Malley et al. can substitute as a placebo control in Longabaugh et al., then the latter findings are reduced by about forty percentage points, although they remain quite large. Yet the possibility arises that the technology for evaluating addiction programs is so impaired that aside from a cobbled and tendentious search for evidence to support the effectiveness of interventions, the findings themselves are chaotic, lacking any ability to estimate the actual effects of treatment.

Connors, Carroll, DiClemente, Longabaugh, and Donovan (1997) conducted an elaborate test of the contribution that the therapeutic alliance—agreement on goals and tasks of therapy and the quality of the relationship between patient and therapist—makes to treatment participation and outcomes. The research proved little except that the benefits of their three twelve-week interventions—twelve-step facilitation, cognitive-behavioral coping skills treatment, and motivational enhancement therapy—were modest at best, ambiguous, and questionable and that the therapeutic alliance was a likely source of patient bias rather than a contribution to therapy.

The therapeutic alliance as measured by therapists may well be a proxy for the anticipated degree of patient loyalty and gratitude for free treatment. Indeed, patient characteristics prior to treatment (age and amount of drinking) were the major predictors of drinking behavior after treatment. Moreover, only the therapists' estimates of treatment alliance enjoyed a consistent but still small ability to predict patient outcomes. Patient estimates of the therapeutic alliance were unevenly associated with outcomes. The customary problems of self-reported measures and the absence of controls discredited the project's reported treatment gains. In light of the many design flaws of the experiment and the uneven findings, it is inappropriate for the authors to insist on the general value of the therapeutic alliance for psychotherapy, especially without addressing the possibility that better alliances with patients produce more falsified self-reports of recovery.

Smoking and Gambling

Recognizing in their very first paragraph that "lies about the extent of the involvement with gambling" characterize the pathological problem, Sylvain, Ladouceur, and Boisvert (1997) then went on to rely on patient self-reports to evaluate the success of their treatments. Their "behavioral and cognitive treatment" provided one or two weekly sessions of between 60 and 90 minutes for a total of thirty hours. The treatment contained four components: cognitive correction of the probability of winning, problem-solving training, social-skills training, and relapse prevention. They reported that there were no statistically significant pretreatment differences between the treated group of fourteen patients and the fifteen on the wait-list. Yet the actual differences between the groups in pretreatment gambling were huge: treatment group patients reported gambling about twenty-three dollars per week, control patients about one hundred dollars. Four of the ten treated subjects dropped out of treatment by the six-month follow-up.

Sylvain et al. (1997) proudly announced that "eighty-six percent of the treated participants were no longer considered pathological gamblers . . . at the end of treatment. Additionally, they had a greater perception of control of their gambling problem as well as an increased self-efficacy in high-risk gambling situations" (p. 731). The authors tempered the findings by admitting that many of the treated patients "did not come back after the first contact, refused treatment, or dropped out early in treatment" (ibid.). Rather than being tempered, the findings are invalidated by attrition, by the intractable problem of unreliable self-reports, and by the large initial differences between treated patients and control patients. Indeed, twenty-three dollars of weekly gambling is a suspiciously low amount for truly pathological gamblers.

In choosing to fund the research, the Conseil Quebecois de la Recherche Sociale and Loto-Quebec obviously ignore its patent methodological weaknesses. Yet a poorly evaluated and feckless cognitive and behavioral treatment is hardly a sincere attempt to handle a serious problem. It is, however, an inexpensive symbol of concern—Scrooge-like charitability without compassion.

The failure of psychotherapy to achieve smoking cessation is more complex. Many people have obviously quit smoking over the past few decades; the sales of cigarettes have fallen off sharply, and civic ordinances that restrict smoking are widely obeyed, perhaps largely because only a minority smoke. Social attitudes have also changed to strongly condemn the tobacco habit. Indeed, a wide-ranging series of "environmental" interventions—information based, health based, legislative, legal, voluntary, and economic—have been expressive, coincidental, and perhaps even causative of the shift in attitudes that attended the reduction in tobacco use, particularly cigarette smoking. Therefore, research testing the effects of psychotherapy on smoking is challenged to document the contribution of treatment to this change and is obliged to employ a credible control for the influences of the environmental interventions associated with decreased tobacco use. It is questionable whether four of the following five experiments—certainly among the best in the literature for the past ten years—achieved the minimal condition of an adequate control, while additional deficiencies compromised their positive findings even further. Overall, the research offers little evidence that any form of psychotherapy provides a routine cure for tobacco addiction. Individual motivation unenhanced by therapy remains the most likely explanation for any reported gains.

S. M. Hall, Muñoz, and Reus (1994) compared eight weeks of supportive group therapy and eight weeks of cognitive-behavioral therapy for smokers with and without histories of major depressive disorder. Patients in the cognitive-behavioral group received almost twice as many hours of therapist attention as patients in the supportive therapy group. Patients in all four groups chewed nicotine gum. There was no nontreatment control. Hall et al. found that cognitive-behavioral therapy was more effective than supportive therapy for patients with histories of depressive disorder—the most successful among the four groups. However, only 34% of these patients were abstinent at one-year follow-up, while only 16% of patients without depressive histories who received cognitive-behavioral therapy were abstinent at one-year follow-up. As is common, this research selected a convenient standard of abstinence—only seven days without smoking before any evaluation point. A more rigorous and medically applicable standard would have wiped out any gain. Coincidentally, the authors cited previous research estimating that nicotine gum was associated with 37% abstinence and placebo gum with 21% abstinence among patients at one year. Thus nicotine gum and placebo effects were more effective than any of the study's treatments. Indeed, placebo effects by themselves exceeded the abstinence rates for two of the four groups. Although the studies are not fully comparable, the authors were conscious of the large contributions of nicotine gum and patient motivation but still neglected to include a nontreatment control. They were also pointedly aware of the different intensities of the therapy. Nevertheless, Hall et al. insisted that "the cognitive-behavioral intervention enhanced treatment outcome for subjects with a history of major depressive disorder" (p. 145).

Diguisto and Bird (1995) may have employed an adequate control for their social-support treatment, although self-help patients, their control condition, probably do not believe that they are in treatment and indeed, may subtly rebel against the notion of being neglected by therapists. In any event, they reported a treatment-group gain of 18% over the control (69% versus 51%) at one-week follow-up. The difference shrank to 7% at six months (40% versus 33%). The findings again become trivial, as the authors conveniently defined abstinence as seven days without smoking. The only reasonable conclusion is to acknowledge that supportive group therapy made no gains over a nontreatment control and that the reported gains, tainted by the research's pitfalls, were most likely the result of patient motivation alone: some people who want to stop smoking do so even without the permission of their therapists.

Although Fortmann and Killen (1995) employed a population-based recruitment strategy, their sample was decidedly not representative of smokers. Apart from purposely excluding those at risk of the treatment conditions (for example, the vulnerability of lactating and pregnant women to nicotine), the sample was self-selected for those motivated to stop smoking and those willing to tolerate a phone solicitation complete with a battery of intrusive questions. However, the convenient measure of cessation—seven days of self-reported abstinence at the data collection point—was corroborated by a biochemical test. They reported that nicotine gum significantly improved abstinence. However, the statistically significant improvement was insubstantial: at one year follow-up, 21% of those using nicotine gum were abstinent compared with 16% who did not use nicotine gum. They also reported that heavier smokers and older smokers were less likely to quit than lighter smokers and younger smokers, findings that underscore the conclusion that the motivation of patients, rather than the treatments, predict abstinence. This point of skepticism is given additional plausibility by the authors' observation that "compliance to treatment regimens was relatively poor" (p. 463). Yet the authors insisted that "nicotine gum increased smoking cessation in this study"; they might have added that the increase was not worth the trouble, especially since they could not be sure that patients actually received the intended amounts of nicotine gum for the treatment.

Killen, Fortmann, and Kraemer (1996) further analyzed the experience of nearly 40% of one-day abstainers in Fortmann and Killen (1995), reporting that increased depression was modestly associated with relapse and weight gain was associated with abstinence, while emphasizing the earlier findings that those who were less dependent on nicotine were somewhat less likely to relapse. However, the design of the study was incapable of disentangling these relationships, that is, whether more depression was a result or a cause of relapse. Nevertheless, the small predictive value of nicotine dependence is puzzling. In any case, the amount of successful abstinence of an initially motivated sample—and therefore, the long-term value of behavioral therapy—was again only about 20%, a figure so low as to be accounted for entirely by patient motivation, especially in the absence of adequate controls and with a meaningful measure of abstinence. Indeed, the most reasonable conclusion of this research project is that psychotherapy has little if any ability to reduce addiction to nicotine. In a similar experiment, Killen, Robinson, Haydel, and Farish (1997) repeated the many methodological flaws of their earlier experiment, which continued to negate their similarly modest findings.

Zhu et al. (1996) reported low rates of one-year abstinence and small but significant differences between the treated groups and the control: 5.4% for the self-help group that served as a standard treatment control; 7.5% for the single counseling group; and 9.9% for multiple counseling. The rates were slightly higher but symmetrical for "those who made a quit attempt" (p. 202). However, the recovery rates are so low as to be explained simply by patient motivation. The differences between the groups may have been created by patient response falsification related to the special demand characteristics of the three treatments. The reports of abstinence are directly related to the amount of contact that patients had with therapists in each treatment condition—self-help only received staff instructions, single-session counseling patients spent fifty minutes with a therapist, and multiple-session patients obviously spent much more time with their therapists. There was no true non-treatment control, which would have been invaluable for estimating natural cessation rates, that is, patient motivation independent of treatment. Such low recovery rates stimulate speculation that treatment in general may harm recovery to the extent that it rewards tobacco dependence with the special attentions of high-status professionals. The additional finding of small-dose effects is also open to reinterpretion as a function of patient motivation rather than the efficacy of therapy doses; patients motivated to stop smoking were also motivated to attend more sessions. Yet the authors never accepted the paltriness of their reported abstinence rates, the serious deficiencies of their methodology, or their obligation to handle obvious points of skepticism. In the end then, they enacted a ritual of treatment—another opportunity for the sinful to repent their civic misdeeds—rather than a clinical cure; a reaffirmation of personal responsibility for continued dependence on tobacco but not either recognition of the customary individual inability to get past this addiction nor the grave social responsibility to prevent tobacco misuse.

Defiance without Reason

It is notable that just these sorts of poorly designed experiments have led to the conclusion that psychotherapy is effective against alcoholism, drug abuse, smoking, and gambling. The false faith in the treatment efficacy of psychotherapy justifies standard treatment controls and the absence of nontreatment and placebo controls, which in turn permit the community of practice to sidestep the issue of accountability. False science produces false proofs that reinforce the continuation of false science. Still, the underlying permission for porous research is given by the society, which seeks a myth of social service rather than effective cures or meaningful improvement.

Nevertheless, these studies of the effectiveness of a variety of psychotherapeutic treatments for the addictions are among the very best ever conducted. Weak and self-serving as they are, the more common quality of research descends to even weaker tests of effectiveness that have even balder professional, political, and ideological uses. The tolerance for misleading research is embedded within the government's grant procedures and the profit taken by the culture in programmatically meaningless gestures that underscore widely held popular preferences.

Still, alternatives to psychotherapy for addiction are no more successful. Even when employing "environmental" alternatives to psychotherapeutic interventions, they still copy its core characteristics: superficiality, ritualism, and, in the end, an insistence on an isolating personal responsibility. Clapp's environmentally superficial minitactics unwittingly parody the influence of changing attitudes toward tobacco on social habits and institutions and the ability of the antitobacco campaign to either mobilize or reflect deep changes in those attitudes. It is never easy to disentangle the causes of social changes from their effects. Indeed, it is impossible because of the inability to run controls for possible causes. Yet the socially efficient interventions of American social welfare, even when they are not psychotherapeutic, recapitulate its essential developmental and institutional emptiness.

The controversy within the alcohol treatment community over nonpsychotherapeutic approaches to reduce drinking among college students seems to fluctuate between an improbable approach that is increasingly discredited (Wechsler et al., 2003) and a deceptive one whose popularity is just emerging. The social norms approach takes its inspiration from the Just Say No to

Drugs campaigns of the 1980s, the Ad Council's approach to social problems, and a variety of cognitive styles of social learning. Social norms programs assume that knowledge of the actual low-alcohol abuse of most college students will reduce the pressure on the others to drink. Similar to psychotherapy, it simply denies the centrality of a culture of alcohol for many college students, assuming that they are pulled by general social norms that are relatively abstemious rather than by peer norms. The social norms logic also imbibes the conceit that the obligation of the culture is simply to provide information—posters, stickers, bookmarks, notepads, and the like—as a spur to sobriety, discipline, and sensible individual choices. Clearly, the social norms interventions are very inexpensive, promoting notions of the minimalist state and by inference moralizing over those who do not conform.

Clapp, Lange, Russell, Shillingon, and Boas (2003) tested an experimental social norms marketing program that failed. This was not a surprising outcome, since at the same time Clapp et al. were running and seeking additional funding for a competitive approach—the Community/Collegiate Alcohol Prevention Partnership (c-capp), a "data-driven, science-based, environmental alcohol prevention" program (Clapp, 1999, p. 22). Yet c-capp and its associated initiatives were not more scientific nor data-driven than the social norms approach. While its interventions were broader, they were no more deep, in the end dramatizing social norms themselves rather than facing the environmental, that is, the cultural structures that encourage many college students to abuse alcohol. Indeed, c-capp may itself deepen the intractability of abusive drinking by insisting that superficial interventions are sufficient. Moreover, it may have as many unintended effects as the approach it seeks to supplant.

Clapp et al. (2003) selected two dormitories on the campus of San Diego State University for their experiment; they randomly selected one for the social norms campaign and samples from both for interviews to evaluate the outcomes. The dormitories were separated by one mile to prevent "the diffusion of treatment" (p. 410). The six-week social norms campaign included a variety of posters and other graphics with "the same basic normative message: 'seventy-five percent of . . . students drink 0, 1, 2, 3, or 4 drinks when they party.'" The statistic was drawn from a survey of students at San Diego State during the year of the campaign. "To add an interactive component to the dissemination . . . , each week during our campaign we sent a research assistant to the experimental hall to ask randomly selected students if they knew the above campaign message or if they were displaying the poster in their room. If students indicated either was the case, they were awarded $5. Students ere eligible to win one prize per week" (Clapp et al., 2003, p. 410).

In the end, Clapp et al. (2003) reported that while perceptions of peer drinking became more accurate among experimental subjects, they actually drank more frequently at post-test than the control students. However, outcomes were measured by self-reported responses to questions about personal drinking, knowledge of alcohol use by other students, and so forth. Furthermore, the data were not collected from a randomly selected group of students; rather, "for a 5-day period during each testing phase, we set tables near the entrance of each hall and solicited volunteer subjects. We offered subjects a coupon for a free slice of pizza and a soft drink (value $2) as an incentive to complete the survey" (p. 410).

Thus their conclusions of ineffectiveness may have been accurate but certainly not on the authority of their uncertain, amateurish research. Moreover, increases in drinking among those who were exposed to the social norms campaign seem to be a gratuitous finding that sustains the hopes of its authors, on unsupported grounds, to endorse their alternative approach. The speculation that the advertised norms campaign perversely condoned up to five drinks per party is counterbalanced by the enormous weaknesses of the research itself: unreliable, self-reported data from students who may have been toying with obviously impaired research, together with nonrandom and therefore probably unrepresentative samples. A foolish intervention evaluated by partisan researchers through a weak design is a test of nothing at all except the appetite of the United States Department of Education and the National Institute on Alcohol Abuse and Alcoholism for expedient science.

The institutionalized tolerance for compatible research is expressed by more than one-half million dollars in funding for Clapp's c-capp, whose effectiveness is reported in a grant application for an expanded program. In three years, students reported that their binge drinking declined by between 2.1% and 3.9% (Clapp, 1999, 2000, 2001). Yet the methods used to achieve this tiny result are as porous as the methods used to test the social norms campaign. Indeed, the alleged gain becomes lost amid the background static of the research. Data were again drawn from the self-reports of questionably representative samples and probably unreliable respondents. It is simply ludicrous to rely on the self-reports of college drinkers who are aware of the researchers' preferences, notably after three years of extensive efforts to demonize alcohol abuse among college students. Indeed, c-capp's activities are themselves elaborate inducements for response falsification.

c-capp and its ancillary programs, based like Clapp in a school of social work, began by organizing a community consensus of more than fifty medical, educational, and civic organizations to facilitate its interventions. Those miniprograms include "Responsible Beverage Service Training, Community

Covenants Sponsored by the the Responsible Hospitality Industry, Removal of Binge Drinking Materials from Campus Outlets, Development of Alcohol and Other Drug Policies, Increased Law Enforcement, Decoy Operations, Enforcement of City Ordinances, and Social Marketing including Billboards, Doorhangers, Handbooks, and Getting the Media Involved" (Clapp, 2000, pp. 18–19). C-CAPP also promised scientific evaluation and a variety of journal publications and manuals to disseminate its wisdom. But three years of experience produced only marginal gains through self-reported data collected from poorly defined and selectively chosen respondents. The results beg for scrutiny of the project's methodological misadventures rather than national funding.

None of the assortment of interventions have had credible successes in other locations, and their evaluations are also deeply flawed. In particular, consensus organizing failed in its principal test: not one of its projects succeeded (Gittel and Vidal, 1998), while the separate C-CAPP programs are improbable public-information attempts on the level of Just Say No to Drugs and questionable regulatory steps. Indeed, prohibiting inexpensive or free drinks ("happy hours") probably delights the local bars by reducing their competition over prices and increasing their profits. In fact, C-CAPP's own evaluation suggests all of its sentimental, over-intellectualized and improbable miniprojects had little effect on binge drinking in college students.

Verbally scorned but deeply accepted, youth drinking is as accommodated by the culture as adult drinking. Large sectors of the economy depend on them. The popular culture ennobles them. Drinking is a rite of passage, a portal into adulthood, for many youth. Rather than consensus organizing, a program is obliged to develop a constituency sizable enough to challenge the institutionalized arrangements that are sustained by the targeted behavior.

Organizational change was not the function of C-CAPP, nor was it the intention of its funding. Rather, it placed the very organizations that needed to change in a position of blocking serious challenges to their convenience by including them on its supervising board. Not surprisingly, in the end they made few accommodations to the problem of youth drinking. C-CAPP advertises its conformity with science and truth but conducts deceptive evaluations. It puts the onus for drinking squarely on the individual while failing to confront the difficulty of mounting environmental strategies. C-CAPP recruited high-status institutions to worry over a perceived social problem but does admit the imperviousness of college students to the risks of drunkenness. For all its invocation of theory, C-CAPP never addressed the persistent misuse of alcohol as a critique of the American culture itself. Americans soften the abrasions of their society through drugs and alcohol; they put themselves beyond the assaults of their culture by dosing their sensibilities; they achieve tranquility through what they ingest rather than through their social arrangements. However, shaking a finger at the culture is not the wisest way of securing funds from its stalwart agencies.

C-CAPP is a Potemkin village of an alcohol-abuse prevention program. Indeed, the prevention of alcohol abuse may be beyond human capacity in a culture with a pervasive attachment to mood-altering substances. C-CAPP avoids the observation that the penalties for alcohol abuse are largely accepted as part of the overhead of American life. C-CAPP, far from being data-driven and scientific, is to the contrary an exercise in socialization, a ceremony of communal values, a reaffirmation of social mores, a reinforcement of governing styles, and a legitimation of the earned, continuing virtues of prominent groups. The problem of alcohol abuse is its incidental excuse; social meaning divorced from defined program outcomes justifies C-CAPP. Rather than questioning the effectiveness of social-welfare arrangements, it actually endorses the voluntarism, social efficiency, and received wisdom of American values. Two important funding arms of the American people have knowingly sustained this ritualism by ignoring its recorded failure to prevent alcohol abuse.

C-CAPP is the high-church modern expression of Carrie Nation's emotional, low-church immediacy. It has supplanted Carrie Nation's ax-wielding rhetoric of sin, damnation, and the sanctity of the family with its own anti-saloon-league message, given status by university auspices and the demulcent invocations of science and social research, which preach sobriety on grounds of health and social wisdom. Yet both forms are prohibitionist, puritanical, and regulatory at heart, while they are devoid of any ability to achieve their avowed goals.

San Diego State University and the many other lower-tier pretenses to higher education write the pulp fiction of America's social preferences. Never very creative, they crank out local adaptations of more original ideas, usually taking their lead from the top-ranked universities and responding only after the ideas have become vulgarized into programmatic comic books. Whether as congressional earmarks or as a competitive research grant from a national institute of some problem, disease, or body part, the point of the program is socialization. Resolution of any social problem is customarily beyond both the capacity of a localized initiative and the national acceptance of institutional change.

A Few Remarks

Psychotherapeutic research employs science as if it were a Hindu's prayer wheel. A nation of lamaseries would assign a few monks to the tasks of revelation, but this very rationalistic nation establishes blue-ribbon commissions and scientific bureaus to study personal adaptation. However, in order to win funding, evaluative research proposals are first obliged to commit themselves to a central American value: happiness is in each individual's hands, and the society only has a small obligation to stimulate the individual toward epiphanies of personal responsibility. The broad consensus that probably defines American culture assumes that the needy individual is willfully deviant from the beneficence and virtue of American society, which is generous, indulgent, and pure of hostility, cruelty, and meanness. The culture is indifferent to the approach—psychotherapy, public information, or environmentalism—so long as it does not cost much and repeats the patriotic mantra of individualism.

There is an equivalence between psychotherapy per se, the cognitive style of social-norms campaigns, and the alternative environmental interventions of C-CAPP: all are superficial, all fail to achieve their goals, all distort evaluations of their outcomes, all neglect social conditions. Most important, all persist as ceremonies of social efficiency, emptied of the resources to address social problems seriously. Yet compared with Ms. Nation, the rationalistic approaches, notably psychotherapy, are the more invidious for employing the science of social proof to connive the reality of social illusion.

4: Eating Disorders, Juvenile Violence, Group Treatments, and Other Problems

The remaining applications of psychotherapy do not improve on any of its earlier failures. Psychotherapy remains a ritual of social preferences rather than a successful clinical practice. In less developed areas, psychotherapy takes on the characteristics of marginal, alternative treatments that justify themselves with frankly empty claims and notoriously unreliable research. As the broader policy-making process shifts to emerging social problems, psychotherapy amplifies its treatments to satisfy social preferences by turning reality into fable. Psychotherapy moralizes personal discipline as individual choice rather than as an habituated response to received social experience, that is, the quality of family, community, and education.

Obesity

Wing, Marcus, and Epstein (1991) acknowledged that it did not make any difference whether obese diabetic patients were treated alone or with their spouses. Both forms of treatment, involving behavioral as well as cognitive elements and provided in sixteen one-hour sessions over twenty weeks, appeared to be equally successful one year after treatment. Yet the more accurate conclusion is that both were equally ineffective.

The patients were on average about 50% or seventy-five pounds overweight and lost about ten pounds at one-year follow-up. However, even this small improvement needs to be discounted by patient motivation—the response of volunteers to newspaper advertisements. The study did not include a non-treatment control nor carry forward the dropouts as failures. Six of forty-nine patients left treatment and were lost to the study. However, after conceding that "this study found no evidence that treating patients together with their spouses . . . was more effective than treating patients alone," the authors ignored the possibility that their assumptions about therapy itself were probably inaccurate. Instead, they speculated that the type of contracting, the assumption of spouse support, self-selection factors, and specific effects (the "together" condition worked for wives but not for husbands) might have diminished the potential benefits of treating husbands and wives together. The authors might have more plausibly speculated on the pernicious effects of therapy—that the attention of therapy for the obese may have actually suppressed the weight loss of motivated patients by reinforcing the role of patient and encouraging them to eat too much. The authors might have also discussed their refusal to include a nontreatment control for an area of treatment with so little evidence of success.

Wadden, Foster, and Letizia (1994) seem to have done somewhat better. They provided behavioral therapy in two conditions—moderate calorie intake or very low calorie intake—to obese women. At the end of one year of treatment and an additional twenty-six-week maintenance program, patients in both groups had lost about twenty-five pounds. However, only 37 of the 49 patients completed the program, and again dropouts were not carried forward as failures; moreover, only 31 of 49 patients completed full body-mass tests. The authors contended that "the results of this study have important implications for the treatment of obesity by behavior therapy," but they never address the absence of a nontreatment control for presumably highly motivated patients who, in typical fashion, were recruited through newspaper ads. The authors did concede that the patients "probably regained more weight after treatment" (p. 169). Indeed, most weight-loss interventions succeed for a short while with motivated patients who customarily regain their weight after treatment, a process of gain and loss that is itself a stress on the body. Rather than therapy, supervision may be the active factor, a very costly and continuous intervention for weight loss.

Similarly, none of the treatment groups in Meyers, Graves, and Whelan (1996) maintained their modest weight loss one year after treatment; even at three months post-treatment, they had regained most of their weight. Each of Wadden et al.'s (1994) behavioral interventions achieved more than thirty pounds of weight reduction at the end of the forty-eight-week programs. Notably, the diet-alone condition did as well as the three other exercise-and-diet conditions. However, the study did not employ a nontreatment control nor conduct follow-up assessments, while again the patients were presumably unusually motivated to lose weight. Moreover, if the diet condition is a proxy for a placebo, then none of the treatment conditions were successful.

Similar results together with similar problems—notably the absence of a nontreatment control—beset Perri, Nezu, Patti, and McCann (1997), Jeffrey, Wing, Thorson, and Burton (1998), and Jeffrey, Wing, and Mayer (1998). It is compelling that supervision itself is the one common, unaccounted condition in almost all of the research, posing an alternative explanation to therapy for the customary, but small and evanescent, weight losses that the research reports.

Binge-Eating Disorder

Wilfley et al.'s (1993) little experiment with obese nonpurging binge eaters is a dark situation comedy. They compared the effectiveness of group cognitive-behavioral therapy and group interpersonal psychotherapy against a wait-list in reducing bingeing. The therapies were provided weekly in ninety-minute group sessions for sixteen weeks. All of the measures—bingeing and ancillary indicators of mood—except presumably weight measurement at pretreatment and post-treatment were self-reported by the patients.

Wilfley et al. stated that at the end of treatment, cognitive-behavioral patients had reduced the number of days of bingeing by 48% (about 2 days), interpersonal patients by 71% (about 3.25 days), and wait-list patients by only 10%. However, at the end of one year the gains were considerably reduced although still substantially less than at pretreatment. Unfortunately, between pretreatment and post-treatment patients gained weight, about 4.5 pounds, in spite of reporting substantial declines in bingeing. At follow-up and again despite substantial declines in bingeing, the interpersonal patients reported a small weight decline (about 6.5 pounds) and the weight of the cognitive-behavioral patients remained unchanged from pretreatment. Either the patients had supplanted their bingeing with steady overeating or their self-reports were grossly inaccurate, considerations that were ignored in the authors' discussion of their findings.

However, Wilfley et al. did address the problem that neither treatment's success was associated with gains in behaviors that were predicted by their separate theories, such as changes in cognitive restraint associated with cognitive-behavioral therapy. They strained their collective imaginations to align their treatments with their theories, in the end concluding that "whether cognitive-behavioral therapy and interpersonal therapy achieve their results through different mechanisms or similar shared mechanisms is currently unknown" (p. 303). They might consider that the mechanism they are searching for is patient falsification, enhanced by the research situation and the authors' subtle demands for patients to report positive results. The research permitted half of their "randomized" patients to select their own assignments, enhancing patient loyalty beyond the customary allegiances created by psychotherapy itself. Moreover, some of their patients were not obese, having body-mass indices in the normal range, but the authors failed to analyze the contributions to their reported gains made by those without serious weight problems or to question why they were included in the study to begin with. Wilfley et al. only recognized their contradictory findings by minimizing the importance of weight loss for the obese: "huge weight losses may not be important because researchers have recently discovered that surprisingly small weight losses can lead to significant improvements in medical conditions" (p. 303). This is an act in a vaudeville science, sustained for its entertainment value—minimal encouragement for patients to reform their eating, along with the assurance that the responsibility is theirs—not its clinical prowess.

Walsh et al. (1997) produced impressive results, especially for patients who received cognitive-behavioral therapy; daily (and sometimes more frequent) bingeing and vomiting dramatically fell to occasional occurrences. Heralding the power of therapy rather than medication, the authors concluded that cognitive-behavioral therapy was superior to supportive therapy and was also superior to medication alone, at least as measured by patient diaries: "cognitive-behavioral therapy is the treatment of choice" (p. 523). However, measured as the frequency of monthly bingeing and vomiting reported during interviews, medication alone was superior to any other treatment. By the end of treatment, the frequency of bingeing and vomiting for patients only receiving medication declined by about thirty-one episodes and thirty-five episodes respectively, and for cognitive-behavioral patients who received medication, the next most successful group, by about twenty-six and thirty-four episodes respectively. It is astonishing that the gains for the medication-only patients were greater than were the gains for the medication patients who received therapy, raising again, although certainly not definitively, the prospect of psychotherapy's harms. The authors' amazement that "surprisingly, the combination of supportive psychotherapy and medication was significantly inferior to medication alone in reducing frequency of binges" is more a tribute to their professional stake in psychotherapy and their selective presentation of data than to their neutrality as scientists in handling the findings of their research.

Importantly, the medication-only group was not controlled by a placebo-only group and the psychotherapy groups (with medication and placebo) were not controlled by a psychotherapy placebo. Thus it is impossible to compare the outcomes against true nontreatment conditions in order to estimate the contributions to outcomes of patient motivation and of the treatment situation itself; but the contributions of medication would seem to be the most substantial finding of the research. Furthermore, the medication was administered orally, a very suspect procedure for patients who routinely induced vomiting.

Additionally, Walsh et al. (1997) found few outcome differences between analyses based on patients who completed treatment and the full sample (which includes the 34% who dropped out), a finding that suggests either that attrition is largely unbiased or that patients differentially falsify their out-comes. In summary, the suspiciously uniform success of all treatments, espe-cially of medication alone; the uncorroborated reports of disturbed patients; and the severe methodological deficiencies cast grave doubt on the efficacy of psychotherapy for bulimic patients who purge. And so it is with Agras et al. (2000), G. T. Wilson et al. (2002), and the rest of the eating-disorder litera-ture: unreliable patient self-reports, amenable samples, attrition, and inade-quate controls.

However, such patently inadequate research, conducted under the auspices of Columbia University's medical school and published in one of the world's leading journals, fortifies the suspicion that the veracity of the findings may not be the point of the experiments. Rather, the drama of social concern involves superficial interventions for very disturbed patients, suggesting that self-help rather than therapy is the motif of its stylized script. The field nour-ishes itself by encouraging a futile sense of personal responsibility and by a marketing prowess for suggesting the individual's strength can overcome almost all adversity. This is very much what to expect if Paul Bunyan had become a psychiatrist instead of a lumberjack.

Violent Children

Echoing the deep social fears of feral children and unsocialized adolescents, psychotherapy is routinely prescribed for youngsters with "a persistent pat-tern of antisocial behavior," ratcheted up in the textbooks as conduct disor-der, oppositional disorder, attention-deficit hyperactivity disorder (ADHD), adjustment disorder, and others. Kazdin, Siegel, and Bass (1992) applied three outpatient conditions to treat them: problem-solving skills training for the children or parent management training or both. Problem-solving skills train-ing "combines cognitive and behavioral techniques . . . (e.g., generating alter-native solutions and engaging means-ends thinking) to manage interpersonal situations (e.g., with parents, teachers, siblings, and peers; at home, at school, and in community)" (p. 736). It provided twenty-five individual sessions last-ing about fifty minutes each. While the individual sessions involved the child, parents were involved throughout the process.

Parent management training was administered in twenty individual ses-sions lasting between 1.5 and 2 hours. Parent training covered the definition of child problems, the logic of reinforcement, assistance in developing tech-niques to be used at home, and so forth. The child's teacher, the parent, and the parent's therapist "developed a reinforcement program to address child deportment and academic performance" (p. 737). Children were actively involved throughout. The third condition provided the full complement of child and parent therapies. All three conditions were provided during six to eight months, although the amount of treatment varied dramatically—more time spent with professionals in the parent training and much more time spent with each family in the combined condition.

The ninety-seven families of the original sample were randomly assigned to the three conditions. Attrition reached 22% by post-treatment, but almost 30% of data were unavailable by the one-year follow-up. More patients dropped out of the parent management and combined conditions than out of the skills training, although the differences were not statistically significant. The authors insisted that the lower IQ of dropouts was the only statistically significant difference between dropouts and completers, although with such small groups other differences may have been important. The sampled children appeared to have serious behavior problems, scoring within the top 10% of the Child Behavior Check List.

Data collection for assessments was impressively broad, utilizing information from thirteen different instruments. Data were collected from the children, their parents, and their teachers, often through interviews conducted by project staff. Great efforts—therapist training, manuals, diaries, and observation—were made to assure that the treatments were delivered as intended.

A large proportion of the enormous number of comparisons between pre-treatment, post-treatment, and one-year follow-up were statistically significant. The combined condition was generally more effective than the two separate conditions. Thus the authors concluded that their "central finding is that treatments can effect change in antisocial and prosocial child behavior and that a combined treatment that addresses cognitive processes and parent-child interaction may represent a viable intervention" (p. 746).

However, the actual changes in almost all measures were quite small across time. In order to get past the seemingly trivial outcomes, Kazdin et al. (1992) analyzed the "clinical impact of treatment" by assessing the degree to which the changed behaviors placed the children within the normal range of the Child Behavior Check List. However, the normal range they chose is simply falling below the 90th percentile. Unfortunately, and despite the authors' claim, the gains are not impressive as indicated by the authors' data. As measured by parents on the Child Behavior Check List, only the mean for children in the combined condition fell below the 90th percentile, and the drop still maintained them close to the authors' very convenient threshold. As measured by teachers, the improvement was more consistent across all conditions, but again the improvements were small. Apparently, when children fell within "the nonclinical range" (that is, they entered the 90% normal zone), they remained very close to the problem boundary.

Other problems with the study erode even these minimal gains. The superior ratings by teachers may well have been more a result of their participation in the treatment, and thus their development of a self-interest in improving the children's behavior, than a true reflection of actual comportment. Moreover, the children, and especially the parents, may have developed affection and a sense of obligation to the therapists and their efforts to help out. Moreover, the parents may also have personalized the outcomes, interpreting any lack of improvement as a flaw in their character—their inability to respond to reason—with the effect of tainting the assessments of their children.

Additionally, the authors failed to employ any nontreatment control, assuming that the effectiveness of each intervention had already been demonstrated. But the prior evidence is as weak, or weaker, than this study. The absence of appropriate controls, particularly in light of the small changes in antisocial behavior, is a critical impediment to concluding that the treatments were effective. Indeed, subtracting even a modest amount for maturation effects and the influence of parents, the teachers, and peers, there are probably few benefits left to redeem interventions. The very small gains may even pose the possibility that therapy exacerbated or prolonged the antisocial behavior. The conclusion of harm is not farfetched when one considers the perturbations caused in family relations by the intrusion of a third, high-status party who in some cases may rob any remaining vestige of authority from marginal parents and thus further undermine the control of their children.

As the authors conceded, the sample was probably not representative of antisocial children, in part because of the eligibility restrictions imposed by the experiment, but also because these children had parents and teachers concerned about their welfare, who applied their energies to improve their children's behaviors. Importantly, the large attrition may further diminish the claims of effectiveness while obscuring the possible harms caused to dropouts lost to analysis. "Our results might only apply to persons who can sustain protracted treatment" (p. 745). Yes indeed, but even in this case the improvements were small, questionable, and possibly biased.

More broadly but quite to the point, the authors stood on their findings to assert the value of psychotherapy for antisocial behavior and suggest that improvements to "optimize" outcomes would emerge from more careful matching of patients and treatments. They ignored a powerful alternative interpretation of their findings reporting that improvements and the superior effectiveness of the combined condition reflected the amount of surveillance rather than the quality of the psychotherapy. Deviant behaviors may have been reduced as attention to the problems increased—a result of general caring rather than the elegance of refined psychotherapeutic skill. Indeed, the alternative environmental concern with social institutions was that much more pertinent as the three conditions of treatment actually failed.

However, the authors' preference for clinical interventions constitutes the core fable of the research and of psychotherapy generally. The culture prefers to view deviance and misbehavior as a result of an errant will rather than as the consequences of inadequate participation in social institutions. In this way, exhortation is the treatment of choice, supplanting the much more costly strategy of equalizing the conditions of family, community, schooling, and employment. In fact, misleading research that falsely boosts the efficacy of psychotherapy is a bulwark against progress, feeding into the culture's parsimony and conceit with high-status reassurances that minimalism is effective and sufficient for the largely poor and lower-status families that constituted the study's sample.

Despite its deficiencies, Kazdin et al. (1992) is one of the most carefully conducted experiments in treating antisocial behavior. The rest of the best is far more deficient. Webster-Stratton and Hammond (1997) largely repeated Kazdin et al.'s interventions, but this time with younger children in far wealthier families and with both parents present, while employing a wait-list control. The results were similarly small, often failing to reach statistical significance; indeed, teacher rating of the children's problems failed to distinguish between treated and untreated groups (perhaps because teachers were not recruited to participate in the treatment as they were in Kazdin et al. [1992] and therefore were more neutral judges). Presumably the most objective measures of outcomes, observations of family interaction made by trained raters, also did not distinguish treated from control patients. Moreover, the study's measures were seemingly open to bias, especially in consideration of the wait-list's incentive to over-report conduct problems in order to remain eligible for treatment. The authors conveniently used mothers' ratings and ignored teachers' ratings (because "only 59% of the teacher reports at baseline were in the clinical range"—in other words, about 40% of the children may not have displayed troubling conduct disorders) in concluding that the outcomes were clinically significant, at least in the home, as measured by mothers but obviously not by the trained observers.

Sanders, Markie-Dadds, Tully, and Bor (2000) employed the Triple P-Positive Parenting Program (really) to treat preschoolers at "high risk of developing conduct problems." They were judged to be at risk because they lived in high crime, high unemployment, poor communities and because their "mothers reported that they were concerned about their child's behavior in response to a specific question" during a phone interview (p. 626). However, after carefully screening out truly troubled families with obvious problems, the final sample was composed of apparently small, lower-risk, stable working families with two parents who had been together for a mean of more than eight years. Not surprisingly, the reported gains were larger than in the previous studies, but still mixed, while the study failed to employ an appropriate control or to assure neutral data gathering. Notwithstanding the wait-list comparisons, the gains seemed to be the logical results of intelligent and concerned parents who take additional time with their rambunctious three year olds. The high arts of the Triple P program remain aesthetically indeterminate.

And so it goes, with the march toward the present gaining no ground. August, Realmuto, Hektner, and Bloomquist (2001) tested the Early Riser's Program but without adjusting for demonstration effects. The study was also marred by potentially biased reports of program participants, imperfect controls, and differential attrition. Still, the outcomes were only small and occasional.

Despite their claims, Henggeler, Melton, and Smith (1992) failed to prove the superiority of family-preservation multisystemic therapy for serious juvenile offenders. Outcomes were small and suffered the same problems of informal house arrest that bedeviled evaluations of community diversion programs for youth in California; that is, the main finding that incarceration was reduced by ten weeks within the year after referral may have been an artifact of the experiment more than a true effect of therapy (Lerman, 1975, on Palmer, 1974). Moreover, attrition was high and measures were uncertain.

In the same way, Jouriles et al. (2001) found negligible and uncertain benefits for the multicomponent family intervention in reducing conduct problems among children of battered women. Most notably, all of the small gains may well have resulted from the unacknowledged benefits of "instrumental support" (concrete resources such as housing, furniture, and the like) rather than from the psychotherapeutic component's uncertain capacity to improve conduct. Even so, the data were largely self-reported from participants, possibly grateful for material assistance, who were well aware of both their special assignment to the experimental condition and the hopes of their therapists for positive outcomes.

Violence is an enormous problem in the United States, particularly among youths. Psychotherapy promises to handle violence inexpensively through clinical treatment without deep and costly attention to the longstanding deprivations of community and family that most likely cause it. Especially because of its ineffectiveness, the continued belief in the curative abilities of psychotherapy states an ideological preference. The preference for psychotherapy ignores America's institutional inequalities by insisting through its implicit tenets that violence is a personal choice—a moral failure requiring voluntary character adjustments—rather than a socially mediated problem requiring family supports and surrogates, greater investments in communities and schools, and opportunities for enriched cultural participation. None of the research had the courage or the will or even an allegiance to the tenets of science necessary to acknowledge that their superficial interventions were incapable of producing substantial benefits and that more intensive, costly attention might be desirable. Psychotherapy's ambition for heroic cure is understandable; the culture's tolerance for the posturing is less readily explained.

Schizophrenia

Stein and Test (1980) demonstrated the feasibility of caring for the seriously mentally ill in the community so long as a variety of concrete support services were provided. They estimated that community care was more expensive than hospitalization, although they argued that in the long run the social benefits exceeded the costs. However, deinstitutionalization as it was worked out during the past decades failed to provide those services; instead, inadequate budgets were repeatedly cut, while some of the limited funds intended for the seriously mentally ill were diverted to more verbal populations compatible with the preferences of psychotherapists. However, psychotherapeutic interventions have not been successful except as they press the fiction of self-reliance, cruelly sacrificing the disabled to a strained social insistence on independence and cost savings.

The recent research suggests that medication paired with a variety of concrete services rather than with psychotherapy are necessary for the successful adjustment of the seriously and persistently mentally ill to community settings (Drake, McHugo, Becker, Anthony, and Clark, 1996; Marder, Wirshing, and Mintz, 1996; Lehman, Dixon, and Kernan, 1997; Hogarty, Kornblith, and Greenwald, 1997; Hogarty, Greenwald, Ulrich, Kornblith, DiBarry et al., 1997; Herz, Lamberti, and Mintz, 2000). It is worth adding that all of these studies were conducted by psychiatrists and that the research customarily employed relatively hard outcome measures (for example, rehospitalization, psychotic episodes, emergency-room visits) in addition to the usual battery of self-reported measures of psychosocial adjustment and patient satisfaction. However, Hogarty, Kornblith, and Greenwald (1997) and Hogarty,

Greenwald, Ulrich, Kornblith, DiBarry et al. (1997) still held out for the benefits of long-term psychotherapy added on to a package of concrete care and medication.

While none of the research estimated the costs of care, it seems apparent that the added services are quite expensive. For example, Lehman et al. (1997) reported that the service staff required to improve the community integration of 77 homeless patients totaled "12 full-time equivalent staff, including a program director with a masters' degree in social work, a full-time psychiatrist and medical director, 6 clinical case managers (social workers, psychiatric nurses, and rehabilitation counselors), 2 consumer advocates, a secretary-receptionist, a part-time family outreach worker . . . , and a consumer advocate" (p. 1039). These costs did not include housing, hospitalization, medical care, and so forth.

Other Conditions

Psychotherapy has also been deployed against a wide variety of other mental and emotional problems with typical results: effectiveness evaporates under scrutiny. Freeston et al. (1997) asserted that they "clearly demonstrate[d] the efficacy of cognitive-behavioral treatment of obsessions without overt compulsions" (p. 410). However, all of their data were collected from patients through interviews or questionnaires. Their study sample of only 29 acute patients—15 randomized to treatment and 14 to a wait-list—resulted from 199 initial inquiries that were highly screened; only 22 patients completed therapy. Moreover, wait-list patients "were informed that treatment would begin 16 weeks after original assessment" and presumably provided them an incentive to maintain their symptoms. Additionally, the insistence on treating patients without overt compulsions nearly eliminated any ability to evaluate gross behavioral outcomes. Ideation is famously amenable to manipulation and response falsification. If obsessive behavior is not amenable to reliable measurement, then it cannot be studied scientifically. All that Freeston et al. could prudently conclude is that a small fraction of those who initially contacted the clinic reported the reduction in their obsessive ideation after going through cognitive-behavioral therapy. Because of the likely wait-list distortions, their improvement, if it occurred, is not evidently attributable to treatment as opposed to natural remission or seasonality.

Franklin, Abramowitz, Kozak, Levitt, and Foa (2000) responded to criticism that randomized samples, because of screening to create diagnostically homogeneous patients as in Freeston et al. (1997), are unrepresentative of customary clinical populations. As a result, the supposedly effective treatments of the best research may not carry over to general clinical practice. Therefore, Franklin et al. (2000) treated patients with obsessive-compulsive disorder who had been rejected for participation in previous clinical trials, who refused to participate, or who had conditions (for example, comorbidity of one sort or another) that would have excluded them from participation. They provided cognitive-behavioral treatment similar to a variety of other randomized studies, but they did not incorporate a control. Franklin et al. reported similarly positive results, which they attributed to the robustness of their intervention. However, their measures, like the measures in their referenced randomized studies, were all dependent on patient self-report in one form or another. None utilized appropriate controls.

It may be instructive in furthering skepticism toward the findings to note that patients who complete treatment and patients who do not complete it typically report very similar outcomes, as in Freeston et al. (1997). Presumably, patients who are deprived of the full dose of treatment should not do as well as those who go through the full course. Yet the elaborate process of psychotherapeutic research is tolerated as a device to create shreds of evidence for a credulous public. A serious clinical science would attend to the credibility of its measures and the appropriateness of its controls while addressing the problems of demand characteristics at least in its discussions, if not actually in its methods.

The Multimodal Treatment Study of Children with Attention-Deficit-Hyperactivity Disorder Cooperative Group, thankfully shortened to MTA Cooperative Group (1999), involved six high-prestige universities and their hospitals (for example, Berkeley, Duke), a cast of principal investigators and coinvestigators large enough for a biblical epic, and two of the nation's most eminent producers of these sorts of events: the National Institute of Mental Health and the U.S. Department of Education. MTA Cooperative Group randomized 579 children with the disorder to one of four groups: medication, intensive behavioral treatment, both, or customary community care. Their principal finding was that all four groups improved greatly, but medication and the combined condition produced the greatest effects.

Yet the research did not employ a placebo or nontreatment condition and obtained almost all of its data from participants (for example, parents and teachers) except for academic achievement, which was measured by a standardized test. It is intriguing that the children's academic performance did not improve, while the greatest gains were apparently reported in the more subjective areas of measurement. Presumably, greater attentiveness should translate into better academic performance. This did not occur, raising the question whether young children were simply drugged into obedience without the excuse of enhanced achievement. More seriously, the MTA Cooperative Group failed to address environmental alternatives to its focused therapeutic interventions, namely greater instructional intensity at school and relatively permanent family and community supports. The chemical imbalances, if they in fact exist, in disruptive children may simply reflect the more compelling inadequacies of schools, families, and communities; to sidestep the issue of institutional inequality by quick recourse to medication seems to insult the Hippocratic oath.

In any event, MTA might have dimmed the glow of its findings with the observation that they may well have been contrived through soft measures and tractable participants. Indeed, the differences between the study's medication intervention and medication within the community treatment condition seems quite possibly to be the result of a town/gown distortion (that is, the university-based MTA psychiatrists substantiating their greater status with compliant patients) rather than a true effect. Any research project of this grandeur and cost—especially when running on public funds—with the ostensible goal of providing credible information would seem obliged to turn over its entire administration to neutral observers and investigators. The failure to do so opens the door to the connivance of professional ambition with public priorities, to the possibility that the public itself preferred the quick and easy over more profound and generous provisions to handle the socialization problems of young children. The narrative line through MTA is not clinical treatment but the Truth of the Tablets.

Cognitive-behavioral therapy has also been applied to anger, irritable bowel syndrome, chronic fatigue syndrome, and insomnia. Chemtob, Novaco, Hamada, and Gross's (1997) mixed findings become even more ambiguous in light of the study's enormous attrition. Seventy-seven patients were referred; of the 35 eligible, only 28 began treatment and only 15 completed therapy. Only two of eleven outcome measures favored the treated group, and even these gains were very small. Still, Chemtob et al. insisted that "anger treatment primarily enhanced cognitive regulation of anger" without any awareness that the cognitive regulation may have only enhanced patient reports, especially after enormous attrition that may have left a small group of accommodating patients who either did not need treatment or were willing to reward their therapists' efforts with testimonials to their improved self-control.

Deale, Chalder, Marks, and Wessely (1997) reported that 70% of patients who completed cognitive-behavioral therapy but only 19% of patients who completed relaxation therapy reduced the severity of their chronic fatigue syndrome. However, the actual improvements were very modest and often not statistically significant; attrition was large; and notably, cognitive-behavioral patients were fully seven years younger than control group's mean age of thirty-eight years.

Rather than proving cognitive-behavioral therapy's ability to reduce late-life insomnia, Morin, Kowatch, Barry, and Walton (1993) documented the treachery of patient self-report. They asked patients and their significant others to document their sleep behavior but also incorporated polysomnography (a sleep machine) to collect the same data. The objective measures consistently, and often to a large extent, undercounted the gains reported by patients and their significant others. Moreover, the study did not involve a true control but only a wait-list control. Again, samples were very small.

Greene and Blanchard (1994) selected only patients who were seeking nondrug treatment for their irritable bowel syndrome and who had not identified a physical cause of their condition. The control, symptom monitoring, was inadequate as a placebo. Measures were self-reported; no objective measures were employed. Samples were very small.

Other psychotherapeutic treatments for other conditions similarly provided inadequate tests of the outcomes: forgiveness therapy for incest survivors (Freedman and Enright, 1996); the cost-effectiveness of psychodynamic-interpersonal therapy (Guthrie et al., 1999); coping and relaxation therapy for cancer patients (Burish, Snyder, and Jenkins, 1991); assertiveness therapy for the disabled (Glueckauf and Quittner, 1992); and bereavement therapy for AIDS patients (Goodkin, Blaney, Feaster, Baldewicz, Burkhalter et al., 1999). All stumble toward the goal of authenticating outcomes.

Cheaper by the Dozen

Group treatment in general is even less well substantiated than individual treatment. Just like the previously mentioned studies, the following research sustains only the conclusion that group treatments are more efficient than individual therapy, producing the same degree of ineffectiveness and possible harm but at lower unit costs, that is, cheaper by the dozen.

Spoth, Redmond, and Shin (2001) compared the ability of two group interventions with a nontreatment control to reduce substance abuse among sixth graders over a four-year period. The program Preparing for the Drug Free Years

> is delivered in five training sessions with an average session length of 2 hour sessions . . . scheduled once per week for five consecutive weeks,

held on weekday evenings, typically at schools. Four of the sessions are attended by parents only; children attend one session with their parents, focusing on peer resistance skills. Essential program content is included on videotapes to ensure standardized delivery. . . . The average number of families per group was 10, and the average number of individual participants per session was 16 (25 for the session including children). (p. 630)

The program assumes that prosocial bonding within the family will diminish subsequent substance abuse and that eleven hours of participation in large groups over five weeks is sufficient to achieve this goal.

In contrast, the Iowa Strengthening Families Program was "based on the biopsychosocial model" that targets poor discipline skills and poor quality of parent-child relationships and encourages resiliency characteristics such as empathy and parent-child bonding. The Iowa Strengthening Families Program

requires seven sets of sessions conducted once per week for seven consecutive weeks; like Preparing for the Drug Free Years, sessions were held on weekday evenings, typically at schools. It includes separate parent and child skills-building curricula and a family curriculum. Weekly sessions consist of separate, concurrent training sessions for parents and children, followed by a family session in which parents and children jointly participate. . . . The concurrent parent and child sessions last 1 hour and are followed by the family session, which also lasts 1 hour. The seventh meeting consists of a 1-hour family interactions session without the concurrent training sessions for parents and children; thus, the total number of intervention hours is 13. . . . Essential program content for the parent and child skills-training sessions is contained on videotapes that include family interactions illustrating key concepts. . . . Group sizes ranged from 3 to 15 families, with an average size of 8 families and an average of 20 individuals per weekly session. (p. 631)

The children were asked during subsequent years to report on their use of alcohol, cigarettes, and marijuana. At the tenth grade, four years after the few weeks of intervention, Spoth et al. (2001) declared victory for both interventions, but notably the Iowa Strengthening Families Program: "Findings showed evidence of intervention-control differences in delayed initiation, current use, and composite use, at a point when students are in high-risk years for substance related problem behaviors. Significant effects detectable 4 years past baseline were observed for both interventions, with a greater number of significant effects found for the relatively more intensive Iowa Strengthening Families Program" (p. 636). Unfortunately, these happy conclusions are unwarranted in light of the experiment's many flaws.

To begin with, the largest benefit of the most effective intervention was small: 18% more of the control group than the Iowa Strengthening Families Program children reported ever having drunk alcohol. Yet even this small gain was undercut by the self-selection of the samples, 35% attrition, and a similar amount of censoring. Approximately 52% of targeted families—perhaps the less concerned—refused to participate in the experiment. In fact, this huge self-selection factor by itself may explain outcomes, although even graver problems mar the research.

All data were based upon the adolescents' self-reports. Aside from problems of memory, these self-reports may have also reflected an amount of falsification proportionate to the notion of family solidarity promoted by the interventions. Indeed, some of the youth, perhaps enough to have created the positive findings, may simply have felt that their responses might be open to their parents. Perhaps too, both types of prosocial training sessions may have encouraged them to report prosocial behaviors in disregard of their actual behaviors. Indeed, Spoth et al. seem sensitive to respondent falsification in making the decision to discount later reports of nonuse in favor of earlier reports of use. Obviously, assuming the reverse—that earlier reports were simply bragging or reflections of peer values rather than accurate statements of substance use—would have greatly diminished their findings. Nevertheless, the authors never conducted objective checks on the reliability of the adolescents' reports.

Furthermore, 85% of the participating adolescents were in two-parent families while the experiment was conducted among rural Iowa families. In short, small findings, questionable data, unrepresentative samples, high attrition, and enormous self-selection are paired with oblivious researchers. The most reasonable conclusion is that short, superficial interventions make no impression on serious personal problems.

In sidestepping attention to the social conditions of neglect that promote substance abuse, Spoth et al. only distinguished themselves by conducting one of the few psychotherapy experiments in which the costs of the evaluation probably far exceeded the costs of the interventions. They failed to provide credible data about the true effects of their programs and carefully avoided attention to the serious flaws in their methodology and the farcical manner in which they measured outcomes. The fact that these two superficial interventions and a woeful research design were taken seriously and sanctioned for testing among a population unrepresentative of the larger problem suggests that national funding agencies are principally concerned with encouraging the modern equivalent of tent revivals to propagate symbols of family solidarity. The National Institute of Mental Health and the National Institute on Drug Abuse are obviously not deeply involved with the institutional imperfections of American life—poverty, broken families, unsupervised adolescents, inadequate schools, and so forth—that are associated with serious drug abuse.

Similar problems undercut all other claims for the value of group therapies: that couples therapy is effective for drug abuse among adults and minimizes the effects of addiction on their children (Fals-Stewart, Birchler, and O'Farrell, 1996; Kelly and Fals-Stewart, 2002; also recall Winters, Fals-Stewart, O'Farrell, Birchler, and Kelley, 2002); that conduct disorders can be forestalled or ameliorated in youths (Webster-Stratton, 1998; Dishion and Andrews, 1995; Barkley, Guevremont, Anastopoulis, and Fletcher, 1992; Dadds and McHugh, 1992); that depressive relapse can be prevented (Jacobson, Fruizzetti, Dobson, Whisman, and Hops, 1993); that rehospitalization for schizophrenia can be reduced (Schooler et al., 1997; McFarlane et al., 1995); that the stresses of chronic disease on patient and parent can be dissipated (Classen et al., 2001; Walker, Johnson, and Manion, 1996); that marriage can be improved (Kaiser, Hahlweg, Fehm-Wolfsdorf, and Groth, 1998); that obsessive-compulsive disorder can be treated (McLean et al., 2001); and that atopic dermatitis can be ameliorated (Ehlers, Stangier, and Gieler, 1995). However, just like unneeded surgery, group therapy may actually exacerbate problems as it intrudes in sensitive and intimate relationships without an ability to improve them.

The common thread through all of this research is efficiency, the ability to achieve difficult behavioral changes through minimal, less costly clinical interventions. The more accurate theme of the research is tacit and largely ignored: unproven psychotherapeutic interventions are pressed in substitution for more substantial attention to social problems.

Conclusion: I Will Act Now

I will act now. I will act now. I will act now. Henceforth, I will repeat these words again and again and again, each hour, each day, every day, until the words become as much a habit as my breathing, that the actions which follow become as instinctive as the blinking of my eyelids. With these words I can condition my mind to perform every

act necessary for my success. With these words I can condition my
mind to meet every change which the failure avoids.

O. Mandino, The Greatest Secret in the World

The mantra of self-help and the texts of psychotherapy express the same Emersonian ideology of self-reliance and self-invention, differing largely in style
rather than substance. The psychotherapeutic emphasis on self-determination
ceremonializes personal responsibility. Whatever benefits are associated with
psychotherapy most likely derive from the patient's embedded character,
notably the motivation to change. Psychotherapy adds little to cure, prevention, or rehabilitation; it may not even sustain motivation. Yet it translates its
clinical inabilities into fables of moral responsibility: the need for the obese,
the beleaguered, the miscreant, the sad, the violent to take responsibility for
themselves and slim down, cheer up, and stop preying on others.

The fact that psychotherapeutic interventions have demonstrated only
a monotonous incapacity to cure, rehabilitate, or prevent is beside the
point. They are cherished fables, elaborate exhortations to virtue and self-
improvement rather than serious clinical interventions. Psychotherapy is a
good stage show whose scripts of behavioral inducement, psychic restructuring, and emotional insight are published in respected scientific journals, tran-
scending popular entertainment with the gravitas of rationality and progress.

5: A Cacophony of Instruments by the Gentlemen-in-Waiting

Obviously, the most fundamental task of research is to develop reliable and valid tools of measurement. Despite an enormous effort, this most basic obligation of any scientific enterprise does not appear to have been adequately fulfilled in psychotherapy outcome research.

In general, clinical judgment—the diagnostic opinions of psychiatrists, psychologists, social workers, and counselors—is customarily accepted as the standard against which interview schedules and patient self-report questionnaires are tested. However, an impressive literature questions the reliability of clinical judgment and even the validity of the diagnostic criteria themselves. Reliability is customarily related to validity; unreliable judgments suggest variable criteria. Indeed, many mental and emotional diagnoses appear to be little more than stigmatizing labels for socially unpopular behavior, the conformity of clinicians with popular opinion.

Kirk and Kutchins have discredited psychotherapy's ability to make clinical judgments. After analyzing the experimental evidence, they concluded that the diagnostic reliability of clinicians' judgments, notably as an extension of the recent editions of the Diagnostic Treatment Manual, has not been achieved (Kirk and Kutchins, 1992; Kutchins and Kirk, 1997). They have reduced clinical boasting that the unreliability problem was conquered to the failures of the research, notably the trials conducted of the Diagnostic and Statistical Manual III (DSM III) (Spitzer, Forman, and Nee, 1979) but also the extensive subsequent literature. "In fact, 'meaninglessness' may be close to what can be claimed about the reliability field trials. Without consideration of the statistical complexities of sensitivity, specificity, and base rates in the DSM III studies, any generalization is hazardous. The lack of data on most specific diagnoses, combined with the small numbers for some classes, suggests that the claims of good reliability were, at best, premature" (Kirk and Kutchins, 1992, p. 158).

Time after time, under the most favorable test conditions for agreement among clinicians who were specifically tutored to apply the same criteria, diagnostic assessments were surprisingly variable. In a study that appeared shortly after Kirk and Kutchins (1992), Williams, Gibbon, and First (1992) reported good agreement among research clinicians on a few disorders (for example, bipolar disorder, bulimia), modest agreement on some disorders (for example, major depression and schizophrenia), and very poor agreement on others (for example, dysthymia, panic disorder). Yet Williams et al. failed to consider that their "test-retest" reliabilities were a product of patient practice—being taught to reply consistently across a battery of repetitive questions over a very short period of time—or to distinguish between inter-rater reliability and test-retest reliability. It is baffling that Williams et al. employed a procedure that cannot distinguish between errors in the clinicians' assessments, inconsistencies in the patients' reports, and actual changes in the disorders themselves.

More recently, Kirk and Hsieh (in review) experimentally confirmed the unreliability of clinical diagnoses. They mailed case vignettes to three thousand experienced psychiatrists, psychologists, and social workers, asking them to provide diagnoses of "a youth engaging in some antisocial behaviors" (p. 10). Fifty-three percent responded. "Even with case vignettes that met the [DSM IV] behavioral criteria for conduct disorder, there was substantial disparity in the DSM diagnoses used by experienced clinicians" (p. 20). Conduct disorder was applied to the vignettes by only 45.5% of the clinicians, rising only to 58.2% when it was grouped together with similar disorders. The vignette method is limited by the amount of information it presents and fails to replicate the clinical environment of decision making. Nevertheless, Kirk and Hsieh's findings, drawn from a representative group of clinicians, are generally robust, confirming similar amounts of diagnostic disagreement even among elite groups of university-based psychotherapists.

In the end, diagnostic judgment in psychotherapy remains unreliable, so much so that it raises questions about the degree to which even highly trained clinicians agree about the fundamental defining characteristics of mental and emotional disorders. Without valid criteria and the ability to apply them reliably among clinicians over time, psychotherapy emerges as a questionable enterprise and outcome research becomes impossible.

The psychometric measurement of the instruments subsequent to Kirk and Kutchins (1992) perpetuates the problem of denial, producing voluminous testimony to reliability that crumbles under scrutiny. Kirk and Kutchins largely assumed that reliability limits validity without actually tracing the relationship between the two. They suggested that clinical assessment error was random, customarily resulting from a variety of technical and procedural irregularities in handling information and perhaps less often from "deceit, fraud or abuse" (Kirk and Kutchins, 1992). However, their interpretation of psychotherapy's role in society sustains a telling source of distortion—bias.

Error drowns true effects in a soup of noise; bias creates unwarranted findings. Indeed, unreliable instruments that produce large amounts of error increase the importance of significant findings, since they must be strong in order to be heard through the background noise. In contrast, bias undercuts the findings themselves, whatever their significance. In fact, bias *increases* reliability and falsely improves the properties of instruments. Statistical power decreases proportionately to error, but measured means do not change. Yet bias changes the means while increasing precision and thus statistical power.

As an excuse for scientific failure, intellectual immaturity is somewhat naive and even willfully self-protective. Bias, however, is subtle—a vehicle for sophisticated and perhaps even unwitting distortions of the clinical proofs that sustain psychotherapy's social prominence. By embracing a scholarship that flouts scientific logic to aggrandize psychotherapy, the field cheapens its clinical role. Instead, it ritualizes the culture's ethos, obediently testifying to the ability of inexpensive and compatible interventions to rectify personal and social problems.

Rather than diagnosis itself, this chapter considers the research instruments that have descended from clinical judgment to provide reliable assessments of mental illness. The process of choosing instruments for analysis has been formidable. The literature is nearly endless, and therefore the present selection of instruments for comment is necessarily limited. Still, the analysis defines a serious problem: the field may not have the ability to measure its defining interest—mental or emotional disease.

The particular threats to the utility of the clinical assessment tools are numerous. It is pointless to validate the psychometric properties of clinical instruments in test situations that are crucially different from the research situations for which they are intended; the demonstration of any instrument's usefulness needs to carry over to its intended purposes. Yet this disparity is common, constituting one of the core threats to the value of virtually all the instruments employed by psychotherapy's outcome research. Researcher and subject motives in the environment in which instruments are validated are customarily different from the motives of researchers and subjects in the tests of outcomes.

Furthermore, neither the validating tests nor the research itself builds in protections against researcher or subject biases. The pervasive problem remains that the findings of the research, whether related to the properties of measurement instruments or to the phenomena they measure, are artifacts of the research situation rather than true, objective outcomes. The ambiguities are deepened by the consistent reliance on patient self-report.

Validating standards are curiously circular. Clinical judgment validates the instruments, which are then offered in later tests to validate clinical judgment. Frequently, the wrong reliabilities are computed: inter-rater reliability is often substituted for test-retest reliability.

Most troubling, there is a lack of recognition that the task of validating a clinical instrument may be impossible. The core methodological difficulty is created by the absence of a true objective standard—a physical or behavior test—to assess emotional and mental illness. Clinical judgment by itself has failed as that objective standard.

The Beck Depression Inventory

The Beck Depression Inventory (BDI) is one of the most widely used scales to measure clinical symptoms. The initial validation of the BDI (A. Beck, Ward, and Mendelson, 1961) has been cited almost ten thousand times between 1980 and 2003 by Social Sciences Citation Index journals; A. Beck, Steer, and Garbin (1988), reporting on its psychometric properties, has been cited more than two thousand times during the same period. These studies have become citation classics, as virtually every investigation of depression—perhaps the most prevalent area of psychotherapeutic practice—employs the BDI either to measure changes in symptoms or to screen patients. The BDI has also been incorporated as a measurement tool in studies of a variety of other problems, notably anxiety.

Its usefulness is widely claimed on grounds of its reliability and validity. Summarizing hundreds of reports of the validity and reliability of the first twenty-five years of the BDI, A. Beck et al. (1988) claim that it offers great internal consistency, high concurrence with other similar instruments, strong construct validity, good ability to discriminate among a variety of conditions, high reliability, and so forth. Nevertheless, in spite of its formal ability to define depression and its reliability under specified test conditions, it fails as a research tool to certify that patients actually suffer the symptoms or the intensities that they report. Large differences persist between clinical judgment and the BDI, while the greater agreement among similar instruments fails to rule out the likelihood that similar biases affect all of them, producing a false confluence and the appearance of independent corroboration. Indeed, the same ambiguities of measurement, notably a result of self-report, that undermine the clinical research also undermine tests of the instruments' value. Just like the outcome studies themselves, the psychometric properties of the BDI are flashy clothes that wear poorly.

The deficiencies of the initial 1961 validation study of the BDI are routinely repeated in later studies. In the most curious way, the BDI was developed specifically because of the great variability of clinicians in making diagnoses but was then validated against clinical judgment: "while there is no reason to assume that clinical evaluation is the ultimate criterion, as long as one is dealing with a clinical phenomenon we will have to rely on expert judgment as our criterion until other measures are developed" (A. Beck et al., 1961, p. 60).

A. Beck et al. (1961) proceeded to use largely the same criteria of depression to develop their instrument and to train a number of psychiatrists. Extensive preparation of psychiatrists in order to reduce the historic variability of clinical judgment involved many meetings to come to agreement on criteria and an enormous amount of practice in diagnosing patients. The research utilized two large samples of patients receiving treatment for psychiatric problems. The BDI ratings were then compared with clinical judgment with findings that the ratings of intensity of depression, although not the diagnosis of depression, were reliable between the two measures.

In spite of their extensive preparation, it is notable that the psychiatrists agreed upon diagnoses only 50% of the time. A. Beck et al. (1961) then fell back on the intensity of depression, rather than diagnosis, to validate their instrument. "The highly significant relationship between the scores on the inventory and the clinical ratings of Depth of Depression and the power to reflect clinical changes in the Depth of Depression attest to the validity of this instrument." Moreover, "it was possible to obtain self-evaluations from the patient that were consistent with the total behavior of the patient as observed by the clinician" (p. 60).

Yet this research situation was designed to nurture a consistent rating among the psychiatrists and the patients. The researchers obviously had an interest in validating the instrument that they had developed. Patients were probably encouraged to report accurately on their current symptoms, at least at their initial testing, and the psychiatrists were aware that they were interviewing clinical populations. At retest, the psychiatrists were aware that patients had been in treatment for two to five weeks and the patients, hopeful of recovery, were aware that they had been receiving treatment. The same psychiatrist interviewed the patient at follow-up. The situation of the research was ripe for symmetrical biases producing concurrence. The concurrence was additionally facilitated by collapsing the four initial judgments of severity by the psychiatrists into only two categories, but the correlations between the psychiatrists and the BDI were still only about .66. "As expected, the most clear cut discriminations occurred when extreme groups . . . were compared" (A. Beck et al., 1961, p. 58). But still, the BDI only succeeded in correctly categorizing 73 out of 83 cases in the first group and 59 out of 65 in the second.

Moreover, the BDI measures only the current mood of the patient, that is, the emotional state at the time of the exam rather than the primary psychiatric or emotional condition. This "state/trait" problem greatly circumscribes the applicability of the BDI, relegating it at best to use as a measure of transient mood.

Evidence published during the subsequent twenty-five years to validate the BDI, exhaustively collected in A. Beck et al. (1988), usually reported presumably adequate psychometric properties: internal consistency that often surpasses .90; stability estimates usually above .65; concurrent validities often above .70; a good ability to discriminate severity of depression; and so forth. But these achievements are diminished by the research conditions in which the data were collected, while some of the data actually contradict the utility of the BDI. Yet throughout the depression literature, both in the clinical outcome studies and in the studies of the BDI's reliability and validity—which are frequently one and the same—there is a consistent failure to protect against serious potential biases. Most notably, researchers with stakes in the outcomes conducted both the tests of the instruments and the tests of the effectiveness of clinical interventions.

The concurrent validity of the BDI (that is, the correlation between the BDI and other scales of depression that purport to measure similar clinical states) is typically only about .67 and is frequently less. Yet with routine disagreements of 50% among clinicians, the value of using clinical judgment as the gold standard for validating the BDI is unclear. Then using the BDI to validate other scales of depression becomes even more questionable, invoking clinical custom rather than scientific proof (see Dobson and Breiter, 1983, as one example). Indeed, deprived of a credible standard, the accuracy of all of the scales will remain uncertain.

Simply asserting the BDI's agreement with other similar instruments does not protect against the likelihood of symmetrical error, that is, of all the instruments being affected by the biases of the research situations in the same way. The fact that the BDI and the Zung scale of depression, as one instance, have a correlation of .75, although frequently less, may seem impressive on the one hand, since few scales tend to correlate this high. But on the other hand, it is worth asking why the correlation is not higher, since both instruments measure the same thing. Indeed, they share many items, but those items often produce correlations only around .50 (Giambra, 1977). The low threshold for acceptable concurrent validities in the social-science literature may be evidence of its capricious standards more than a compelling reason to accept such imperfect measurement tools. In fact, a less self-protective discipline might impose a frank rule of modesty, an explicit warning to psychotherapy patients that they are about to undergo a procedure of uncertain effectiveness. But this sort of "set" might create very unwanted patient responses on the BDI.

A. Beck et al. (1988) went too quickly past the issue of "fakeability," with only two references to the ease of falsifying responses to the BDI: "Beck and Beamesderfer (1974) discussed how easily the BDI can be distorted with respect to faking, and Whitmell (1978) has reported that community mental health patients were able to describe themselves as either depressed or not depressed according to the set given them in advance" (p. 81). Thus patients responding to researcher cues may be influenced to report consistency with clinical ratings in the validation studies and improved scores in tests of psychotherapy's effectiveness. Indeed, Beretvas and Pastor's (2003) conclusion that in studies of the BDI's reliability "test-retest time was not a statistically significant predictor" of reliability coefficients across studies cannot simply be interpreted as endorsing its reliability (p. 87). For one thing, the finding does not account for memory bias, or subtle demands for consistency in spite of symptoms, or even perhaps for the possibility that the measures should have varied more as the state of depression changed.

The problem of response falsification is not simply an interesting sidebar but the principal threat to the validity and reliability of the BDI. It is routinely ignored, notably by research that does not include a true placebo control for psychotherapy but only a wait-list control. Wait-lists apparently motivate patients to maintain their symptoms or at least the report of their symptoms in order to remain eligible for service (curiously, Propst, 1980, reported that the BDI was the *only* score that changed for wait-list patients). None of the research isolates the obvious demand characteristics and expectancy biases that are created by clinicians doing research on their own interventions. None of the research even makes the concession of handing over the conduct of measurement, let alone design and auspices, to neutral raters and judges. Indeed, the clinical experiments seem to cherish "fakeability" as a protection against confronting findings of ineffectiveness.

More generally, A. Beck et al. (1988) accept the findings of the literature without any scrutiny of the credibility of study designs. As a few examples, Giambra (1977) tested three depression scales by administering all of them to students in a single session. The problem remains of separating out true reports from a desire for consistency. Still, he found only modest agreement even in items that were identical. Either mood fluctuates almost instantaneously in late adolescence or there is a problem of concurrent validity.

Strober, Green, and Carlson (1981) found a "high" 5-day test-retest reliability (.69) for the BDI among *patients*. However, unless depression is an extremely volatile condition with rapid rates of spontaneous remission, .69 does not speak favorably to the consistency with which the BDI measures the same condition. Here as in A. Beck et al. (1961), the researchers expended considerable time to assure consistent clinical ratings, but in the end the ability of the BDI to discriminate between major depression and a diagnosis other than depression was only .72. Characteristically, the actual extent of disagreement was not reported.

Gallagher, Nies, and Thompson (1982) found that the test-retest reliabilities of the BDI among the elderly were "reassuring" (p. 152). Still with six to twenty-one days between test and retest, it is not clear whether the reliabilities reflected the stability of the reports because of the stability of mood or in spite of the stability of mood. A baffling circularity is created when mood is assumed to be stable in order to test a scale and then proven to be stable when the scale is stable.

Byerly and Carlson (1982) were unusually forthcoming in questioning their own results, although in this case they were explaining the failure of the BDI and other instruments to discriminate among different diagnostic groups. "Failure to find consistent differences among diagnostic groups for all three scales may be due to (a) unreliability in the diagnostic criteria; (b) specific individual scale insensitivities; (c) response biases on self-report for certain patient groups; or (d) finally, a combination of the three possibilities. The design of this study does not allow a specific answer to this issue" (Byerly and Carlson, 1982, p. 803). Nor does the design of any other study that raises the question of why research is conducted before serious threats to its credibility are addressed. The other studies that A. Beck et al. (1988) rely on, notably for proof of reliability, stability, and concurrent validity, share similar problems.

A few of the studies suggest considerable problems with the BDI. In particular, Tanaka-Matsumi and Kameoka (1986) question its fundamental validity, whether it assesses depression or "general emotionality," whether it can distinguish anxiety from depression, and most important, whether social desirability influences the self-report of depressive symptoms. While the research was conducted on college students, its findings raise broader concern with the common use of the BDI to screen subjects for research.

Hatzenbuehler, Parpal, and Matthews (1983) found that initial scores for mild or moderate BDI scores routinely fell without any therapy, an effect that cannot be attributed either to the objective state of mood or to falsified reporting. Perhaps college students are a unique population of the depressed, although Hatzenbuehler et al. pointed to similar effects with other groups. The fact that "repeated administrations of the BDI result in significant decline of high scores" suggested far more than a simple corrective by assessing "depression immediately prior to conducting an experiment" but rather that "studies using BDI change scores would clearly have to control for the effects of repeated testing" (Hatzenbuehler et al., 1983, p. 364, 365; see also Sacco,

1981; Hammen, 1980). The routine reduction in BDI scores among those screened as depressed poses a considerable challenge to research, reprising the imperative for placebo controls to estimate changes in reported depression that are unassociated with treatment.

The problem of transient scores is compounded by research designs and validation studies that repeat the application of the BDI. Atkeson, Calhoun, and Resick (1982) found that by itself, repeated application of the BDI diminished the degree of reported depression.

The research subsequent to A. Beck et al. (1988) did not repair the methodological pitfalls of the earlier studies nor clarify their ambiguities. However, many recent studies, including quite a number that Aaron Beck himself has authored, have reported increasing reliability (Steer, Brown, and Beck, 2001; A. Beck, Brown, and Steer, 1997; Winter, Steer, and Jones-Hicks, 1999; Buckley, Parker, and Heggie, 2001; Leigh and Anthony-Tolbert, 2001). At the same time, anomalous findings are reported; as examples, the application of the BDI seems to have an effect on mood (Raag, Pickens, Bendell, and Yando, 1997), while it fails to adequately identify depression among Alzheimer's patients (Wagle, Ho, and Wagle, 2000).

In short, none of the research adequately protects against the expectancy biases of the researchers, while the problem persists of continuing to validate the BDI against uncertain clinical judgment. Moreover, only rare commentary addresses the clinical meaning of employing scales that explain little more than 50% of the variance and consistently make numerous errors of judgment. It seems, however, that the field is generally pleased with the BDI and similar instruments. Yet in the absence of effective protections against researcher biases to confirm their expectations, that very satisfaction may be transmitted subtly as the principal cause of reliability among patients whose self-reports are not corroborated against objective criteria.

The Eating-Disorder Examination

The frequency of bingeing and, in many cases, weight change measure the success of any intervention to treat anorexia nervosa and bulimia nervosa. Associated attitudes, for example, body image, may be important components of eating disorders, but they are not determinative of successful outcomes. Instruments that fail to reliably measure the focal behaviors of treatment are not useful for research.

The Eating Disorder Examination (EDE), administered through an interview, relies entirely on uncorroborated patient self-report. This unaddressed problem of reliable measurement is compounded by the sensitivity of pathological eating behaviors. "Many individuals with eating disorders . . . hide their disorders. Most individuals with bulimia nervosa, for example, will binge eat and purge only when alone. The eating disorders are also associated with high levels of deception and resistance to treatment" (Anderson and Williamson, 2002, p. 292).

While the EDE appears to have achieved great reliability, the tests are flawed in a variety of ways. The psychometric properties are established in situations that are crucially different than the research situations for which they are intended. They do not employ objective checks on the self-reports. Particularly relative to bulimia nervosa among the nonobese, it is often uncertain whether a true pathology exists. In the end, the frequent preference to measure outcomes in terms of the EDE, especially where weight change itself is crucial, reveals more about professional introversion than successful treatment.

Cooper, Cooper, and Fairburn (1989) set out to test the EDE's ability to provide "clinicians and research workers with a detailed and comprehensive profile of the psychopathological features of patients with eating disorders" (p. 154). They applied the EDE to groups of patients with eating disorders and to a group of people without eating disorders, finding that the EDE discriminates well on almost all measures. However, it did not discriminate well on items relating to the respondents' perceptions of subjective bingeing, that is, their feelings of overeating rather than the actual amount that they ate.

Cooper et al. (1989)—a typical test situation for validating the EDE—obviously wished for patients with eating disorders to report disorders and normals to report no eating dysfunction. However, the typical situation in clinical research is apparently different when the effectiveness of psychotherapy is being tested. In the clinical setting, the therapist-researcher obviously hopes the patient reports less disorder after treatment. Indeed, the very sensitivity of the behaviors, together with voluntary patients' stake in successful outcomes and their presumed sense of obligation for treatment, predisposes clinical research toward reduced reports of eating dysfunction after therapy and at follow-up.

Cooper et al. (1989) set up a situation naturally disposed to great patient self-report accuracy. All of the patients were referrals for eating disorders, that is, they had allowed themselves to be identified as having an eating disorder by reporting the criterion behaviors prior to the administration of the EDE by the researchers. They were obviously seeking treatment for a condition that they had explicitly recognized. In contrast, the normals in the control had been screened for people who would not report eating disorders. But the EDE was not validated in a situation in which the deceptiveness of reporting, perhaps after unsuccessful treatment (even recognizing that success cannot be measured apart from the patient's reports) or in the belief that treatment was administered, would be most relevant. Thus Cooper et al. simply tested whether people who tell a story at one time would be likely, shortly after, to retell it in similar circumstances. It is worth recalling that Wilfley et al.'s (1993) obese, nonpurging bulimic patients reported improvement after treatment on the EDE but continued to gain weight. Either they cut out the time between meals, eating small portions constantly, or, more likely, they misreported their binges and caloric intakes.

There is also a problem with false positives—normal-weight patients who otherwise seem to be bulimic—reporting distorted body images, frequent bingeing and purging, and so forth. In a still undefined number of cases, people will exaggerate their symptoms (perhaps like depressed patients on wait-lists) for a variety of motives—to receive treatment, to participate in the treatment of a fashionable flaw of the soul, for professional attention, for recreational vengeance on their feckless and meddlesome therapists, in expression of their depression, or due to other emotional problems. Anderson and Williamson (2002) acknowledge "evidence that self-reporting of binge episodes may be an overestimation of the actual frequency of their occurrence" (p. 293).

Rosen, Vara, and Wendt (1990) compared "the EDE with self-recorded eating behavior in order to determine if various ratings of binge eating . . . on interview agreed with more objective and detailed information about the subject's intake" (p. 521). Their subjects were college students and women with bulimia nervosa. With a straight face, they defined subject logs as "primarily behavioral," providing more objective and detailed information than interviews (p. 520). The authors never addressed the obvious problem that the eating disordered who distort verbal reports will also distort written reports. Instead they stated with no evidence at all that patients "recorded all food and liquid intake for the seven days prior to being administered the EDE" (p. 522). Not surprisingly, the agreement between the EDE and the patients' logs in reporting episodes of vomiting was high (.81). However, the other reported concurrent validities were modest at best and, for purposes of treatment and research, very poor. The correlation between the overeating items of the EDE and patient logs was only .40, but the authors still concluded that these two sources were "related closely" (p. 524).

Presumably, the patients underreported their bingeing in the interviews. A correlation of only .40 between EDE interviews and logs for the most critical items raises a serious concern with response falsification even under these optimal conditions of reporting, when subjects knew their responses were to be compared with their logs. It is worth wondering whether the difference between the EDE interviews and the logs represents a measure of shyness, deception, or faulty memory. It is perhaps worth speculating that a sense of caloric values is related inversely to falsification of the logs, that is, patients who were aware of the calorie count of their food tended more often to distort their logs.

Moreover, Rosen et al.'s (1990) finding that EDE interviews are useful indicators of actual behavior was reached in a study of largely normal subjects, not those with diagnosed bulimia nervosa, the patients in the clinical studies. It is simply misleading to apply the reporting behavior of people without bulimia nervosa to those with the problem. Rather than an endorsement, the findings of Rosen et al. indict the EDE as a useful research tool.

Rizvi, Peterson, Crow, and Agras's (2000) claims for high test-retest and inter-rater reliability repeat previous problems. Their subjects had similar incentives at each point of testing, whereas in the research application of the EDE, patients experience different pressures on their responses before and after their therapy. Rizvi et al. repeated Cooper et al.'s (1989) findings as well as their biases, with the reliability of the subjective bingeing items much lower than the others, again suggesting the reactivity of eating behaviors to research situations.

Other Instruments

Heatherton, Kozlowski, and Frecker (1991) offered a rare instance in which a self-report scale was compared with truly objective measures. In this case, the Fagerstrom Tolerance Questionnaire (FTQ), a popular measure of smoking intensity, was validated against saliva tests that measured cotinine and carbon-monoxide levels. Eight different models of the Fagerstrom instrument rarely predicted more than 30% of the variance in the laboratory tests. The authors still insisted that the instrument "is a valid measure of heaviness of smoking" in comparison with objective biochemical measures. However, the utility of an instrument that predicts objective criteria so poorly is questionable. Yet it is not clear whether the unexplained variance in the laboratory measures was due to response falsification, poorly designed questions, or the unreliability of the lab tests themselves. The experience of the FTQ as an indicator of the accuracy of self-report documents a severe problem of measurement in psychotherapy.

In the absence of objective measures, Sobell, Sobell, and Riley (1988) were able to achieve great reliability for their time-line method to assess recent drinking. However, the time-line procedure was validated with normal drinkers. The two tests were separated by about twenty-five days. Reported test-retest reliabilities were very high, with 63 of 79 computable correlations exceeding .85. While time line seemed to improve over the "quantity-frequency" method, neither employed any objective standard. Yet the study only validated the time-line procedure with normal drinkers, while it was intended to be employed with heavy drinkers. Addicts and heavy users are notoriously unreliable, especially when reporting use and particularly under the conditions of therapy, which frequently involve serious criminal sanctions.

Unfortunately, Sobell et al.'s (1988) claims for the validation of time-line self-reports among abusers also suffered debilitating problems. The patients were aware that their self-reports were to be checked against corollary sources of information. However, in its typical use in research on psychotherapy for alcoholism, the time-line method was applied without the corollary procedures. This is similar to the fallacy that because self-reported use among heroin addicts is reliable when paired with urinalysis, it is therefore reliable by itself (Winters, Fals-Stewart, O'Farrell, Birchler, and Kelley, 2002).

Many other instruments share the fallacy of validating themselves in conditions that are markedly unlike the situations of their intended use. Customarily the instruments, intended to measure particular patient conditions after the delivery of psychotherapy, are validated when patients do not receive therapy. Both the instruments and the clinical research itself routinely ignore the malleability, or more precisely, the reactivity of patient self-reports, that is, the sensitivity to research "sets." However, research conducted without a therapeutic component ignores the likelihood that depressed patients in therapy will suppress the report of their negative thoughts in order to avoid the depressing thought that they failed to benefit from therapy. In just this way, neither the BDI (A. Beck et al., 1961; A. Beck et al., 1988) nor the Hamilton Rating Scale for Depression (M. Hamilton, 1960, 1967) acknowledges the special conditions of psychotherapy that may distort patient responses to the state of their depression.

Studies that have attempted to validate an instrument in the conditions of therapy suffer a similar problem in the absence of objective measures. Shear et al. (1997) attempted to validate the Panic Disorder Severity Scale (PDSS). They applied it to 186 patients who were diagnosed with panic disorder and a subset of 89 patients of these patients after short-term treatment. A further subsample received two independent assessments. The authors reported moderate to high measures of a variety of psychometric properties. However, all the results only showed agreement by the clinicians on the patients' symptoms, which were, again, self-reported during clinical evaluations. The consistency among raters says very little about the plausible consistency of biases and demand characteristics that may have encouraged patients to report consistent improvements after treatment. Once again, clinical judgment itself has not enjoyed any great reliability except when great efforts are made to train a select group of clinicians in similar procedures. Nevertheless, the convergent validity between the PDSS and another similar scale was only modest (.55), while correlations between separate items on the two scales that probed the same symptoms were surprisingly imperfect. For example, panic frequency, asked in both scales, only correlated .69. Rather than a demonstration of convergent validity, the disparity between the reports of equivalent items on different scales raises many questions about response falsification and the design of instruments. Instead of concluding that the scale was sensitive to change because clinicians' ratings were consistent, the authors might have raised points of judicious skepticism: that the demand characteristics of treatment, rather than treatment itself, created the consistency or even that the "set" of an item or question, that is, its situation in a scale and not just its content, influenced responses.

Hollon and Kendall (1980) attempted to measure automatic thoughts, a central component of the cognitive theory of depression. As they noted, despite the widespread use of cognitive-behavioral therapy in treating depression, "there appears to have been little systematic effort to assess changes in cognitive content and process as a function of treatment" (p. 384). Yet a direct physical marker of specific cognitions has been elusive, with the result that self-report instruments attempting to assess identified cognitions are difficult to validate.

Hollon and Kendall (1980) validated their Automatic Thoughts Questionnaire (ATQ) with college students utilizing the BDI, among other scales, to test for concurrent validity. They found that the ATQ both is reliable and has acceptable levels of concurrent validity in identifying specific automatic negative thoughts associated with mild to moderate depression. However, the ATQ itself suggests thoughts to the subjects—its questions are not open ended—while test-retest reliability, the critical concern in measuring the occurrence of automatic thoughts after psychotherapy, was not probed. Hollon and Kendall (1980) excused the omission on grounds that retesting the ATQ needs to be compared to retests of self-reported levels of depression. Yet again, the procedure may be pointless, as the ATQ shares many items with tests of depression and the retesting procedure cannot separate out training effects (memory rather than accurate report), the transitory state of depression, and the confirmatory pressures of the research. Indeed, without an ability to handle these problems, the psychometric properties of the ATQ appear contrived and misleading.

Similarly, patient and therapist agreement on the Working Alliance Inventory (WAI; Horvath and Greenberg, 1989) and the Session Evaluation Questionnaire (SEQ) does not provide "a useful bridge between psychotherapy process and outcome" (Stiles, 1980, p. 176). Based on self-report and without objective validation, agreement can be interpreted as an index of the demand characteristics of psychotherapy itself. Responses to specific items may reflect little more than the patient's expression of satisfaction with therapy and the therapist. The metaphorical "bridge" between process and outcome has yet to be objectified as a valid tool for exploring the determinants of outcome. It is worth pondering the fact that the outcomes in these studies are measured by instruments validated through similarly ambiguous processes, suffering similar problems of patient motivation and self-report.

The Global Assessment Scale (GAS) of overall functioning, like many other scales, is validated without any reference to the objective facts of its own criteria even when those facts can be checked. Based upon interviews alone, judges assess whether subjects "need constant supervision for several days to prevent hurting self . . . , [are] unable to function in all areas . . . , [are] generally functioning with some difficulty . . . , [show] good functioning in all areas" (Endicott, Spitzer, Fleiss, and Cohen, 1976), and so forth. Many of these possibilities are amenable to objective verification. Thus inter-rater reliability and concurrent validity reflect the state of clinical judgment rather than the objective truth of an individual's functioning. In this way too, the GAS is more sensitive to the biases of clinicians in the research situation than to the objective situation of patients. Rather than objectifying and validating clinical judgment, the GAS simply codifies its ambiguities. Still, the concurrent validities remain quite modest at crucial points, ranging from only .42 to .67 (adjusting for sign), reflecting a great amount of disagreement over issues of improvement in treatment.

The diagnostic inter-rater reliabilities reported by Silverman and Needles (1988) for the Anxiety Disorders Interview Schedule were high. However, test-retest reliability is the crucial property to establish for the research situation.

Conclusions

The conclusion seems compelling that in addition to the poor methodological quality of the psychotherapy research itself, the field has not successfully developed adequate instruments to measure its outcomes. Adequate measurement is the most fundamental requirement of quality research in any field. It is worth considering that some combination of measurement unreliability and bias have contrived the evidence for psychotherapy's effectiveness. Research statements about the outcomes of psychotherapy are profoundly meaningless as clinical statements.

The BDI, EDE, WAI, GAS, ATQ, FTQ, time-line and quantity-frequency methods, PDSS, and so forth are probably among the best researched instruments employed in clinical studies. The more common instrument, sometimes even a one-off, ad hoc compilation, is less well understood, with psychometric properties estimated casually along with its use as an outcome measure. The invalidating flaws of the best instruments suggest that the field does not reliably measure its outcomes. Yet the huge attention to instrumentation, particularly in depression research, may appear to be a tribute to the scientific commitments of psychotherapy. However, the actual conditions for validating the instruments, the common exaggeration of their utility, and their common abuse in clinical studies imply that the rush to clinical research, if not professional self-promotion, may be the determining motives. Such failure could not persist for so many decades without the quiet complicity of the culture itself.

While the literature considers reliabilities of above .65 or so to be acceptable "for purposes of research," the meaning of reliabilities and concurrent validities at that level may be problematic for clinical decision making. The studies of instruments routinely ignore the actual error rates in assessment while emphasizing their impressive significance levels even more than the discovered relationships. Yet by explaining only 50% of variance but, more importantly, containing many errors in judgment consistently across studies, the instruments fail to provide credible evidence that any psychotherapeutic procedure is effective. Moreover, marginal reliabilities would be acceptable for research purposes if the subjects were monkeys and the outcomes were not taken up as clinical truths. However, the findings of the research are quickly incorporated into clinical judgments that affect the well-being of patients.

Test situations to validate the instruments do not generally reflect the methodological threats to credibility—demand characteristics realizing the researchers' expectancy biases—that exist in the experimental situations in which they are employed. Bias is not addressed by attention to reliability. The customary refusal to incorporate true placebo controls in order to assure symmetrical motivation among research subjects encourages misleading findings.

The problem of measurement persists even though some of the underlying behavioral phenomena associated with mental and emotional problems can be measured objectively (for example, days lost at work, weight, perhaps even sleeplessness, time out of bed, illicit drug use, and so forth). But the difficulties of measurement in no way excuse the buoyant optimism of the research. In the spirit of first things first, the research agenda might attend to true measurement before it presumptively attempts outcome research.

The fact that better procedures may not be possible does not improve the usefulness of the instruments nor dictate the acceptance of weak research. Some problems remain intractable despite the best intentions of researchers. The conclusion, for the present at least, may be that scientifically credible research on the effects of psychotherapy is impossible.

The shaky research constructs a moral imperative to disclose the tenuousness of treatment, particularly to patients but also more frankly to the culture and to the credulous audience of clinicians. Yet abstract moral imperatives rarely create political imperatives or affect social institutions. The reverse is more common. The reality of clinical practice—indeterminacy, probable ineffectiveness, and possible harm—is crowded out by psychotherapy's utility as fable. There has yet to be a tool, let alone a measurement instrument, that protects its own use or can impede its interpretation as metaphor beyond its actual production function. In abiding social mandates for policy minimalism, psychotherapy ritualizes dominant preferences for individualism and self-sufficiency. Clinical outcomes are ignored, as clinicians and patients perform an elegant pageant of moral instruction.

"But he doesn't have anything on," said a little child . . .

"He doesn't have anything on!" the whole populace shouted at last. And the emperor shuddered, for it seemed to him that they were right. But then he thought, "Now I must go through with the procession." And he carried himself more proudly than ever, and the gentlemen-in-waiting carried the train that wasn't there at all. (Andersen, 1987, p. 71)

6: Magic, Bias, and Social Role

There is not a single tenet in the logic of scientific discovery that psychotherapy research has failed to distort, disobey, or subvert. Rather than the challenges of diagnosis and measurement, the field might first attend to the biases that—through the collusion of obliging and seductive clinicians—create the illusion of reliable instruments and effective treatment. It is supremely ironic that psychotherapy's exquisite sensitivities to the patient construct the very vehicle of its biases. From the concerns of psychoanalysis with transference and countertransference to the far more directive therapies of the contemporary field, the literature is consumed with explaining and controlling the practitioner's verbal and nonverbal influence over the patient. Yet the attention to therapist influence stops conveniently short of skepticism toward the accuracy of patient assessments of the effectiveness of treatment. The therapeutic alliance—the defined vehicle of psychotherapy—powerfully conveys the demand characteristics of the therapist, made all that more profound by the quality of the established relationship, a discipleship of self-discovery. Indeed, many patients probably guard their relationship with their therapists more than they pursue the remission of their symptoms.

Quite clearly, psychotherapy does not employ physical cures, although its insistent parallel with medicine has improved the social authority of the field. Nevertheless, psychotherapy is not a medical treatment but, as acknowledged by the core of the field, is more akin to a religion, a credo, a philosophic investigation, even a "comprehensive ideology" to ease the troubled psyche and change unwanted behaviors (Zeig, 1997, p. 35). The process of becoming a communicant in a rite of self-discovery is guided through interpersonal belief, the patient's relinquishing doubt and accepting on faith the power and wisdom of the therapist. The successful relationship itself, the most essential requirement of therapy, creates powerful incentives for the patient to deny his or her failure in the therapeutic process, risking the therapist's displeasure.

The potential researcher biases have long been recognized and listed if not actually tested. In fact, the extent to which the outcomes of psychotherapy are artifacts of the research situation rather than the results of psychotherapy undercuts the authority of the field. Orne (1959, 1962) explored the subtle "demand characteristics" of research situations that might account for behavior under hypnosis. Rather than the motivations of the subject to act out particular roles, or increased suggestibility, or "an altered state of consciousness,"

Orne (1959) argued that patients actually responded to "explicit and implicit cues provided by the hypnotist and the situation" (p. 277). In short, subjects may respond to the researcher's preferences to confirm his or her hypothesis rather than to the substance of the experiment itself, "the experimental variables." Orne argued that the demand characteristics of an experiment take

> place within the context of an explicit agreement of the subject to participate in a special form of social interaction known as "taking part in an experiment." Within the context of our culture the roles of subject and experimenter are well understood and carry with them well-defined mutual role expectations. A particularly striking aspect of the typical experimenter-subject relationship is the extent to which the subject will play his role and place himself under the control the experimenter. . . . Just about any request which could conceivably be asked of the subject by a reputable investigator is legitimized by the quasi-magical phrase, "This is an experiment," and the shared assumption that a legitimate purpose will be served the subject's behavior. (Orne, 1962, p. 777)

The therapeutic relationship in an outcome experiment is even more demanding than Orne's supposedly neutral laboratory investigations of hypnosis. The patient presumably desires the same ameliorative outcomes as the therapist. At the same time the patient's goodwill—the tendency to endorse the therapist's skill by exaggerating positive outcomes—is nourished by the therapist's skill in establishing emotional authority of one sort or another, by the patient's stake in succeeding, by the obligation imposed by usually free clinical care, and perhaps even by a sense of symbolic representation, the notion that the patient succeeds not just personally but for all others with similar problems. To fail for himself or herself is to fail for all who suffer.

Rosenthal and Rubin (1978) provided a more systematic and quantitative dimension to demand characteristics, referencing them as "interpersonal expectancy effects." They concluded that in the interactions most similar to psychotherapy, the researcher's expectations probably account for about .70 standard deviation of the reported improvements and perhaps more than 1.0, large amounts that probably unmask the pretense to effectiveness in psychotherapy. These estimates of expectancy effects exceed the average benefit of psychotherapy reported by Smith, Glass, and Miller in 1980 and greatly exceed the average benefits that they reported for studies employing placebo controls. While there may be some controversy concerning whether therapist expectancy is a legitimate psychotherapeutic technique (a "nonspecific factor") or a placebo effect, therapist expectancy probably leads to the patient's falsified reports of recovery more often than to clinical improvements. Yet Rosenthal and Rubin's (1978) base of studies may not have included many that were direct tests of the influence of psychotherapists. Still, Rosenthal's later (2003) discussion of covert communication, one of the vehicles of researcher expectancy biases, provided a compelling point of skepticism. The burden lies with the researcher to assure that patient outcomes are real rather than mirages brought about by the researchers' love of their hypotheses. Unfortunately, expectancy-bias precautions have not been taken in the research. There is hardly any evaluation of psychotherapy that employs neutral, independent observation of patient outcomes or that even collects the reports of patients by interviewers unaffiliated with the research organization.

Similarly, Kintz, Delprato, and Mettee (1965), and more recently Nickerson (1998), have offered exhaustive support for the likelihood of ubiquitous "experimenter effects" and "confirmation bias," their synonyms for the illegitimate influence of researchers and experimental situations on research subjects but also for the frailty of researchers in sustaining their skills by ignoring disconfirming evidence. Nickerson collects a number of explanations for confirmation bias: the desire to believe, faulty information processing, a preference for positive outcomes, simple credulity, the desire to avoid errors, and educational effects, that is, the influence of culture in predisposing certain outcomes. All of these threats to the integrity of research are probably live during psychotherapy, in which the patient, the therapist, and the researcher usually desire similarly positive outcomes. The pressures on patients, especially when they are the sole judges of outcomes, may constitute undeniable demands to confirm researchers' expectations and perhaps even to image therapeutic benefits. Nickerson's droll final suggestion that his conclusion of ubiquitous confirmation bias may itself be an instance of confirmation bias is not a fateful conundrum. Rather, it suggests that the problem might be better handled in psychotherapy if the community of researchers frankly acknowledged the deficiencies of the research and then proceeded to institute substantial protections for objectivity and neutrality. Yet if the expectancy cues in therapy are inseparably embedded in the research situation, then the outcomes of therapy—to the extent to which they rely upon self-reports—become permanently indeterminate. Nevertheless, the incorporation of multiple controls, and notably placebo controls, along with a variety of measurement conditions including blinding and neutral assessment would seem to be minimal requisites for credible clinical-research efforts. These protections, however, have not been routinely adopted, and the ubiquitous pitfalls of methodology force speculation about the field's motives, its stakes in perpetuating the appearance of its clinical prowess.

The possibility that the research situation creates reports of positive outcomes independent of actual clinical outcomes seems central to the very nature of the therapeutic relationship. The therapeutic relationship is a coercive medium of trust and belief that promises relief from psychic discomfort and affirmation of personal worth to a needy patient. The power of the therapist is imposed on the patient through the role of psychic healer whose abilities are certified by the authority of science. The responsibility for successful therapy subtly shifts to the patient, creating a situation that encourages the denial of failure in order to remain worthy of the affirmations of therapy itself. Most notably, the relationship demands unquestioning belief by interpreting skepticism as rationalized resistance. It is a wonder that any patient would have the temerity to confess, even indirectly, an inability to live up to the therapist's expectations or to challenge the therapist's authority with persistent reports of failure. In failing at therapy, the patient risks the stigma of being irresponsible and, therefore, undeserving of national communion by stubbornly maintaining a flawed character, that is, by refusing to marshal the necessary self-control to reform his or her behavior.

Bias in the Psychotherapeutic Relationship

With near uniformity, psychotherapy's different schools routinely define the patient's relationship with the therapist in terms of deep trust, dependence, reliance, openness, spontaneity, truth, and psychic importance. The therapeutic relationship conveys the healing truths of therapy itself. It is predicated upon overcoming any resistance of doubt in the patient. It is also inseparable from true belief and cultish communion, achieving a deeply emotional faith in a transformative process without the hesitations that test prudent doubt. The therapeutic relationship is built on the patient's profound vulnerabilities, his or her need for evidence of existential superiority and of psychic growth toward the sublime satisfactions of timeless insight, self-discovery, compassion, and wisdom. Patients who achieve an appropriate alliance with the therapist have suborned their ability to assess their clinical progress properly.

The patient's commitment to therapy often transcends any objective process of treatment (such as the removal of a wart by a dermatologist), becoming an emotional acceptance of a new faith. The literature of psychotherapy is deeply suspect, as it largely ignores the patient's conversion experience, that is, the emotionality of individual commitment to the therapist as healer and to therapy as revealed truth. It also ignores the dependent narcissism of the relationship, the patient indulging the heroics of personal rebirth and self-invention and the therapist the histrionics of psychic salvation. Indeed, the required discipleship should devalue the patient's objectivity as well as the assessments of collaterals who participate as informants and judges. It is worth considering that reported treatment successes may be better explained by the degree of the patient's absorption into the discipleship of therapy than by any magic of treatment. The blind faith and distorted self-reports would, of course, be minimized by credible proof of the ability of profound devotion to dispel unwanted behaviors. Unfortunately, no proof exists that the acceptance of Christ as a personal savior leads to Heaven or that a course of psychotherapy leads to personal improvement.

The centrality to psychotherapy of the relationship between therapist and patient is routinely described in terms that discredit the neutrality of either participant. These descriptions become even more vivid when the leading clinicians and theorists summarize their own work. The following comments are drawn from papers published in the *Evolution of Psychotherapy: The Third Conference*, edited by Zeig (1997), who also contributed a paper. (The conference was held in 1995.) The contributors fervently justify their subjective methods and their clinical brilliance through moving vignettes of patient recovery, with little if any recourse to more systematic evidence. Notably, each claims that his or her success emerges from successful relationships with patients. None consider the possibility that those intense relationships induce fictitious reports more than actual behavioral change or that they are playing to patients susceptible to cultish belief.

Marmor's description of Alexander Lowen, the first "mind-body therapist" of "bioenergetics" and the founder of the Institute for Bioenergetic Analysis, serves as a general ideal for the therapist. Marmor presents Lowen "as a warm, caring, passionate man with powerful convictions who unquestionably inspires strong feelings of positive tranference in most of his patients" (Zeig, 1997, p. 145). He offers reasons why Lowen's patients respond positively to treatments that emphasize releasing muscular tension. The question is notably appropriate given Lowen's theoretical notions, for example, "grounding" ("the degree to which an individual is connected to the ground or earth energetically and with feeling") and the "objective criterion" for determining "an individual's contact with reality": "when one studies the feet and legs of patients one can observe how alive the foot is from the quality of the tissue, the skin tone and motility. Flat, pale-looking feet that are relatively immobile indicate a lack of feeling and denote an absence of real contact with the ground. That lack of feeling is due to a diminution in the feet's energetic charge" (p. 137).

With this sort of theory—a phrenology of the foot—any positive outcomes are probably due more to the therapist's skill at inducing positive transference and distorted patient reports than from any curative skill. Marmor, however, is largely the believer, not the skeptic, insisting on the therapist's influence over the patient through the subtle reinforcements of operant conditioning. "I wish to make it clear that in emphasizing the role of suggestion and persuasion in Dr. Lowen's method it is not my intention to denigrate it. My research over the years has clearly indicated that suggestion and persuasion are part of every psychotherapeutic technique" (p. 147).

Indeed, Marmor might also have included the possibility that the wellspring of suggestion resided as much in the therapist's demands for *reported* change to sustain his theory and, of course, his practice as in the patient's motivations for change, relief, or understanding. Lowen's "powerful inspirational quality," operating through "powerful positive transference" and "skillful metaphors," inspires religious conversion instead of behavior change. Whatever rituals of belief they may script, Lowen's techniques apply a near irresistible pressure for his patients to falsify their actual behaviors.

Gendlin describes the therapist's relationship with the patient as uniquely intense and deep, more "than was ever possible through the forms of traditional society. Many therapists connect so deeply with their clients that their other relationships cannot compare with that depth. But that is because the therapist-client relationship is fenced in and limited as to action so that it can be deep and real within its narrow channel" (p. 209).

But the specialness of Gendlin's relationship is all the more remarkable, or perhaps all that more facilitated, by the deep impenetrability of his basic therapeutic assumptions about "focusing." "Focusing helps to let a person become a continuous inside at that zone between consciousness and the unconscious that is the body; at that edge is where concrete change and novelty arise. And it is at that edge that we can feel what is in the way of being inwardly continuous" (p. 206).

Gendlin's use of the therapeutic relationship for "finding each other's individuality" competes with a more skeptical view that interprets the therapeutic relationship as the critical ploy of cultish cohesion. The very insistence on intense relationships requires a recognition of their proportionate distortion of perception, the likelihood that the psychically born again are improbable witnesses of their lingering imperfections. Indeed, Gendlin's dramatic heroics begin to convey the emotive pressures of the therapeutic relationship to unmoor the patient from even a modest objectivity.

I am here to say, "Don't fall for the omission of the person. I know you [the patient] are there struggling, and if I can help you with that, then what I am doing is real." Processes double when two of us [therapist and patient] are in contact. The therapy process is larger than either of us can think or predict. It takes us both along with it. That huge process would scare me off, if I had to manage it. If it required certain qualifications, I know I would not have them. But the process requires only a person, and that is fortunate because I am a person. I don't know how I made this status; I must have snuck into the wrong line somewhere. But I am sure that I am a persona. And that is all that is required. If I sit down in this chair opposite the person, then the large process will happen. (Zeig, 1997, p. 198)

And so it is with psychotherapy generally: the therapeutic "relationship is the soil that enables the techniques to take root" (Lazarus, personal correspondence, December 19, 2003). However, it is an unusually intense relationship in which the therapist is not a neutral caregiver like a dental hygienist or a nurse. If the relationship is sustained through therapy, the patient has revealed his or her vulnerabilities, establishing the therapist in a uniquely powerful position to bribe congenial reports of therapy's success with affirmations of the patient's worth, progress, sensitivity, and so forth. Indeed, many schools of therapy, particularly the behaviorists, argue that the therapist's ability to modify the patient's dysfunctional behavior is precisely dependent on this vulnerability. The patient's vulnerability to the therapist's approbation or disapprobation presumably creates the conditions in which the therapist can directly reinforce alternative, more adaptive behaviors. It is the authority gained by the therapist's unusual access to the patient's vulnerabilities that makes the presentation of suggestions and techniques acceptable to the patient.

Unfortunately, the therapist's powerful authority has led to ethical lapses and probably also to a frequent dependence on therapy that is itself a clinical problem. It has also led to a predatory arrogance of psychotherapists, who assume they have the professional right if not the duty to gain emotional access if not control of their patients. Indeed, the naive belief in the value of a defenseless relationship as the avenue to emotional cure has been the portal for much abuse. Yet even under optimal conditions of genuine therapist concern, the defenseless relationship has not been endorsed by evidence of positive outcomes.

The essential problem of the outcome studies lies in the likelihood that the behavior most frequently influenced by the therapeutic relationship is the patient's reports. Patients unable to change their behavior may dissemble in order to maintain the esteem of their therapists; they may exaggerate their recovery; they may even deceive themselves into believing that they are better. The stronger the relationship, the greater the distortion of reported behavior. Thus the more skilled the practitioner in gaining trust and establishing a strong bond with the patient, the greater the likelihood that the patient will find pleasure in the relationship and, thus, the greater the likelihood that the patient will seek to protect that relationship with reports of positive outcomes. Indeed, the psychotherapeutic enterprise, taken as a complex organization, may be a telling instance of Weber's notion that bureaucracy institutionalizes charisma. However, in the case of psychotherapy it is charisma itself, devoid of any consequential production function in clinical treatment—the institutionalization of an affirming relationship but devoid of cure, prevention, or rehabilitation.

Without objective and independent measures of behavioral change over time, it is nearly impossible to separate biased reports from accurate patient self-assessments. The problem of response falsification is gigantic generally and not simply in psychotherapy. For example, respondents in the National Election Surveys typically over-report their voting behavior by about 50%. Voting is a relatively low-key behavior. Distortions are often greater for more sensitive questions that probe sex, substance abuse, health, and income (Epstein, in press). Issues of therapy are possibly the most sensitive, involving socially obnoxious behaviors, self-esteem, core happiness, and the like. Therefore, it is likely that self-report in the therapeutic relationship is even more unreliable than usual, especially since the respondent (the patient) after therapy is not truly as anonymous. The patient, in comparison with the randomly dialed respondent to a phone interview, has established a deep, relatively long, and presumably endearing relationship with a therapist who is being evaluated at least in part by the patient's assessments.

Yet psychotherapy has largely ignored the problems of self-report, preferring to accept, with little testing of the data's value, findings that complement its clinical value. However, the larger interest lies in the society's acceptance of the porous research and its institutional reliance on psychotherapy. Indeed, the research may be more a ceremony of the society's preference for rational forms rather than for the real thing; social preferences accepted with the assurances of rational choice rather than rational evidence; scientism rather than science; research as a rabbit's foot rather than as a rational test; apotropaic charms rather than elusive searches for unsettling possibilities; rituals of social value rather than the frightening voids of impaired social arrangements; social integration, coherence, and adaptation rather than social change. Instead of a production function in clinical treatment, psychotherapy is a ceremony of social values, a ritual in the process of acculturating the American citizen. Psychotherapy inevitably bends toward the acceptance of those core values, preferably expressed as behavioral change and emotional satisfaction but at least as verbalized conformity—obedience to social authority.

Psychotherapy as Religion

The therapeutic relationship as the vehicle for bias acts through the stakes of the profession to exaggerate clinical effectiveness. However, the simple tie between the needy patient and psychotherapy exists in a far more complex social envelope that determines its characteristics. Rather than a misadventure of an aberrant group of practitioners, the therapeutic relationship is a deeply sanctioned, socially intended vehicle for dramatizing and affirming social values. There is little about mainstream psychotherapy—the interventions that enjoy the approbation of the best of the literature—that is liberationist, novel, avant-garde, or revolutionary. The dominant therapies, those that serve the greatest number of patients and have been accepted by central social institutions such as universities, hospitals, and clinics, are obedient to central social values. The observation may even be tautological. Indeed, the conformity with institutionalized American preferences is so close that psychotherapy constitutes a powerful expression of America's civil religion. The relationship between therapist and patient is the same as the relationship between minister and parishioner, with the same implied pressures for straying members of the flock to return to the virtues of conventional belief. Even more powerfully, in both instances the methods of teaching, learning, and knowing are spiritual, not rational. For all its scientific trappings, psychotherapy is cognitive only in the sense of appealing to thought, but not to rational, objective information. Even its most rational form, cognitive therapy, is mere metaphor in the same way that Christian Science is not really scientific. Both are metaphysical.

Through a gnomic, immediate, and personal experience of the communicant and the patient with the ineffable, the American religion and psychotherapy both transmit the same core values: a heroic individualism; a sense of chosenness; a cultural loyalty similar to patriotism and, occasionally, chauvinism; and a preference for nonrational, spiritual, transcendent, immediate, sublime forms of knowing.[1] Indeed, psychotherapy, together with its ecclesiastical institutional support in the university, its professional societies that act as curias, and its extensive parish organization in clinics, social-welfare pro-grams, and private practices, constitutes America's most important civil reli-gion and civil church.

Heroic Individualism

Heroic individualism differs from common, egalitarian individualism in several ways. Common individualism undergirds institutions of liberal democracy. It implies individual rather than group justice, freedom of expres-sion, personal privacy and protections against an intrusive state, the moral equality of individuals, at least ethical claims on common resources for per-sonal growth and even certain social protections, universal suffrage, and per-haps also equality before the divine in the sense of the Protestant Reforma-tion. The most important consequence is that individualism necessitates personal responsibility, a relationship of stunning complexity and dispute in the face of external forces that appear to determine behavior.

In contrast, the heroic form is not merely a statement of formal equality or rights but a dogma of extreme personal responsibility, the assumption that the hero can vanquish all foes and all challenges through transcendent effort, wisdom, dedication, insight, virtue, and will. Heroic individualism stresses a mythic obligation for grand achievement to fully credential the ideal human being, the evolutionary apogee of American culture as an exemplar of self-creation. It demands Bunyanesque feats of personal triumph over evil, temp-tation, adversity, inheritance, family, poverty, alien culture, and the rest. Rather than resulting from social factors, heroic achievement results from the individual's self-invention in the sense of both Fichte's self-positing ego and Nietzsche's will to power. In this way, heroic individualism and the achieve-ment it inspires come to measure moral worth, not simply success.

The tradition of heroic individualism rejects the Enlightenment impulse to reason. It seeks spiritual and emotional transcendence; it is proof of chosen-ness, divine favor, and both national and personal exceptionalism. It is not reasoned, reasonable, or rational but mystical, an epiphany of the true and the good. It is both deeply Romantic and romantic; it is nostalgic for an imag-ined past, often pastoral and communal, of pioneer heroics on the frontier and in millenarian pursuit of the virtuous. It is grounded in the socializing myths that the tradition has produced and its concordance with embedded private attitudes and choices, not simply public policy.

The heroic form pervades the myths and legends of America: Paul Bun-yan, Johnny Appleseed, the poor immigrant who achieves a fortune through hard work, the pioneer on the frontier, the martyrs of the Alamo, the patri-archs of the American state, the sod breaker, the lone inventor, the autodidact and the self-trained athlete, the plucky cancer survivor, the nation's social and political martyrs, the redeeming heroes of the Revolutionary War and the Civil War, and on and on. However, the heroic form is less distant than it is in fairy tales; in America it is transmitted through most social institutions, and notably psychotherapy, as immediate expectations for all Americans and is customized to the near infinite dramatic possibilities of everyday life. Yet even in its demotic, everyday expression, it maintains a passion for personal responsibility and extraordinary effort.

The generosity or meanness of American social policy balances personal and social responsibility in a material form, notably, the benefit levels for recipients but also most other program characteristics of eligibility and service organization. Heroic individualism is realized in American social-welfare policy as the very meager provisions for people in need. American social policy imposes great burdens on individuals under the mythic assumption of each person's capacity for heroic effort, his or her ability to overcome personal impediments largely by individual efforts. The myth persists in spite of obvious disparities in life's situations (for example, some children raised in indulgent homes and many others in deprived homes) and the obvious interdependence of the culture and the economy.

Heroic individualism, like all ideologies and binding social beliefs, persists despite contradictions in its logic and apparent discontinuities with actual social conditions. It is a form of blind faith, unquestioning belief, personal epiphany, spiritual excess, and social custom. Thus the society chooses to judge recipients of public welfare as morally deficient, not simply unlucky, impaired, unfortunate, or inexplicable. The poor exist in defiance of the nation's virtuous character by indulging their passions, failing to discipline themselves to study or work, and stubbornly continuing to be improvident, inattentive, disrespectful, cunning, promiscuous, and dishonest. They refuse to take responsibility for themselves. Thus against a standard of heroic individualism, a meager provision is a just necessity in order to stimulate the lazy, provide a disincentive for failure, and encourage personal heroics in overcoming poverty. American socioeconomic stratification becomes justified as moral stratification, with lower-status and poorer Americans deferring to more successful Americans not just in buying power but in claims on leadership and power.

A distorted and suborned social science, obedient to these preferences, obscures the fact that the assumptions behind the judgments are ideological, not rational. Social-science research commonly expresses the deeply held values of the American people rather than any credible estimate of actual economic relationships between penury and work, effort and outcome, and so forth. In this way, the pseudoscience of psychotherapy that testifies to its effectiveness serves to endorse psychotherapy but, more importantly, to smooth its social acceptance as ideology by a society that accords science and technology the reverence of inscribed, revealed truths.

Heroic individualism is a persistent, dominating Romanticism of American culture and even perhaps the most distinctive feature of the American ethos. Emerson's passionate individualism and transcendentalism, although not his disdain for the businessman, are deeply embedded American values that continue as central expectations of role models in movies, theater, athletics, poetry, fiction, and, most tellingly, in the personal interactions of Americans with each other, performing their tasks as parents, children, workers, citizens. It is a tribute to the vitality of the heroic myth that Americans have sustained a nearly raw passion for their beliefs for such a long time.

The core of Emersonian personal responsibility was better elaborated, notably for psychotherapy, by Fichte. His "self-positing ego" taken to operatic extremes by Nietzsche's superman, is America's powerful metaphysical assumption behind its approval of social neglect. Fichte argued that people create themselves in essential moral ways and that human consciousness entails obligations for personal responsibility. He largely discounted the influences of society. The self-positing ego is a fixture of Freudian psychoanalysis and of the largest number of psychotherapies. Indeed, psychotherapy must assume a self-motivating and self-determining human consciousness if it is to maintain a core process of verbal reasoning that ignores the patient's material circumstances except as they become psychologized during the therapeutic sessions. The isolation of the dialogue between therapist and patient in the emotional Skinner box of therapy reinforces the imperative for the patient to take responsibility for his or her behavior and thus leads to the therapeutic denouement, akin to Freud's catharsis. At the dramatic climax of therapy, the patient acknowledges his or her personal and social sins—dysfunctional behaviors—and at least commits to change; the therapist then rewards the commitment, providing absolution, by congratulating the patient for psychic progress toward transcendent emotional maturity, a superior consciousness, a more noble and reflective existence, and so forth.

Not coincidentally but with little effect, Freud was frustrated but never discouraged by the obdurate neuroses of his patients. Indeed, he may have even been peeved that they refused to endorse his most rational expectations for their recovery from neurosis by simply changing their behavior. Yet the exasperation with patients never obtruded the least slip of doubt into the Freudian psyche, the thought that perhaps his approach to their problems needed a bit of adjustment. Contemporary psychotherapy is equally oblivious, ignoring the absence of credible evidence of systematic patient change. Still, psychotherapy persists along with a continuing enchantment with Freud and the treatments he inspired.

Yet successful behavior change may be beside the point. Proselytizing the civil religion, a social role rather than a clinical one, is the point. Psychotherapy provides the tyranny of an impossible standard visited on a psychologically frail population deprived of the demulcent supports of family, secure employment, or accepting communities. The patient as sinner is purified for communion and fellowship with the American congregation through the sacraments of the therapy, rites that are administered through the communion of a defenseless believer and a manipulative guide. The attractiveness of psychotherapy lies in the patient's acceptance of the necessity and virtues of heroic individualism in a public way, that is, by going for therapy. Thus psychotherapy is a cautionary folktale, a morality play with a missionary role in conversion that affirms the culture's preferred identify and self-image. Behavior change when it occurs is a nice bonus, but it is not necessary to sustain the performance of the field's crucial social role. Psychotherapy's prime audience is the larger society, and, only as a matter of convenience and theme, the patient.

The same preference for heroic individual responsibility defines America's reformed religions, where the sinner accepts Christ into his or her life and demonstrates the acceptance by personal change, that is, virtuous behavior. But again, the baptism or rebirth—a public avowal of faith—is more important organizationally than in the actual remission of sin.

Heroic individualism is deeply sanctioned by mass consent. It is accepted by rich and poor, blacks and whites, the religious and atheists. It is implicit in social policy and explains its categorical stringencies and many inadequacies. American political ideology has always been to the right of center, with the free market maintained at the core of electoral debates (Lowi, 1995). The American liberal argues for a bit more industrial regulation and a tittle more for workers and the poor; the American conservative—in actuality the European liberal rather than the tory—prefers a bit less regulation and lower taxes on business and the successful. Even the most contentious terrain in the culture wars, abortion, enjoys a surprising amount of agreement, with the real divide between the pro-choice position and the center rather than between the pro-choice and the anti-abortion positions (Dimaggio, Evans, and Bryson, 1996).

Thus heroic individualism appears bound up with America's deep preference for a free market and its indifference to need. While a sizable portion of Americans state that they favor a more communal notion of responsibility, that voiced preference has not led to legislation or supportive actions in the private sector. Union membership is way down; few candidates in even the poorest districts run on platforms of substantial increases in governmental outlays; for decades there have been no sizable demonstrations of popular unrest over national fiscal policy or expenditures; women, racial minorities, the elderly, and environmentalists, perhaps the largest and best organized social movements of the past several decades, have refused to press egalitarian agendas. The "maternalist" state of supervisory programs is institutionalized in preference to the egalitarian or redistributive state, with its heavy taxing and large financial redistributions (Gordon, 1992).

There is a price for propogating a myth that excoriates and excommunicates the nonhero and vilifies the nonheroic. It is probably not the violence in the media that propagates youth violence but the society's commitment to heroic achievement and transcendence that provokes kids to kill, especially those isolated from this romantic ideal who are humiliated by parents, peers, and caregivers—high-school jocks who torment their more uncoordinated and bookish peers, successful parents who torment their unsuccessful children. These humiliations are not the superficial media insults of television and movies, which can be readily edited, but rather the deep messages of the culture itself. Youth violence and violence in general are inevitable results of cultural conditions, and heroic individualism may be one of the most pernicious.[2]

The Other Elements of Psychotherapy as Civil Religion

Wide acceptance of heroic individualism as the core metaphor in the American myth and the communion it provides within the American culture provide the ecstacy of chosenness. Both as an individual and as a collective experience, chosenness is an important binding force in ethnicity, nationality, and nationhood that can also engender patriotism, chauvinism, ethnocentricity, and authoritarianism. The individual is motivated; the society is coalesced. The process is gnomic, that is, it proceeds not through coherence and reason, let alone a rational and objective discourse, but through an ineffable spiritualism that far exceeds the naive esprit de corps of teams and squadrons.

Psychotherapy proceeds in a similar fashion. The therapist builds toward the patient's ecstatic insight—acceptance of his or her own heroic individualism—through processes of transference, identification, support, "cognitive" endorsements, behavioral reinforcement, peer pressure, and the like. Not coincidentally, the tool bag of psychotherapy is much like the tool bag of the mystic, the religious missionary, and the cult as well as the salesman, the quack, the trickster, the booster, and the con artist. The tools are the socio-emotional techniques of recruitment. The so-called cognitive forms of therapy are not rational but rather the rationalistic metaphors through which therapists and patients with a preference for the rational style establish an allegiance in order to emotionally communicate a series of social values or perhaps to negotiate the patient's capitulation to at least a verbal acceptance of those values.

While psychotherapy denies its ineffectiveness, the field largely acknowledges that it has still not been able to identify the precise elements of supposedly successful treatment. Indeed, it insists that placebo controls are no longer necessary and that moneys should best be spent on research controls that vary only the internal conditions of therapy in order to discover the variant that contains the essence of cure, prevention, and rehabilitation. However, "non-specific factors" and "yet to be specified" factors apparently account for the bulk of change in the controlled outcome studies. These factors constitute placebo treatments, nonprofessional activities that are unrelated to psycho-therapeutic techniques. The success of placebos would weaken the hold on professional status and social authority if, in fact, psychotherapy's crucial role were clinical instead of religious. The field's attempts to redefine placebo effects as treatment successes—patient motivation transformed into therapist skill by professional edict—speaks to its institutional insecurities and clinical fears.

Patriotism, belief in God, and belief in the efficacy of psychotherapy are muddled through a self-certifying faith that is sustained by a variety of non-rational forms: personal testimony, peer pressures, assurances from social authorities, mystical transcendence, and so forth. These are also the common forms of psychotherapeutic proof and evidence. While the small number of controlled studies pretend scientific rigor, they shrink under scientific analysis to soulful communal affirmations of group chosenness, the ideological statements of believers. Even the best of the research is little more than a fable, stylized in the custom of science but without its essential methodological rigor.

However, the overwhelming portion of the field continues the unscientific mood and even a self-absorbed scholarship in the manner of Freud and the first circle of his devotees, Adler, Jung, and Rank. Their works and those of contemporary theorists of psychotherapy are metaphysical, with endless numbers of case examples pressed forward in testimony of wondrous cures and the healing insights of the therapist. They are little vanities, and because there is hardly ever any independent corroboration of their facts, they are the sweaty exaggerations of believers that go uncontested in a credulous society content with itself.

The central psychotherapies write separate fables on the theme of psychotherapy as social religion. Each embodies a distinct metaphor and even separate rituals, but each shares the catechism of the religion. In this way, cognitive-behavioral therapy is defined by the metaphor of thinking, that is, cognition; behavioral therapy, predicated on preconscious or subconscious action, is defined by the metaphor of man as animal and instinct; psychodynamic therapy is defined by the metaphor of emotion. Each is a different stylistic adaptation to a different social subculture in the broad process of socialization, and each is often prescribed more for its symbolic value than for any relevance to clinical problems. It is not coincidental that the supposedly more intelligent, reasoning, and successful social classes engage in psychodynamic therapy and cognitive-behavioral therapy, while welfare clients, foster children, and other lower-status groups, especially in congregate settings, are prescribed behavioral therapies that emphasize "consequences" for nonadaptive behavior.

The Functions of Psychotherapy

Psychotherapy's social roles rather than its clinical prowess sustain practice. Psychotherapy proselytizes, although in a secular idiom, the core elements of standard American religions: the central value of heroic individualism, gnomic processes of personal knowing and of institutional development, and cultural affirmation, that is, the chosenness of both the patient and American society. The civil religion is part of the broader socialization that attends to deviants and deviance, guards boundaries of acceptable behavior, invents symbols of civic virtue and civic sin, and justifies economic and social stratification. Psychotherapy as civil religion contributes to the organizational integrity of American society, its coherence and social efficiency. Thus deprived of proven clinical effectiveness, that is, a production function in cure, prevention, or rehabilitation, psychotherapy's role becomes entirely ceremonial. Without any deep rationality either in choosing goals or pursuing them, psychotherapy performs the social and political rituals that affirm the national ethos.

The near uniform refusal of the field to discipline itself with scientific proofs and the absence of even the basic communal values of science suggest that psychotherapy, like America's passion for heroic individualism, is a Romantic form, an instance of the anti-Enlightenment and anti-intellectual in American life. Despite much research that appears superficially to conform with scientific dicta, the case study—evidence from the couch, personal testimonies of therapists and patients—persists as the frequent logic of psychotherapy's proofs of effectiveness. The case vignette is much like a folktale, a little morality play, a sermon, and a literary fable, standing for proof of effective treatment in startlingly similar ways to the public testimony of God's immediacy in many reformed churches. It is indeed personal testimony, presumably the patient's but the recording therapist's, and it fulfills the full drama of sin, struggle, and redemption (of course, through the guidance of the therapist). The cases appear innocent enough as the theorist presents them at conferences, in papers, and in books to illustrate some point of disorder or treatment. However, the camp style of the meetings and the true belief of the audience converts simple description to tenets of faith through the seduction of dramatic identification.

There is little that is ingenuous in a skilled orator presenting stories that an audience takes as sagas of salvation from personal turmoil. But there is nothing rational in the cases: no independent scrutiny of their facts, no counting of incidence, no control for natural cure or unassisted, spontaneous salvation, and no credible identification of determining factors. Indeed, the critical obligation of therapy is first to establish a relationship that is so strong and so impervious to "rationalization"—the dismissal of prudent doubt as psychological defense—that the therapist's truths and conveniences become the patient's beliefs. Rather than cure, the therapeutic relationship serves to distort reports of true outcomes by inducing a near religious blindness, a heroic miasma, in the patient.

> The Sages of Antiquity kindly invented a way of telling people the truth without being rude to their faces: they held before them a singular mirror in which all kinds of animals and strange things came into view, and produced a spectacle as entertaining as it was edifying. They called it "A Fable," and whatever foolish or intelligent thing the animals performed there, the human beings had but to apply it to themselves and thereby think: the fable alludes to you. (Andersen, 1987, p. 33)

Psychotherapy appropriates science as a metaphor, a rhetorical device, and a prop in a play in order to induce belief and faith. Psychotherapeutic science is only a heroic fable: a deep problem of psychic suffering, a deep communal commitment to find a solution, deep thoughts of the wise, experimentation, decisive proofs, success, and the propagation of liberating treatment. The psychotherapeutic researchers and clinicians are the scientist-heroes (or researcher-clinicians) in this fable of learning and virtue, of hard work, dedication, introspection, and insight. The fable enables the application of their disciplined cognition to experience, a eureka moment, and a cure. The resulting success and fame for psychotherapy's scientists and clinicians underscore their virtue and the justice of the American system of rewards, its social and economic stratification.

A commercial enterprise—for example, a skill, a factory, an industry—that loses its production function (its material reason for being, its market share, its ability to prosper by what it creates) will shut down or be reduced to a tourist attraction, a sport, a handicraft, a museum display, or a footnote in the history of human productivity. Such were the fates of hand typesetting replaced by linotype; the horse, horsemanship, horse lore, and the horse business supplanted by the car; hand weaving yielding to the automated loom; hunting and gathering by agriculture; the sail by steam power; and the near endless parade of other technological innovations by their replacements. But psychotherapy and psychoanalysis never had a production function, and Eisner (2000) and Dufresne (2000), as two examples, are probably incorrect in predicting their demise simply because they cannot achieve their formal goals of behavior change, insight, and personal psychic growth.

All psychotherapies, from those on the fringes of credulity to those in the center of customary practice, are ceremonies of social belief. Unless psychotherapists bait society with confessions of their ineffectiveness and then go on to demonstrate it credibly, there is no reason to conclude that the happy concordance of psychotherapy and social convenience is in danger. Rather, as society changes so will the tenets of personal reformation. This has been the story of the passing of the ceremonial batons from psychoanalysis, in order, to ego psychology, to behavioral forms, and currently to cognitive-behavioral therapy. Each transfer came along with its own rituals of insight, proof, adherence, popularization, institutionalization, and then competition among new subjectivities vying for mastery as rituals of socialization.

Eisner (2000) goes through the clinical evidence in each of the contemporary therapies, demonstrating their distance from credible science. He concludes in the spirit of obsolescence: "The most fundamental symptom pointing the way to the death of psychotherapy is the total lack of adequate scientific evidence that it is effective. Despite the amount of clinical research that has been conducted, because of the severe methodological flaws, including generalizability, irrelevance of expertise and lack of fidelity to methods, few psychotherapy modalities will likely survive more than a decade or two" (p. 205).

Dufresne is more profound. He deconstructs the deconstructionists along with the original constructionists of psychoanalysis, concluding that they lied, distorted the historical record, insulated themselves from reality and criticism, were blind to reason, were narcissistic, and trampled on the logic of human rationality and good philosophical discourse. Moreover, "given the devastating critiques of Freud and psychoanalysis now available . . . , Freud's continuing popularity must be seen as a function of ignorance, naivete, religiosity, and the politics of the psychoanalytic movement . . . ; which is to say that it is a function of the transmissibility of holy doctrine from generation to generation, and from analyst to patient" (Dufresne, *Tales,* 2000, p. 186).

Yet Dufresne neglects another, more functional explanation for the "transmissibility" of the field: its ceremonial role, played out with little regard for rationality and bounded by only one concern—it dare not confess its fecklessness and destroy the dramatic illusion of the character it portrays. So then, Dufresne's announcement of annihilation is only a welcome curse, a bit of hope: "Psychoanalysis is dead, and burial and obituary get the last word at the end of the psychoanalytic century" (p. 186). Yet the annihilated psychoanalysis is spitefully robust. Psychotherapy and even psychoanalysis are not zombies but flourish as vital social expressions of widespread preference, impertinent evidence of the intellectual's ability to take permission from the culture to reason away the inconvenience of reality. The demise of psychotherapy is as wildly inaccurate as Marx's withering away of the state under communism, a confusion of hope with history.

It seems quite likely that social preferences are selectively combined into cultural institutions without conscious choice as the familiar becomes exalted into the sacred, necessary, and true. The connivance of social incentives with professional convenience has overwhelmed the small amount of skepticism in psychotherapeutic research. The culture conducts a market competition for symbols of its central values, and psychotherapy is delighted to offer evidence of social efficiency that superficial interventions incorporating those values are effective against a range of individual problems. Despite the monotony of its grand epiphanies—invariably, revolutions in human consciousness—psychotherapy has rarely supplanted the heroic form with more modest treatment philosophies. The small critical tradition in the field—Eysenck, Wootton, Rachman, Gross, Masson, Dawes, Zilbergeld, and some others— is unpopular and ignored. Imagine the incongruity of nonheroic psychotherapy, during which a patient is told week after week that his or her ambitions are probably unattainable because he or she is an imperfect human being: try to enjoy what you are, not what you want to be. Perhaps any patient this well defended should not have sought therapy in the first place.

Much of the American culture remains actively antiheroic and simply respectful of individualism. Yet its influence does not dominate in either public policy; the popular culture; the high culture of reflection, creativity, and education; or, decisively, the private, personal, quotidian choices that create social institutions. America is heroic and superstitious, yet its wonder may lie in the restraint of its own primitive Romanticism. Nevertheless, those restraints dominate neither the society's strategic choices nor its prevailing expressions in mainstream psychotherapy. Thus it would be a cheap shot to evaluate psychotherapy against the antics on its margins—past-life therapy, est, alien space-abduction therapy, among many others—even if the professional margins absorb more patients than the center. The fact of mainstream psychotherapy's adherence to the tenets of the American religion and notably heroic individualism says much about the actual role of the field. As with stage illusions, the magic of psychotherapy is not unearthly at all but concrete human manipulation, a social entertainment with institutional importance.

Attempts to define social role are speculative. They can never be rational, and their reasonableness rests on the sensibilities of the reader as well as the probity of essentially weak evidence. The analyses in the next three chapters, respectively, of psychodynamic therapy, behavior therapy, and cognitive-behavioral therapy, gain their authority from three sources: first, the absence of credible evidence of a true clinical production function; second, their internal conformity with important social values; and third, their coherence as folktales, fables of social virtue, rather than as objective scientific theory. These are the core treatments of psychotherapy, characteristically prattling on about self-positing consciousness and becoming clinically inchoate, that is, socially meaningful but deprived of any ability to address the personal dysfunctions that define the field. "In our world, storytelling (like so many other arts that were once practiced by everyone) has become a specialty" (Appiah, 2003, p. 51). Irony is destiny but unfortunately rarely in consideration of justice, decency, or consciousness itself.

7: Psychodynamic Psychotherapy

Freudian psychoanalysis has had a pervasive influence on the humanities and psychology but less as a clinical practice with testable effects than as a profound statement of heroic individualism.[1] Psychodynamic psychotherapy (PP) persists as ideology in spite of its plangent claims to scientific authority. Yet psychoanalysis in particular but also PP are quintessential antisciences, relying on gnomic belief and the metaphysics of self-invention rather than on a scholarship of consecutive empiricism to sustain their critical tenets, the psychodynamic assumptions.

PP's failure as clinical science emerges from a single observation: there are no scientifically credible tests of its effectiveness.[2] The very best of the contemporary clinical research is porous, naive, and biased. However, the field's insistence that these obviously compromised proofs substantiate its claims to scientific practice call attention back to the society that sustains its practice. Indeed, PP has squirmed in its weakness, frequently denying that behavioral cure—therapy—is the goal. Instead, the field retreats to insight and notions of maturity—"nonneurotic autonomous adulthood"—to justify frequently interminable treatments and uncertain outcomes (Wallerstein, 1995, p. 293).

Psychoanalysis as a journey of self-discovery rather than a corrective for inappropriate and unwanted behaviors is reserved for the wealthy to pick through autobiographical minutiae four or five days per week over as much as a decade and longer in order to find in themselves at last the gold of insight, creativity, and emotional grandeur that has eluded discovery for much of their adult lives. Psychoanalysis and PP are the platinum and gold status symbols and the fables of heroic individualism. Indeed, analysis and extended PP are so expensive, customarily exceeding the tolerances of even generous private insurance, that by practice if not by intent, the evidence from the couch on which PP theory is constructed has come from a highly screened group of patients. Quite importantly, the "analyzable" patient is not only self-absorbed but also credulous and "psychologically minded," that is, amenable to accepting the myths of psychodynamics.

Psychoanalysis and even PP are intended for "a special groups of patients," largely neurotics who are "intelligent, articulate, motivated for analysis, highly cooperative, rational and reasonable" (Wallerstein, 1995). Recalling Gross's (1978) YAVIS types, PP screens for patients who may not need PP at all. In fact, some definitions of analyzability seem to restrict it to those who are not emotionally impaired at all, making it a pure religious experience for the well-adjusted. "Is it our belief that only those patients are analyzable who have the capacity for transference-free relationships. . . . Patients who lack this capacity . . . require preparatory psychotherapy. This means they need to be helped to build an object relationship based on reliable and predictable perceptions, judgements and responses. They require more than interpretation and insights" (Wallerstein, 1995, pp. 276–277).

PP exposes psychotherapy as a religious movement that seeks out converts—the analyzable—who are primed for its message and dogma. Needy, anxious, and unsure people are drawn to a practice of soul cure that advertises itself as scientific and medical, that promises to discover the hidden exceptionalism of the patient, that provides a heightened consciousness of superior existence through processes that unlock consciousness and pierce the veil of reality, and that remains available only to the select few—the intellectual elite, emotionally sensitive, and sufficiently brave to endure the rigors of self-exploration.

PP has done what every successful movement does: it satisfies psychic needs with fantastic ritual and untested, actually untestable theories, pressing the convert to internalize hope and metaphor as literal truth. Conversion and commitment to a religious movement are intensified when the reality of needs is reflected in interpersonal failures, communal blame, and emotional unease. Doctrinaire assurances of exceptionalism—the believer's sense of divine favoritism, personal superiority through religious faith, and ultimately some form of salvation or redemption—become emotionally credible when the religious experience assuages anxiety, fear, loneliness, and impulses toward violence with fellowship and communion, compounding irrational faith with irrational social pressure. Magic and fable for the psychically vulnerable are epoxy bonds to religious faith. For many patients, the extraordinary length of their analysis and therapy is probably better explained by their need for belief than by the value of their insights. Freud may have invented some of the most powerful social fables to accompany the transformation of the industrializing West into its present form. He certainly perfected the myths that accelerated the transformation of the cult of psychoanalysis into the present institution of psychotherapy.

The Psychodynamics of Pyschodynamic Psychotherapy

All forms of PP largely accept the same family of underlying assumptions about human development, the source of emotional and behavioral problems, and the logic and role of treatment. Heretical assumptions about any of the basic dynamic assumptions of Freudian theory have customarily expressed themselves as distinct therapies, notably cognitive therapies that displace the central role of emotionality in PP with thoughtfulness and behavioral therapies that emphasize the external contingencies of learning. Nevertheless, as the next two chapters argue, the two other dominant schools of psychotherapy frequently return to Freudian assumptions, notably concerning the therapeutic relationship and the role of early learning, but recast them in their own vocabulary.

Freud's psychoanalysis is intended to resolve the problems that impede psychosocial development. It is largely restricted to common adult neuroses—frequently anxiety, compulsive behavior, and depression—that are presumably the consequence of traumatic failures in handling the challenges of early childhood. Those challenges result from the inadequate socialization of infantile sexuality (a novel Freudian invention), which actuates different erogenous zones—anus, mouth, and genitals—at different times. Neurotic problems emerge from unresolved Oedipal conflicts, occurring between three and one-half and six years of age, during which instinctual drives, perhaps for security or dominance, impel the male child to wish the death of his father so that he can marry his mother. The female child goes through mirror-image conflicts, desiring the death of her mother so that she can marry her father. More serious adult problems such as narcissism, borderline personality disorders, and psychoses result from poorly resolved conflicts of pre-Oedipal stages. As Malcolm's (1982) analyst insists: "If you take a person's adult life—his love, his work, his hobbies, his ambitions—they all point back to the Oedipus complex. That's a fantastic thing to say. And we have found this out" (p. 159).

Both boys and girls are customarily frustrated in their narcissistic desires. The traumas of frustration—unresolved or poorly resolved conflicts—emerge in adulthood as emotional and mental problems. The adult personality is formed as the ego attempts to reconcile instinctual drives (the id) with social expectations for appropriate behavior (the superego) and with the importunities of reality itself. The superego represses the antisocial impulses of the id into the unconscious, a hidden repository for early traumas. The ability of the ego to function appropriately in the creation of an autonomous adult personality is impaired by the intrusions of insistent unconscious impulses to resolve earlier traumas through current relationships and behavior. These neurotic and psychotic reenactments—essentially symbolic behavior—cannot succeed, since current relationships are obviously not the causes of childhood traumas.

Expectations for psychic healing are built on reliving developmental experiences and gaining insight into their meaning through the analyst's guidance. Psychoanalysis attempts to make the unconscious conscious by regressing the patient through the techniques of free association, dream interpretation, and analyst guidance. Adult problems are resolved by insight into the patient's futile attempts to resolve early traumas through symbolic behaviors. Insight is gained through the therapeutic relationship and presumably leads to behavioral change, even character change, but at a minimum softens "misery into common unhappiness" (Malcolm, 1982, no page).

Some considerable dispute occurs regarding whether the vehicle of change resides with insight alone, the relationship with the therapist, or both. However, the argument is pursued through hermeneutics: analysts interpreting the hallowed principles of their field, made sacred in the prophetic texts of Freud and others, through their own clinical cases. It is stunning that analysts and even therapists persistently discuss, with hardly any empirical grounding, the metaphysics of transference, countertransference, Oedipal conflicts, and the rest (as one example, see Chessick, 1996). The field's hermeneutic preferences and its indifference to empirical testing have facilitated the accumulation of uncertain techniques and theories of practice—a clinical practice with pretenses to science but without any of its substance.

Psychoanalysis was compromised both in duration and in depth to provide two basic types of psychodynamic therapies. Supportive psychodynamic therapies were aimed at the suppression of clinical symptoms and involve "such devices as inspiration, reassurance, suggestion, persuasion, counseling, reeducation, and the like and avoid[s] investigative and exploratory measures" (Wallerstein, 1995, quoting Knight, p. 37). On the other hand, expressive psychodynamic therapies "utilize such devices as exploratory probing through questioning, free-association, abreaction, confession, relating of dreams, catharsis, interpretation, and the like. All with the purpose of uncovering and ventilating preconscious and unconscious pathogenic psychological material" (Wallerstein, 1995, quoting Knight, p. 38). However, unlike psychoanalysis, PP only has the goal of providing specific symptom remission through insight rather than a thorough character reconstruction through "exhaustive" probing and the recovery of infantile memories. These nonpsychoanalytic therapies may last up to a few years. Briefer forms of PP can be either expressive or supportive and are designed to achieve specific symptom remission within weeks or months.

All forms of expressive and supportive psychodynamic therapies accept basic psychoanalytic dynamics, although updated to accommodate new preferences. However, in light of the field's committed hermeneutic style, Levenson's (1995) summary of those adaptations marks changing cultural preference rather than new scientific findings, which in fact do not exist. PP refreshed its symbolism to maintain its social significance. In this way, the abbreviation of the expected length of PP from the many years of analysis to the few months of brief PP did not follow on the heels of credible evidence of clinical effectiveness but rather signaled a compromise between two values that are largely unrelated to effectiveness: limited insurance coverage and persistent demands for psychotherapeutic care. The demands seem to be unconstrained by the actual effectiveness of psychotherapy but related more to psychotherapy as symbolic attention, even status. The majority of changes in the style of PP still accept the basic structure of the Freudian session—patient drives, therapist role, transference, countertransference, interventive techniques, and assumptions about the patient—but now include a more democratic view of the therapist's role and a more relativistic assumption about truth. Thus the therapist's emotionality is acknowledged on the assumption that "neutrality" and abstinence are impossible. As another example, insight and the "expansion of consciousness" are now seen in postmodern terms as "shared analytic reality" and "social construction" (Levenson, 1995, pp. 32–33).

PP is an emotional rather than a rational process. Its insights are supremely subjective, that is, the understandings and explanations of analysis and therapy are intuitive: they make sense to the patient. The entire intellectual structure of PP theory is essentially offered to the patient not as a clinical or rational proof but rather through the emotional test of whether its insights are satisfying, that is, whether the patient is comfortable in belief.

The patient is typically resistant to understanding, since confrontation with earlier traumas is deeply threatening and unpleasant. Indeed, the traumas have been repressed precisely because of the patient's reluctance to confront them. Analysis and therapy are processes by which the patient gains the strength to finally resolve these fears.

Classical psychoanalysis assumes a universal goal—adult autonomy—pursued through unique individuals. In its purest and longest form, the "abstinent" analyst provides the security for the patient's self-exploration, offering only the rarest guidance through suggested interpretations of the patient's free associations and dreams. The patient is encouraged to "transfer" his emotions and behaviors onto the therapist, who is guided by the patient's actions while remaining alert to the potential intrusions of his or her own emotional reactions—countertransferences—to the patient. Many analysts themselves go through analysis in order to gain better insight and therefore control of their countertransferences. Whether real or neurotic, one of the many endless ruminations within the field, the transference is the major portal through which the analysis occurs.

The therapeutic relationship, either one of abstinent subtlety or more directive interpretation and guidance, is the vehicle of psychotherapeutic treatment. The patient gains insight through the relationship, testing perceptions as well as new behaviors and attitudes. For PP, the therapeutic relationship has changed in a variety of ways over the decades. Initially, the transference was assumed to contain only the irrational contents of neurotic behaviors, but later analysts concluded that it could also encompass the objective elements of the nonneurotic therapeutic relationship. The basic assumptions still remained the same: the patient's relationship to the therapist accurately mirrored characteristic relationships with others; the source of the neurotic behavior resided in earlier failed development challenges, notably in Oedipal conflicts; and most important, some form of personal change, either modest insights or heroic transformations of character, would be engendered by PP.

The emotionality of PP, the charged catharsis associated with insight, inculcates an extreme individualism—adult autonomy, self-determination, self-actualization, self-invention—that is achieved through an obligation to explore personal motive. By offering up unconscious compulsion to conscious control, PP underscores individual responsibility for personal behavior. "Psychoanalysis [and PP generally] is in practice an attempt to extend the area of rational control and therefore of responsibility. The contribution it makes at the theoretical level is that of assisting in showing that the indefinite extension of causal discoveries in the realm of human behavior in no way of itself necessarily narrows the limits within which we assign human responsibility" (MacIntyre, 1967, p. 252).

Yet in this context "rational control" implies consciousness and awareness rather than scientific truth or even objective fact. Indeed, the expansion of human responsibility, at least as treatment but also in fathoming human problems, explains the attractiveness of PP and of psychotherapy generally (despite their cost and probable futility) as a symbolic armament in America's struggle against public liability for private failure. The heroic individual is infinitely responsible for his or her behaviors. The impulses, conditionings, and imprintings of hidden dynamics are no excuse. The individual's choice between awareness and oblivion itself tends to absolve society of responsibility for its wayward citizens.

The journey back to early developmental stages, notably to the Oedipal conflicts, are the mythic journey of self-creation and self-reinvention that the courageous embark on to become the modern hero—the autonomous adult. Like the imperative for Christians to be reborn by the confession of their sins and acceptance of Christ, analysis pursues character change through the confrontation of individuals with their psychological creation, a process that commands them to accept responsibility for their actions.

Freud Reconsidered

It is a measure of the phenomenal influence of psychoanalysis that a thorough debunking of its claims took longer than fifty years in a scholarly community that considers itself to be both scientific and astute. The criticism of psychoanalysis has been profound but not necessarily influential. The recent inspirations of PP—expressive and supportive therapy as well as their shortened forms—have accumulated an impressive experimental record of failure (covered in earlier chapters). Nonetheless, a large proportion of psychotherapists claim a psychodynamic orientation, while an even larger proportion employ psychodynamic theory in the guise of other therapies.[3]

Grunbaum (1984) criticized psychoanalytic theory against a deep background of support for the evidence from analytic sessions themselves, mediated through the analyst into the literature but without rigorously objective or controlled designs. Following Freud himself, the field held that its hermeneutical style of investigation, involving the impressions and internal logic of the analyst, produced profound insights and credible evidence and largely without professional bias or the natural distortions of patient self-report. Grunbaum cited two prominent analysts who claim that "analysts possess a unique store of wisdom . . . that far more is known now through clinical wisdom than is known through quantitative [that is, controlled] objective studies" (p. 101).

Grunbaum (1984) made his argument in refutation of Popper (1962) but still relied on Popper's demarcation of falsifiability. Grunbaum insisted that Freudian theory was falsifiable and not "immunized" against testing. He demonstrated that Freudian theory did indeed produce a variety of assertions that could either be falsified by clinical observation or, indirectly, by epidemiological comparisons. As one example, if repressed homosexual longings are necessary precursors of paranoid delusions, then the easing of strictures against homosexuality should lead to a reduction in paranoid delusions. Still, if the homosexual longings could not be specified or if the theory allowed for reinterpretations of their apparent absence (or presence), then the theory would maintain the hermetic, self-validating qualities of nonscientific theories. If the theory was hermetic, then the presence of paranoid delusions would *prove* the prior existence of homosexual longings; if homosexual longings were undiscovered, then their unconsciousness testified to their relevance—the fact that they were repressed. Similarly, the belief in prior homosexual longings must be inaccurate, confused, imagined, or a twist of unconscious motives if paranoid delusions were not present (or the longings subsided). These were the qualities of circularity and untestability that Popper claimed barred Freudian theory from being a science.

However, by rejecting Popper's argument, Grunbaum pressed a far more devastating criticism of Freudian theory: that it failed to accept and apply the canons of clinical science by relying for methodology on the weak premises of clinical data and insight. Specifically, Grunbaum refuted what he termed the Tally Argument of psychoanalysis—that successful analysis proved the assumptions of analytic theory. The Tally Argument relied on a variety of methodological assumptions: clinical data were credible and uncontaminated by suggestion; there was a crucial difference between analysis and other treatments that operated by suggestion; retrospective methods were adequate; untreated controls were unnecessary; and the patient's introspective reports were accurate once repressed conflicts were resolved.

In refutation of the Tally Argument, Grunbaum repeated the standard reasons for clinical testing that are broadly accepted in the scientific community. He specifically rejected alternative formless, hermeneutic methods of interpretation that are frequently reduced to the observation that "each researcher is left with his own opinion" and therefore that data have no probative value (Rubovits-Seitz, 1998, p. 174). In doing so, Grunbaum also rejected tenets of psychoanalytic theory, namely free association, repression, defense mechanisms, and the unconscious itself. Grunbaum's debunking of psychoanalysis for its failure as science stopped short of indicting the field's motives, which may be irrelevant if the issue is simply one of its clinical knowledge, its role in treating emotional and mental complaints. Yet the motives of the field and the society that sustains it are central to explain the graduation of a failed clinical form into a social institution.

If in fact any positive conclusion about PP can be drawn from Grunbaum's analysis, it resides in the realm of hopeful conjecture and faith more than in clinical science. Rubovits-Seitz (1998) insists on a Panglossian conclusion in Grunbaum that "the scientific methodologies of psychoanalysis, dynamic psychotherapy, and clinical interpretation can be better; they are improvable" (p. 209). But in fact progress has been illusory, and the recurring retreat of psychoanalysis in particular into hermeneutics and insight abandons the claim to clinical efficacy, at least in a modern scientific sense. More than simply Freudian psychoanalysis, both PP itself and psychotherapy in general have been "incredibly oblivious to the contaminating effects of suggestion . . . the power of pure suggestion to effect impressive even if only temporary remissions," that is, patient expectations and self-reports sustained and distorted by irrelevant feelings about the therapist and the therapeutic situation (Grunbaum, 1984, pp. 129, 131).

Grunbaum's criticisms are themselves falsifiable by adequate methodological testing of the tenets of therapy as well as by credible evidence of the field's effectiveness. Yet neither body of research exists. The early criticism of the field is still the prudent point of skepticism: therapists "induce their docile patients by suggestion to furnish the very clinical responses needed to validate the psychoanalytic theory of personality" and the efficacy of practice itself (Grunbaum, 1984, paraphrasing Wilhelm Fleiss, p. 130).

Grunbaum's critique has been extended and deepened by others who question the internal logic and clinical abilities of psychoanalysis as well as its standing as science and philosophy (Macmillan, 1997; Crews, 1993; Dufresne, 2000, 2003). The same criticisms apply to PP and psychotherapy in general. The apparent methodological progress of the field continues to ignore the basic problems of credibility that beset Freudian theory. In fact these problems of evidence and meaning have become structural characteristics of the psychotherapeutic enterprise rather than the transitory barriers to progress in a subcommunity of scholars dedicated to neutral, objective inquiry. PP's defiance of standard clinical science and accountability protects its social role as civil religion, with its accompanying institutionalized benefits.

Changes in the definition of the transference, the countertransference, the earlier development stages and the source of neurotic behavior, the goals of analysis, and so forth were not occasioned by systematic clinical evidence but rather by a growing consensus of analysts at prestigious psychoanalytic training institutes. In the entirety of his long and impressive review of psychoanalysis, Wallerstein (1995) references systematic data in only one short chapter devoted to outcomes. There is no example of consecutive argument over any aspect of psychoanalysis that is impelled by clinical trials or even systematic evidence. The development of psychoanalytic theory proceeds chapter by chapter, theorist by theorist, concept by concept with little reference to clinical evidence except the very unsystematic impressions of the analysts themselves. The field was built largely on the satisfaction of clinicians with their own outcomes, which is perhaps the most antagonistic situation for the advance of any scientific enterprise.

This is no small point. Psychoanalysis was never scientific, despite the constant invocation by the community of psychoanalysts of the science of psychotherapy. Its forms of knowledge were hermeneutic and continue to be subjective, literary expositions of the basic texts of the field sifted through the semiconscious imaginations of the scholars. The sacred scrolls start with Freud and his early disciples, such as Ferecnzi, Adler, Jones, and Jung, and the second generation of analysts, such as Horney and Sullivan. The contemporary period of analysts—Kohut and onward—build their arguments from metaphysical differences over treatment and the internal consistency of arguments guided by their own experience but rarely if ever by data that tests their theories.

Philosophical interest in psychoanalysis is understandable in light of its moral weight rather than its scientific accomplishments or commitments. Impressions from the couch, shaped into fables of appropriate behavior, compose the core of psychoanalytic scholarship. As a moral statement, PP does not abide any concern with what actually exists but only with the probity of what ought to exist. Objective systematic evidence never disciplined psychoanalysis or dimmed the self-proclaimed brilliance of the analysts themselves and their epiphanies of introspection. Even the current literature of psychoanalysis is willfully ignorant if not actually contemptuous of objective evidence that discredits most of its assumptions, at least to the extent to which they can be specified for testing. The force of Oedipal conflict, resistence, childhood sexuality, unconscious determination, the technical value of free association and dreams, and the rest of the psychodynamic baggage persists as the metaphysics of a community of scholars in denial of science. Freudian dynamics might even lead to the insight that the strength of psychoanalytic denial is in proportion to the need to maintain faith under siege.

The Effectiveness of Psychoanalysis and PP

Wallerstein's (1995) pride in "how far the field has come" (p. 331), reflected in endless compendia of PP practice and "research" organized to display the progress of treatment and the increasing clarity of concepts, does not measure a scientific advance. The changing face of PP—its adapted concepts and the decreasing length of treatment—did not proceed because older concepts became discredited by newer evidence. Rather, newer ideas and procedures displaced older ones because they were more socially acceptable. The field's hermeneutics mediated changing moral styles. Older notions of childhood sexuality and Oedipal lust, as two examples, were unseated by more compatible notions of many developmental stages and age-necessary learning tasks. Compatibility is a political claim, not a scientific truth. Heroic individualism persists as the central metaphor of PP because the social preference for heroic individualism persists. The failure to accept scientific rationality becomes apparent in the defining pitfalls of the field's research and notably in its compromised tests of effectiveness.

In fact, many if not most of the propositions of the field have bypassed rigorous scrutiny in becoming regnant clinical truths and articles of social faith. Wallerstein (1995) quotes Pine on the inseparable necessity of relational factors and interpretation in the therapeutic alliance:

> Certain specific relational factors of the psychoanalytic situation have an essential and general role to play in relation to interpretation. By contradicting the patient's wish, fantasy, or expectation at the moment of interpretation . . . they add a direct experiential impact to the already affectively laden cognitive impact of interpretation. And by producing a reliable context of safety, they permit the patient, at the moment of destabilization or mini-disintegration, to reintegrate in progressive ways. (p. 317)

Apart from the fact that most of PP's concepts enjoy a literary power and suffer a vagueness that frustrates specification for research, tests of the clinical relevance of the dynamics of therapy have not taken place. Pine's professional insights are at best reasonable conjectures, assuming of course agreement with the underlying assumptions of the analytic process, but they are not scientifically tested. The alternatives that Pine posits—relational factors versus interpretation versus both—have not been experimentally manipulated. They probably cannot be given the contentiousness of PP differences and the customary failure of the field to specify its operations, even though it has manualized procedures for a few research projects.

> Whether the therapeutic alliance as described in its maternal, caring aspects of Zetzel, the primary transference of Greenacre, the basic trust of Erikson, the positive transference of Freud, the diatrophic relations of Spitz, the anaclitic relations felt necessary by Gitelson, the holding environment of Winnicott, the real relationship of Greenson and Wexler, or the listening with empathic immersion described by Kohut, and the followers of self psychology, all of these fall under the rubric of the necessary empathy and basic humanity of personal relationships which cannot be excluded from the analytic bond without harsh consequences and self-defeating results. (Wallerstein, 1995, p. 317)

Each of PP's adaptations over the past few decades recasts myth in response to fashions in human relations. However, the assertion that the adaptations constitute necessary interventions to prevent "harsh consequences and self-defeating results" (whatever they may be) has not been credibly tested. They probably cannot be, but this time because it would require an experiment of Nazi cruelty. Nevertheless, the actual clinical importance of the assertion has not been established, with the result that a far more modest statement is required. However, Wallerstein is not quoting a scientific claim but rather an ideology of personal and social behavior based on little more than metaphysical dissatisfaction with previous notions and a subjective, undisciplined, and untested reading of experiences with a highly selective group of patients.

In the common pattern of the field, Wallerstein traces the research in psychoanalysis through three methodological periods in an attempt to substantiate increasingly positive outcomes. It is notable, however, that even in his descriptions, the most powerful research is seriously deficient, sustaining Grunbaum's broad indictment of the field as unscientific rather than Wallerstein's pride in the field's consecutive, objective, systematic progress.

Wallerstein acknowledges that the first studies, conducted until the 1960s, were seriously flawed. They relied on the "necessarily biased" retrospective evaluations of the therapist's own patients, which were made without standard agreement on diagnosis or outcomes. The second period of studies was designed to repair these flaws.

The Columbia Psychoanalytic Center project (Weber, Bachrach, and Solomon, 1985a; Weber, Bachrach, and Solomon, 1985b; Weber, Solomon, and Bachrach, 1985; Bachrach, Weber, and Solomon, 1985) reported on two cohorts of more than 1,500 patients treated during a twenty-five-year period. They compared patients who had gone through psychotherapy with patients who had received psychoanalysis. While they found that most patients benefited, those receiving analysis fared better (although they started out at a higher level of functioning). Further, the benefits exceeded initial estimates of the patient's analyzability, suggesting the unreliability and theoretical ambiguity of clinical judgments. However, the research was seriously impaired: patients were highly screened for each therapy and were decidedly not randomized to the different treatment conditions. Thus the improvements, noted largely by the therapists themselves, were probably biased in the first place. Additionally, the "independent" judges were tied to the treatment institute and were hardly neutral on the issue of the effectiveness of their craft. Blinding could not have been maintained. More important, the absence of a placebo control prevented any estimate of natural remission, the degree to which the improvement would have taken place without analysis or therapy, and even the degree to which patients deprived of analysis or therapy might have improved even more and more quickly than treated patients.

In a similar but much smaller-scale study, Erle (1979) reported that 24 of 40 analytic patients "benefited substantially" (Wallerstein, 1995, p. 493). But again, there was no control, patients were screened for treatment, and ratings of patient conditions initially and at outcome were highly suspect, being made largely by the analysts themselves.

Although included in the second period, Pfeffer (1959) seems more akin to the first period, involving only nine patients, lacking controls, and relying on suspect measurement procedures. However, Pfeffer found that transference neuroses "were rapidly reactivated" long after analysis had terminated, suggesting that analysis had largely failed. These findings were corroborated in other similarly impaired research.

Third-period research, according to Wallerstein (1995), measured outcomes at follow-up, "the postanalytic phase." Third-period studies, although contemporaries of the second-period research, also attempted to account for the outcomes, combining group statistical designs with deep case studies. Unfortunately, even the best of the third-period studies do not repair the imperfections of the previous research but simply add another layer of obfuscation and illegitimate support. Kantrowitz (1986) and Wallerstein (1986) lack appropriate controls, independent measurement, and reliable measures. Analysts and patients make assessments of progress that are not compared against equivalent untreated patients. Ratings are neither blind nor neutral.

Typical of the numerous enterprises to marshal evidence of the effectiveness of contemporary PP and the pertinence of its processes, Bornstein and Masling (1998), on behalf of the American Psychological Association, assemble the state of the art but without improving on the underlying weaknesses of the research itself. The metanalyses of PP similarly fail to get past the pitfalls of the primary research (Anderson and Lambert, 1995). While occasionally employing randomized controls, the other problems of measurement neutrality, attrition, follow-up, and the rest block any positive interpretation of even the best of the primary research (see, for example, Blomberg, Lazar, and Sandell, 2001; Piper, Joyce, McCallum, and Azim, 1998; Piper, McCallum, Joyce, Azim, and Ogrodniczuk, 1999).

Loftus (1994) and Dineen (1996) have compellingly detailed the ease with which vulnerable people internalize suggestions from therapists and other high-status interrogators such as police. With tragic consequences, graphic reports of sexual abuse are contrived by people who were never victimized at all. The implications for impaired recall from the couch are profound. If phantom trauma can be created through the patient's suggestibility, then the more mundane recollections of patients are perhaps even easier to induce.

Yet in the end, PP is not pointless scholarship but merely pointless science, maintaining an enormous fable of self-invention and heroic overcoming through the art of storytelling—the cunning of myth simulating reality. It

constitutes a core religious tradition in the secular church of heroic individualism. PP does not simply operate as if it were a religion; it *is* a religion, complete with a founding prophet, a founding myth of a central God (Oedipus
and his unique magic of conflict) that gives meaning to existence, a continuing procession of faith-based revelations that work out the myths, an intricate series of rituals and ceremonies to bind communicants to the faith, and
inevitably, a professional priesthood to maintain sacred practice, the purity
of the rituals, and the adaptations of dogma to current social imperatives.

"It's All How You Want Your Life to Be"

C. M. Hall (1998) went right to the heart of the matter with little flutter
about science and knowledge:

> Heroic self is the most vital nucleus of human character and agency. It
> consists of peoples's most cherished values, which predictably guide
> and direct their behavior; their deepest convictions and belief; the sub-
> stance of these values, convictions and beliefs, and mechanisms for
> ordering priorities. . . . Heroic self transcends mundane realities and
> moves towards societal contributions which go beyond selfish desires.
> When individuals live according to the core altruistic principle of
> heroic self, they produce creative solutions to life's problems. Heroic
> self transforms banal routines into extraordinary accomplishments by
> committed action. (p. 3)

According to Hall, people can be heroic individuals but customarily are
not. The transformation of the banal into the heroic is the role of PP and the
rest of psychotherapy. However, the reconciliation of existence with aspiration—what is with what ought to be or what might be or what one would
wish to be—elevates psychotherapy into the role of mythmaking. PP's removal
of heroism from the realm of the fantastic would be more believable if the
outcome research of the field credibly testified to its success. Yet the field has
not demonstrated this ability, nor is the far less heated insistence on personal
improvement—the mantra of the field's more modest promises—all that
credible. In fact, people most often fail to fulfill their heroic possibilities even
after intensive self-scrutiny but instead dispel their disappointment through
the illusions of psychotherapy.

Still, C. M. Hall (1998) defines the democratization of the heroic—every
person a transcendent individual—as the mission of psychotherapy. Both
expressive and supportive therapies intend to elevate the mundane to the

noble, an illusion of individual behavior that probably defines therapy itself. Belief in heroic fulfillment in both lengthy and short-term PP takes place through the therapist's insistence on gnomic precesses of belief—the essential emotionality of PP, that is, patient feelings as the criteria of the real—that build on psychological mindedness, the patient's susceptibility to myths of the self. For Jurjevich (1974), "Freudwashing" is conscious; "most psychotherapists overtly recognize their purpose to be a guided change in the subject's attitudes and beliefs . . . that enables the subject to live in greater ease with himself and others" (p. 462). However, the guided change, often a narcosis of denial, is hardly neutral but rather predicated on self-invention, the pretense that personal change takes place outside of social values. In fact, the notions of personal novelty and self-creation are the essence, and indeed the falsity, of heroic individualism that pervades therapy.

P. Crits-Christoph, K. Crits-Christoph, Wolf-Palacio, Fichter, and Rudick (1995) reported a patient's epiphany of personal responsibility ("agency"), "a dramatic change," at the eleventh session of brief supportive-expressive therapy, in which the patient "decided to give up his initial wish (as revealed in earlier sessions) to be taken care of":

PATIENT: I started to interview for a new employee. . . . How am I going to deal with a conflict and all that? But I am not going to let that stand in the way of finding someone. Finding somebody will sort of pull, push me through the pipeline that I have to deal with.

THERAPIST: So you have some anxiety, but it's not an anxiety that stops you from doing what you have to do?

P: Trying not to. Trying to refocus, get focused, do something, stop sitting around. Not focus on being depressed, woe is me, because that's really not going to change anything. I mean, coming here and trying to figure out where it stems from might change it, but sitting at home lying in bed, reading, or whatever, and not going to work doesn't change anything. So.

T: That sounds like somewhat of a change in your feelings. What do you think may have precipitated that change?

P: Um, I don't know. Deciding that I better do something about this. I can't keep telling myself: I'm depressed, I'm getting more depressed, I'm not going to get better. Only I'm going to correct the situation at work. Nobody is going to step in. My employee is not going to come to me tomorrow and say, "You know, I decided this conflict that we've had is really all my fault, and I'm going to work more hours now, and really see your point of view and what happened, and let's go forward."

т: Right. (pp. 66–67)

The patient had responded to an ad for psychotherapy to handle his anxiety. He was a successful professional and husband who felt compelled to take over the family business. The reluctance to give up his own career for his family apparently created his anxiety. The exchange demonstrates that therapy leads to the patient's accepting responsibility for his actions in the family business. Yet there is no demonstration that the patient is better off taking control of the business as opposed to selling it or hiring a manager and pursuing his own career. Indeed, his anxiety—a tussle perhaps between his obligations to his wife and his obligations to his mother and siblings—may be quite appropriate, a natural condition that is not easily amenable to resolution and, from a different perspective, should not be.

The initial problem with the employee led the patient and therapist to consider deeper causes of anxiety, or as the patient states it, realizing "what I was doing." Insight and control are the elements of heroic individualism; in the patient's words, "It's all how you want your life to be." The therapist refuses to encourage the patient to sacrifice himself for his family, which might seem quite reasonable since the pay is probably good and his cherished wife seems content with the arrangement.

> P: I've got to change my way of dealing with people, my way of thinking about things. So, you know, the biggest thing is the realization if I want my life to change, if I want to be more positive, if I want to have a personal life, I've got to do something about it. And not go through being depressed and victimized. Because that's not really going to get me anything. . . . I still get depressed and anxious.
>
> T: So there is a lot of stress even if you were not going to be overwhelmed by the fear of—
>
> P: Dying. You die anyway.
>
> T: You die?
>
> P: You get hit by lightning, and all of sudden you're dead anyway.
>
> T: Mm-hm.
>
> P: You've got to look at things to see a positive outcome of them. It's like building a house, right? If you don't see, if you don't plan in your mind how to build it, you can't physically build it. You die anyway. It's all how you want your life to be. But I can't say that I'm still not dreadfully fearful of someone dying or something like that. But I didn't call my parents immediately to see if they're still breathing.

Because I guess on one level I know, I guess if you realize that, you
can sort of stop doing it if you decide that you don't buy into it
anymore.

T: Mm-hm. It gives you more choices.

P: Right. Or become more responsible for your own outcome of things.

T: It must be a relief to know that it's not really about what other
people are doing to you, that it's something that you can change.

P: And stop buying into that, you know, these outside forces are what's
causing it.

T: Mm-hm. Exactly. (pp. 68–69)

Here is someone who has made a life out of complaining, acting the victim and getting on quite well, it seems, except for some anxiety, perhaps an
existential structure of complex modern relationships. The truly successful
therapy might demonstrate that there are leaders and followers and that the
patient is a follower, who might best ease his psychic pain by accepting the
subordinate role. Indeed, the therapist might invoke the ancient nobility of
family loyalty and sacrifice for blood relatives.

Personal fulfillment rather than communal obligation is the obvious focus
and force of therapy, a process through which personal isolation and self-
obligation are elevated, notably within a social context that promotes these
values. The therapy does not point to the fundamental neurosis of allowing
personal desire to consume life, the *wanting* of greater personal recognition
and control. Surrender to others in the patient's safe environment might be
far more fulfilling. Yet therapy presses the Freudian assumption of unresolved
Oedipal (or developmental) conflicts as the defining elements of anxiety and
neuroses. Anxiety is probably all that more fearful when people assume that
it is an unnatural condition rather than the necessary reality of human development itself. It is useful to stress that this patient was never overwhelmed
by anxiety or morbid thoughts but sought therapy the way many seek
Scotch—a cheaper and perhaps more successful solution.

Yet through therapy, the patient and the therapist work "through the more
primitive wish . . . by making a transition to a more modified adult-level
wish":

P: I think that there's part of me that wants someone else to take care
of me. . . . a warm comfortable feeling. That [feeling] fights changing myself, reahing out, becoming competitive. Breaking out of that
shell or whatever.

T: I think the other side of this is that as a person who's taking over
some of the responsibility for keeping that raft aloft, so to speak, it's

almost as if part of you needs to succeed so that you could create that secure, childlike sort of haven. And when something feels like it's getting screwed up with that, it just messes up the feeling you have that you can create the security for yourself and the others. You know, that's the fear that you would have if you failed someone.

P: Yeah, and that things will get out of control . . . and you die. . . .

T: What made you want to jump back into the womb? What were you feeling? (p. 72)

The therapist assumes that "the roots of the patient's difficulty accepting his sister's death and accepting his grief are not clear, he understands that his reaction of wanting to be taken care of, 'jump back into the womb,' certainly intensified after the death" (Crits-Christoph et al., 1995, p. 73). Yet the PP literature cannot sustain any statement of this sort. There is no clinically credible evidence that ties sibling death to passivity under any circumstances. Rather, the patient comes to believe in the fable of early familial conflict as a plausible explanation of his own troubles through the emotionality and dependencies of the therapeutic relationship. The psychologically minded are prime candidates for PP, because they are susceptible to gnomic explanations; they have a need to believe in magic. However, belief gained through emotional need constitutes conversion, not cure. In fact, there is a constant ambiguity throughout the previous dialogues and throughout therapy in general regarding whether the discussion is metaphorical or real, whether the desire for the womb and death are metaphors for passivity or actual ambitions of the patient. Perhaps the tolerance to negotiating between metaphor and reality—a susceptibility to fantasy—constitutes psychological mindedness.

Barber and Crits-Christoph (1995) refuse to consider that a patient motivated to seek therapy and one who comes in with a considerable record of personal achievement might be better off going through the sadness and stress of personal decision making, free of the interference of a therapist. In this way, the outcome would clearly be the achievement of the patient and would provide concrete encouragement for further autonomy. The literature cannot speak to this point since, in addition to its many other pitfalls, it has failed to institute appropriate controls or adequate follow-up. In fact, the sessions are written like a soap-opera script, with dialogue interspersed with stereotypical descriptions of the patient and therapist and heroic summaries of the patient's progress. Enter troubled, speak deeply and revealingly with therapist, exit smiling. The exchange is moralizing and theological but not evidence of scientific cure, prevention, or rehabilitation.

Barber and Crits-Christoph (1995) extend PP to a variety of severe psychiatric problems, even schizophrenia and drug addiction. In one of the chapters, Luborsky, Woody, and Hole (1995) offer empirical evidence in support of treating heroin addicts with PP, concluding that "opiate addicts were both interested in the professional psychotherapies and benefited from them" (p. 155). In one instance, the authors present a case example of a heroin addict who takes drugs because he feels "deprived and angry" when others do not give him the recognition he deserves. The authors seem to accept the accuracy of this statement and claim to be able to work through it successfully. However, in each case the clinical research is severely impaired and the interpretations are self-serving. Indeed, to accept the addict's reasons for his addiction at face value is bizarre. An inverted motivation seems more reasonable: the addict has found an excuse to justify his addiction, that is, the anger and sense of deprivation are contrived as excuses for taking heroin. Neither a lack of respect and recognition, which may in fact be appropriate, nor feelings of anger and deprivation are probably propelling the addiction. An inability to control physical and psychological demands of euphoria may have much more to do with addiction than an addict's self-pitying and juvenile excuses. Yet the addict is enjoined through therapy to realize an epiphany that leads to a heroic overcoming. Nevertheless, cure rates for any psychotherapeutic intervention for addiction, schizophrenia, and less serious disorders remain negligible at best. Therapy and the droll little melodramas of clinical investigation remain skits in the social drama of moral instruction.

An interminably undetermined if not indeterminate literature transforms the basic assumptions, assertions, and scientific claims of PP into literary forms. A picture is painted, a fable is devised, an ethos is underscored, and good behavior is idealized by the fundamental principles of PP. The audience is less the patient and more the culture itself, ever desirous of encouraging institutional forms that press its central ethos. PP in the United States underscores heroic individualism, inviting conversion and rededication through a process of realigning, reaffirming, or simply reimagining character through the emotional experience of therapy. The cathartic quality of the PP experience and its insights is quite similar to the epiphanies of a camp-meeting revival—a bit less hysterical but still emotional. Being visited by the Holy Ghost or one's own awesome unconscious may be quite the same thing.

Throughout, the therapist is selling a theory of human action to psychologically minded patients softened up for the pitch by the culture itself, that is, through their own experiences in the culture. The same biases and expectations that have corrupted the basic clinical research also intrude themselves into PP through the uniquely trusting relationship with the therapist. Especially in light of transference dependency, the patient is only too willing to accept the subtle directions of the therapist in achieving heroic status through PP's special insights into human development and clinical cure.

The process of achieving belief is emotionally dependent on the imposed discipleship between therapist and patient—the suggestibility of the patient. The therapist is only too happy to have his or her assumptions accredited through the not-so-free associations of patients and their testimonies to achieving autonomy, that is, through their reports of personal change. The convenient testimonies from the couch become the field's evidence in one way or another. That is, either through the frank hermeneutics of psychoanalysts or through the impaired clinical research of expressive and supportive therapies, biased data are offered as credible testimony to effective clinical practice.

Psychoanalysis, PP, and psychotherapy in general are better placed in the tradition of Aesop, the Grimm brothers, and Andersen than in the company of Newton, Darwin, and Einstein. The philosophic lineage of PP descended in modern times as the reaction against the Enlightenment from Fichte and Hegel through Nietzsche and others to the postmodernists, including the subjectivist, introspectionist, self-positing heroism of Freudian theory and its offshoots in PP and psychotherapy. Even while its practitioners sedulously reaffirm its scientific status, its scholarship is testimony to the reverse. In fact, psychoanalysis and PP are scientific in the same sense that theosophy and Christian Science are science, that is, not scientific at all. The practice of psychodynamics is consistently religious in both form and commitments. PP has its roots in Freud's romantic inventions rather than in the spirit of the Enlightenment. The impulse for revelation, conversion, and psychic healing through gnomic processes of belief rather than objective evidence—knowing as insight and introspection that supplant skepticism and rigorous testing—has substituted an ineffable unconscious for the frankly supernatural and spiritual causative agents of modern religions. Psyche for PP and soul for the religious are the same metaphysical devices, distinguishable only by their associations with distinct social institutions but not by their functions.

Psychoanalysis and PP lack any rigor of objectification and testing; they have never redeemed their basic constructs and relationships, their dynamics, from the murk of the fantastic. It took almost one hundred years for Freudian psychoanalysis to reach even a slight acknowledgment of its deficits, but PP still persists in practice in spite of its clinical inconsequentiality; in fact, its own stubborn persistence is a fine example of the basic Freudian defense mechanism of denial. The rest of PP's forms will likely endure until the demand for its social utility changes, that is, until a less heroic individualism and a more cooperative, supportive ethos become popular.

Theosophy and PP

The culture and scholarship of Freudian psychoanalysis and PP in general lead inevitably to an obtrusive question: How can so much be written without acknowledging, let alone insisting on, the tenuousness of treatment? Freud's near contemporary, Madame Blavatsky, may have provided the key to the answer. She gave Freud a run for his money as a theorist and a cult figure even while psychoanalysis beat out Theosophy in the game of market share. Truth is not the issue; belief and fable are. Only one small section of humanity, in devotion to one medium-sized area of human activity—science—has committed itself to the objective, systematic testing of assertions. The rest is content with faith and inner reality. Magic and superstition may even be a necessary balm of social coherence and tranquility.

A sociological marvel, Theosophy is a fanaticism of occultism, astral souls, levitation, magic, and reincarnation, never having grown into mainstream religion or philosophy in spite of its parallels with Fichte and Hegel's metaphysics. Yet its similarities to PP and the early psychoanalytic movement are striking. Its inspirational prophet and revelator, Helena Petrovna ("Madame") Blavatsky (1831–1891) was a Russian émigré who either sincerely believed in her magical, mystical, and prophetic abilities as medium and adept or was one of the nineteenth century's more successful charlatans.

Theosophy, like PP, pressed an ideology of extreme individualism, which may account for its attractiveness to nineteenth-century Americans. "Man's best guide, religious, moral and philosophical, is his own inner, divine sense. Instead of clinging to the skirts of any leader in passive inertia he should lean upon that better self—his own prophet, apostle, priest, king and saviour. No matter what his religion, he will find within his own nature the holiest of temples, the divinest of revelations" (Blavatsky, 1972).

In fact, G. M. Williams's (1946) synopsis of the importance of Blavatsky's career could easily be applied to Freud, his voluminous correspondence, his relationship to the inner circle of the early psychoanalytic movement, and psychodynamic theory itself.

> Madame's Theosophical career offers an intimate picture of the strange, secret process of creating a cult. She left a mass of confidential writings that show with the vividness of a biological moving picture the process of breathing life into the dry dust of a new evangel, the creation of an atmosphere of authenticity, the manufacture of legends, and evidence, the casual enunciation of a new theory, and its evolution into a sacred principle venerated by the faithful. (p. 8)

Like Christian Science's Mary Baker Eddy, her contemporary,[4] Blavatsky promised her followers "spiritual first aid," basing much of her ritual and theology on obscurantist Eastern religious doctrine, notably karma, reincarnation, the power of the mind over physical reality, discipleships, and ancient inaccessible magic. Self-denial and meditation were regimens for her disciples, who were required to give up meat, smoking, sex, and liquor (even while Madame smoked something like two hundred cigarettes per day). The spirit world contained Mahatmas and Masters, a brotherhood that had achieved great wisdom on their way to the maximum allowable number of reincarnations. They returned to impart their wisdom to the worthy, that is, to Theosophists, but only through the intercession of Blavatsky, God's one true medium and greatest adept. Blavatsky was the only path to the hidden cosmos and the lost wisdom of the ancients, who were revered to the point of suggesting that since their time, human civilization if not human evolution had reversed themselves. She demonstrated her unique powers through paranormal miracles: seances to materialize the dead, levitation, magic, and the rest.

Her fame continued to rise even after the Society for Psychical Research in London concluded that Blavatsky was "one of the most accomplished, ingenious and interesting impostors in history" (G. M. Williams, 1946, p. 10). Even then she attracted many prominent people—for example, Alfred Russell Wallace and Thomas A. Edison—and her teachings drew a sophisticated audience. Williams exposes Blavatsky's spiritualism to the same logic that reduces Freud's psychoanalysis to ludicrous science and fanciful contrivance. However, in both cases, "such an estimate misses the point: Madame's greatness, which makes her a vital force to a limited public even today, lay in her power of suggestion. After hurling defiance in the teeth of the polite world, she whirled around and forced it to take her seriously. She compelled susceptible intellectuals to believe in her and try to do what she wished. She had uncanny power over people" (p. 11).

Blavatsky's psychic world is much like Freud's unconscious, and both are expressed through the convoluted symbolism of dreams, their disguised messages from the psychic world, only unraveled with the interpretive assistance of an adept. Blavatsky's infinite panorama of long dead Masters can be understood metaphorically in equivalence to Freud's psychic structure of id, ego, and superego. That the functions of the Freudian psyche may occur in specific areas of the brain does not diminish their mystical causes nor testify to their material source (Solms, 2004; Hobson, 2004). After all, Blavatsky's incarnations and materializations took physical form but from supernormal, "astral" causes. As Blavatsky (1972) observed, "in these fantastic creations of an exuberant subjectivism, there is always an element of the objective and real" (p. 59).

Communication with the psychic world through a medium is much like making the unconscious conscious through a therapist. "The true Adept, the developed man, must, we are always told, become—he cannot be made. The process is therefore one of growth through evolution, and this must necessarily involve a certain amount of pain," that is, self-confrontation and personal analysis (Blavatsky, 1972, p. 92).

PP patients are instructed in the dynamic processes of personality and the psyche much as Blavatsky's "chelas" went through their discipleship at the foot of the grand adept. In both theories: "over-anxiety" needed to be treated through explorations of the psyche; ego was central; insight or "spiritual wisdom is entrance upon a higher plane of existence," resulting in "a new man" (Blavatsky, 1972, p. 94); the "only mission is to rekindle the torch of truth" (ibid., p. 95), which for both Freud and Blavatsky pretended to science; however, truth is very uncomfortable and is consistently resisted; psychic progress needs to overcome resistance through trust and faith in the master and in the processes of psychical progress; esoteric knowledge is taught through a discipleship of great obedience and self-denial. A notable difference from Freud, however, resides in Blavatsky's assumption that the "higher mind" processes "true knowledge" of the spirit, which transcends science; Freud emphasized emotionality and the scientific qualities of the process.

Both appropriated science out of its context. Yet Blavatsky seemed to refer more to content—the substance of science, the material of its discipline, for example, chemistry, biology—than to the process of discovery. Freud, on the other hand, ventured introspection as a substitute for rigorous objective testing. In fact, Freud is the more hermetic and self-absorbed in his assumption that knowing thyself is knowing the world; Blavatsky deferred to external powers, although she was imaginative rather than scientific in her affection for "Esoteric" forces.

The plausibility of psychic progress for both PP and Blavatsky comes from the evidence of practice. "Enough has been given, it is believed, to show that the existence of a Secret Universal Doctrine, besides its practical methods of Magic, is no wild romance or fiction. The fact was known to the whole ancient world, and the knowledge of it has survived in the East, in India especially. And if there be such a Science, there must be naturally, somewhere, professors of it, or Adepts" (Blavatsky, 1972, p. 112).

Freud and Blavatsky both invoked science in the same sense of authoritative information but not objective, systematic experimental facts. Testimonial evidence from the couch and the redemptive powers of conviction certified by anonymous sources are on about the same level; both invoke an authority of belief, and both use contemporary social forms to induce credulity.

An unfalsifiable, unshakable belief was required of chelas, just as "analyzability" appears to be essential for PP patients and psychoanalysts in training. Indeed, suggestibility—the emotionally fertile soil that cultivates expectations—may be the actual medium of belief needed by patients and chelas to materialize their redeeming uniqueness and existential heroism.

The astral soul informs Blavatsky's ego in a way that is quite similar to the combination of the id and the superego: a conflict between primal, selfish urges and the morally acceptable that Blavatsky discussed, many decades before Jung, as emanating from the "collective consciousness" of culture (Blavatsky, 1972, p. 59). In this regard, however, Freud seems a bit short on imagination. Blavatsky improved upon man's mystical "triune" of body, soul, and spirit with variations on the mystical number seven: seven dimensions of man, which are themselves each divisible into seven parts. The psyche as the unconscious represents

> the existence of a personal spiritual entity within the personal physical man. . . . There are external and internal conditions which affect the determination of our will upon our actions. They rejected fatalism, for fatalism implies a blind course of some still blind power. But they believed in destiny, which from birth to death every man is weaving thread by thread around himself, as a spider does his web; and this destiny is guided either by that presence termed by some the guardian angel, or our more intimate astral inner man, who is but too often the evil genius of the man of flesh. . . . When the last strand is woven, and man is seemingly enwrapped in the network of his own doing, then he finds himself completely under the empire of this self-made destiny. It then either fixes him like the inert shell against the immovable rock, or like a feather carries him away in a whirlwind raised by his own actions (that is, karma). (Blavatsky, 1972, pp. 48–49)

Like Freud, Blavatsky conferred immense power not on the material world but rather on psychic forces—for her the Occult, for him early sexual experiences and the unconscious. However, Blavatsky's mind-over-matter specificity, in the manner of Christian Science's "radical reliance" on faith as a cure for physical disease, placed both in peril of falsification. Perhaps Freud's greatest advantage over cults such as Theosophy and Christian Science, then and since, has been the untested and perhaps untestable inscrutability of his theories, their defiance of predictive specificity, and their frequently circular self-certification. Alas, Blavatsky could not communicate with dead souls, let alone dead Mahatmas, and many of Eddy's followers suffering childbirth, tooth pain, and debilitating disease began to doubt, like the maiden thrown off the Maya mountain, that belief was either very satisfying, sufficient for their conditions, or profitable in the long run.

The defining precepts of both Theosophy and PP are barriers to science. They are hypothetical, defying probative empirical tests. The fields remain undisciplined by objective reality but vulnerable to the distorting ideological imperatives of society. It is intriguing that despite its fascination with oriental religions, Theosophy did not preach a Zen-like peace and acceptance but the very self-invention that characterizes PP. Both sought an overcoming of unhappiness with an assertive heroism. In neither form was insight an end in itself, but rather it was a vehicle for worldly ambition—the psychic in service to the material. It is difficult to fathom the objective reasons why Blavatsky is assigned to the historical sideshow as a crackpot and fraud, while Freud is hailed as perhaps the twentieth century's most influential thinker. Apparently, style counts.

So What's So Bad?

PP may simply be a form of occult science, that is, not a science at all but a mystical, vaporous belief in magic that seeks to quell the terror of inevitable extinction. Its similarity to Theosophy is not disturbed by credible evidence of clinical success. Put another way, Theosophy, PP, and psychotherapy in general, if they provide any benefit at all, do so as psychic comforters in the manner of religious hope rather than as clinically engineered, reliable remedies for a variety of personal and social complaints.

Freud and Blavatsky dug deeply into the occult to produce contemporary myths of human existence. Freud's Oedipal myth stood the test of time; Blavatsky's occultism was alien to modern sensibilities. Both were gurus; one in a lab coat, the other in robes of the East. Both were charismatic, skillful adepts with little patience for intellectual challenges, let alone heresy. But the symmetry of psychodynamics and Theosophical metaphysics affronts any conventional principle of modern science. Neither Freud nor Blavatsky inspired a credible scholarship of objective learning; rather, they relied on introspection and hermeneutics to develop their truths. Insight in both was self-evident, a function of right thinking and the faith of discipleship (a giving over of trust on the basis of emotional need rather than credible evidence). Both attracted true believers, cultivated practitioners, therapists and adepts, and built communities of the faithful, although the more successful

scientific pretensions of PP may explain why it flourished. A different generation, gone for a hundred years, sought transcendence from the yellowed
texts and mysticism of long-gone prophets. Science as symbol—scientism—
has replaced the occult as the modern source of belief, magic, and wonder.
The society prays to a personal god of vulgarized science through the many
churches of psychotherapy.

This religion, that religion, what's so bad? PP provides false hope, divert-
ing many from dealing with the reality of their situations. In fact, PP may be
a form of retreat. As a corollary, clinical intervention may be undesirable for
most human moods; the blues pass and are probably a necessary human
experience. In fact, many situations should provoke displeasure, and some
people should indeed be unhappy in consideration of their mischief. Moreover, many people might do better by not seeking professional advice for
their psychic problems. The therapeutic relationship is not therapeutic but a
folie à deux that propagates heroic individualism through customized myths:
a creation myth, an existential myth, and a myth of personal change through
self-invention. All are centered on heroic overcoming and extreme personal
responsibility. Troubled people might more profitably learn to accept their
own imperfections, changing, if at all, through the painful abrasions of social
intercourse.

Finally, and most problematic, PP and psychotherapy in general foster a
response to personal problems—seeking advice and affirmation from authority—that is the antithesis of the autonomy and self-direction that the theology of psychotherapy preaches. PP is not simply a myth in its grand sense of
ontological reconciliation, an instructive compromise between aspiration
and reality, but a crummy series of vain lies, that is, myth as contrivance and
illusion. A more useful heroism might be built around a tolerance for reality
rather than an insistence on psychological rebirth.

8: Behavioral Therapy: The Owl and the Mule

The precise, scientific terminology of classical and operant conditioning theory is not equivalent to its use in contemporary folklore as learning by association and learning by carrots and sticks. While the common usage provides some insight into the careful experimentation of behavioral conditioning in the laboratory, it defies the controlled comparisons of science. Instead, the tenets of science have been appropriated by intuition and tradition to endorse personal experience and sustain cultural values. Behavioral therapy (BT) speaks as though it has inherited the wisdom of the laboratory science of behavioral learning theory, but it is actually a product of social and political imperatives trespassing across the borders of scientific meaning. Behavioral therapy is not a clinical expression of an underlying scientific rationality of behavior science but rather its metaphor, shaped by broadly popular social preferences to ratify institutionalized American values. The metaphoric use of BT is particularly troubling, tending to stigmatize the most needy Americans as less than fully human by way of justifying both inadequate public and private provisions and frequently the contempt in which they are held.

For relatively functional patients, who usually seek treatment voluntarily, behavior therapy promises painless, quick miracle cures for their fears, anxieties, and quirks. But for poorer, marginal, and sanctioned groups—the poor, foster children, prisoners, the demented, the retarded, the regressed, the primitive, and so forth—BT takes on a sinister meaning as it is substituted for interventions such as cognitive and psychodynamic therapies predicated on reason to modify either thought or emotion through frequently coercive procedures. In application to less favored groups, behavioral interventions signify the need for external restraint, as though these people were feral animals lacking higher sensibilities and incapable of learning from reasoned discussion. Indeed, the process of applying behavioral methods may actually deprive people of the fundamental human capacity for thinking, that is, rationality and reasonability, as a concomitant of therapy itself. In this way, behavioral therapy ritualizes, formalizes, and justifies deprivation and coercion. In a chapter that repeatedly contradicts itself, James and Gilliland (2003) trip onto the actual social role of behavior therapy while meaning to praise it for its adaptability and specificity.[1]

[Behavior therapy's] scientific method of changing behaviors and developing problem-solving skills is suited for diverse cultural populations whose members are sometimes offended by catharsis and the open expression of personal feelings and concerns. Eysenck, Eysenck, and Barrett (1995) noted that the behavioral system views and responds to client gender, age, and socioeconomic differences in unique and appropriate ways. . . .

Behavioral counseling works for mentally limited clients because of its behavior modification and management techniques that successively approximate their goals and do not rely heavily on the cognitive domain for that clientele. The approach also works for many patients and students of inner city schools and rural environments where clients are conditioned to operate on short-term contingencies and where concrete, clear, structured formats are desired. In these cases, the client is not dependent on the counselor. Progress is visible and evident because clients can tell when beds are made, cigarette consumption is diminished, pounds are lost, and money is saved. They may have real trouble discerning when they are doing better, thinking straight, or improving their attitudes. Measurable goals and attainments put immediate and short-term reinforcements within the grasp of clients who can neither wait for long-term rewards nor delay gratification.

People of color as well as people from other diverse backgrounds, such as those with language disadvantages, physically disabling conditions, economic and educational disadvantages, and diverse sexual orientations often face social, political, and other environmental influences and problems that require more than one-to-one talk to resolve. (James and Gilliland, 2002, p. 195)

Apparently, BT is the fail-safe, default treatment of choice for the unreasonable, who more often than favored groups are minorities, rural residents, physically and mentally disabled, uneducated, poor, and gay. Yet the reservation of BT for miscreants, deviants, and the depraved of the lower classes is one of the very few descriptions of the deployment of behavioral therapy in the literature that gets past the clinical obfuscations and polite professional jargon of "appropriate treatment," "stepped care," and "evidence-based practice" to define its intended role as a metaphor to discredit less favored groups rather than as a serious clinical intervention.

Yet no form of BT enjoys credible proof of effectiveness; the drama of bypassing cognition for coercion and soothing talk for conditioning scripts a fable of social labeling and sanction. The society's attitude to its poor, dependent, and disabled citizens is summarized in the use of BT that denies the patient's capacity for free will—cognitive independence. In fact, the calving off of cognitive-behavioral therapy (CBT) from BT is occasioned more by demands for flattering regard in the treatment of supposedly rational, wealthy, and largely successful populations than by any provenance of clinical ability. Rather than individual considerations of effective intervention, behavioral methods are often applied on a moral schedule: more deserving groups merit cognitive interventions; the less deserving need to be conditioned, and frequently through punishments rather than inducements.

Not coincidentally, the language of behavioral therapy pervades social work, the occupation most concerned with social deviants and socially marginalized groups including the poor. In recent decades, as general enthusiasms for pure behavioral interventions have given way to therapies with greater cognitive content, BT seems increasingly reserved for lower-income working people and the inhabitants of the putative underclass. The divide in therapies further emphasizes the puritanical divide in worth between the owls and the mules—those who prosper through intellectual pursuits and those who struggle to make a living through routinized labor.

Yet even in the case of BT, heroic individualism plays a central role. The BT patient is expected to internalize conditioning and generalize it to other behaviors. Indeed, the patient's continued resistance to behavioral ministrations is interpreted as willful defiance even in the face of the initial assumptions of conditioning that seem to deny volition.

Behavior Therapy without Behaviorism

BT was initially predicated on the insights of conditioning theory with animals, an expression of behaviorism that disputes the usefulness of inner states and hypothetical constructs as scientific explanations of behavior. Yet BT has come to include a series of interventions largely ignorant of those principles and even the basic tenets of behaviorism except for a vulgarized, rudimentary, and superficial commitment to measurement. Indeed, BT mocks science, accepting the authority of studies that are caricatures of sequential, objective, coherent, careful, and controlled experimentation.

Wolpe (1958, 1973) carefully grounded behavioral treatments in classical and operant conditioning theory. His notion of reciprocal inhibition built clinical interventions on the specific pairings of stimuli in classical conditioning and operant reinforcement. While his treatments are uncertain applications of those principles, the theory of learning allows for a theory of clinical practice. Indeed, many current behavioral interventions—behavioral contrasting, role playing, assertion training, aversion therapy, flooding and implosion therapy, satiation, self-monitoring, self-management and self-regulation, behavioral modeling, behavioral rehearsal, and even token economies and systematic desensitization—maintain only the vaguest ties to basic learning theory. They are usually formalizations of the conventional wisdom of human development rather than the precision tooling of careful experimentation, analysis, and clinical trials.

The tenets of behaviorism have been specified oddly in the contemporary understanding of BT. Behaviorism implies a commitment to the determinism of human behavior in measurable terms that reject mystical, unknowable forces such as "mind"; a recognition of the near impossibility of reliably measuring conscious states; a rejection of hypothetical constructs as causative of human behavior; and, specifically, a denial of introspection as a source of credible information. Behaviorism assumes that measurable events outside of "mind" can be functionally related to measurable outcomes. In defining BT, Bellack, Hersen, and Kazdin (1982), one prominent example among many, violated these behavioral principles in a manner that blunts Wolpe's precision and commitment to conditioning theory.

> (i) A strong commitment to empirical evaluation of treatment and intervention techniques; (ii) A general belief that therapeutic experiences must provide opportunities to learn adaptive or prosocial behavior; (iii) Specification of treatment in operational and, hence, replicable terms; (iv) Evaluation of treatment effects through multiple-response modalities with particular emphasis on overt behavior. (p. 287)

However, Bellack et al.'s definition actually subverts the scientific rigor of behaviorism. The assertion of a commitment to empirical evaluation is undercut by the near characteristic employment of single subject designs, that is, "multiple response modalities." While BT appears committed to objective measurement, in practice it accepts a series of interventions that cannot be specified for replication. BT relies frequently on patient self-reports in order to devise idiosyncratic treatments based on individual case histories. Moreover, in its current forms many BT interventions, and not just CBT, employ a variety of cognitive techniques that are often little more than introspective devices, the epiphenomena (for example, hypothetical constructs) excoriated by behaviorism.

Sidman (1960) elaborated the experimental logic of single subject designs. Yet at the same time he provided the grounds that undercut them. Sidman noted that

In any experiment, there is much behavior that goes unrecorded and even unobserved. Because such behavior has not been selected for observation, we sometimes make the mistake of ignoring its possible systematic or technical importance; yet it may play an important mediating role in the processes we are investigating. To ignore such behavior in our explanatory scheme is a misapplication of the operational principle. If the behavior is potentially observable, then it cannot be excluded from consideration because of an arbitrary decision, in a particular instance, to leave it unrecorded. (p. 364)

Further, Sidman contended that the number of alternative explanations for conditioning experiments outside of the controlled laboratory increases with more advanced animals. As the prime example, humans bring complex memories and behaviors that may not respond directly to research cues. "Much of the variability [that is, among research subjects and patients] stems from the considerable and largely unknown behavioral history that higher organisms bring with them to the laboratory" (p. 385). These include "the effects of uncontrolled historical factors" and the fact that "they do not remain in a controlled laboratory environment for the duration of a lengthy study" or treatment (ibid.).

Therefore, the decision to compare the behaviors of research subjects to their own baselines rather than to randomized controls opens the door to alternative explanations for treatment outcomes: patients may be self-selected and highly motivated to change their behaviors and might well change through any process of treatment or even without any treatment at all; patients may simply be adapting to the research situation itself, with little ability or desire to generalize their responses outside of the clinic; even without specific motivation to change, patient problems may be seasonal, with the most amenable portion of the cycle being presented during treatment; the patient may be responding to expectancies (his or her own and those of the researchers) rather than to the treatment itself; and finally, accurate baseline measures may be impossible to obtain, with the result that estimates of problems are greatly exaggerated.

Randomized placebo control procedures are necessary to handle these threats to the credibility of treatment. In Sidman's (1960) own terms, randomized placebo controls are "techniques for determining whether our experimental results are actually a product of our explicit manipulations, or whether they stem from the operation of some other known or even unsuspected factors" (p. 342). Indeed, randomization is precisely the technique to assure that experimental and control groups are equivalent in factors that are *unknown.* Nevertheless, Sidman failed to explicitly compare the apparent limitations of multiple response modalities against the logic of randomized controlled experimentation. He only addressed controlled experimentation as a brief aside. Yet following the logic of behavioral experiments with animals, single subject designs are accepted and even preferred with humans. However, fashionable enthusiasms for single subject designs to evaluate BT have produced more self-deception than reliable evidence of effectiveness. Without randomized controlled procedures, clinical science is not science and will never mature.

The sanction of debased research and a conveniently lax application of behaviorism has encouraged the BT community to frequently ignore the principles of conditioning in promoting a long list of interventions. The problem of applying core scientific requirements to BT is further thwarted by a fundamental theoretical problem. Even when not explicitly acknowledged in its clinical applications, conditioning theory may not be readily testable though the effectiveness of behavioral interventions themselves may be. Conditioning theory can predict an event and its opposite. Thus testing the application does not certify its theoretical antecedents, with the effect of marooning BT as essentially a series of ad hoc and commonsense fables. BT and psychotherapy persist not for any proven clinical virtue but rather as expressions of cultural preferences, little more than folksongs orchestrated as Italian opera.

For each application of Wolpe's reciprocal inhibition, a corollary conditioning situation can be defined that is diametrically opposed to the initial prediction of behavior change. Wolpe's (1973) case explanation of the process of systematic desensitization is one among many examples.

> If the child fears a visitor's long black beard, he is quite likely to become reconciled to it by deconditioning events that may occur if he sits on his father's lap while the latter speaks to the visitor. The child may at first intermittently glance at the beard so that the anxiety arousals are smaller each time. Since they occur against a background of warm and pleasant responses to the father, these small fear arousals are presumably inhibited; and, gradually, as the fear subsides, the child tolerates lengthening looks at the beard. (p. 95)

Following Wolpe's theory of reciprocal inhibition, sitting on the father's lap relaxes the child in the presence of the beard and thus "counterconditions" anxiety with comfort, eventually replacing the pairing of the beard with anxiety. This classically conditioned absence or lessening of an anxiety response to the stimulus of the beard operantly reinforces the comfort that the child now feels in the presence of the formerly anxiety-producing stimulus. According to Wolpe (1973), "if a response inhibiting anxiety can be made to occur in the presence of anxiety-evoking stimuli, it will weaken the bond between these stimuli and the anxiety" (p. 17).

However, conditioning theory also predicts the reverse. The comfort of the lap positively reinforces the child's anxiety, since the anxious response to the beard may be positively reinforced by being drawn onto the father's comforting lap. The child's anxiety response is further reinforced by the departure of the stranger. In these ways, the child's anxiety response to the beard may be strengthened by the "deconditioning." To impute motive, the child may learn that anxiety is useful in ridding itself of the anxiety response and in achieving a pleasurable response from the father.

Like much social-science theorizing, the actual outcomes of an intervention are largely the consequences of observed events rather than the predictions of theory. This problem for conditioning theory is created by the field's hasty application of laboratory animal conditioning—for example, the work of Watson and Skinner—to clinical therapies for humans but absent the laboratory rigor. There is no Skinner box for BT. The painstaking and gradual experiments that led to explanations for the association of isolated stimulus-and-response conditions of animals in highly controlled settings are not replicated by BT's lineage of experimental development. BT's identification of the conditioned stimuli that become paired with unconditioned stimuli when it occurs at all and the processes of stimulus generalization are pure speculations. In the same way, it is not at all likely that even the most careful clinical histories will unearth the conditioning processes that created unwanted habits, even assuming that the initial cause has much relevance to sustaining those behaviors.

Because of ambiguous theory and failed testing, BT is not scientific conditioning. The elegance and precise operationalizations of classical and operant learning, in their application to BT metaphors for the real thing, become appropriations of science for social ends. The science that forecasts the reactions of animals in laboratory learning experiments has not been adapted successfully to human behavior. Perhaps the problem lies with the large amount of cognition that human researchers are willing to grant their subjects in departure from a strictly observable science. The social insistence on a prominent role for human cognition in psychotherapy seems to have overwhelmed prudence in developing clinical science. Concern with effectiveness was pushed aside by demands for compatible metaphor. Yet the favored methods for evaluating BT and the research itself confirm the ad hoc, weak, and failed clinical ability of BT. Furthermore, the poor quality of the outcome research reprises questions about the conditions of science in the field.

Skinner anticipated the temptations of hasty extrapolation of simplistic models of animal conditioning to complex human behaviors. Skinner (1938) concluded *The Behavior of Organisms* with cautions and challenges that, in the subsequent sixty years or so, BT has blithely ignored.

> The reader will have noticed that almost no extension to human behavior is made or suggested. . . . But it is a serious, though common, mistake to allow questions of ultimate application to influence the development of a systematic science at an early state. It is possible that there are properties of human behavior which will require a different kind of treatment. But this can be ascertained only by closing in upon the problem in an orderly way and by following the customary procedures of an experimental science. (pp. 441–442)

BT is still at an early stage, but it is not science. Skinner did not need to ask his pigeons about their history, preferences, and progress in training. The custom of orderly experimental science implies experimental controls in evaluating BT. "Because it is experimental, a science of behavior may justifiably claim greater validity than popular or philosophical formulations" (Skinner, 1938, p. 434). And because of its failure to achieve Skinner's "conspicuousness" or to develop a credible experimental science, BT and psychotherapy in general are best understood as popular formulations.

In CBT, reinforcers became ever more cognitive but ever more elusive. BT's attenuated but continuing popularity has little to do with clinical success but much to do with the degree to which it frequently fulfills a social role, rather than a clinical one, that disparages various groups for deviance, disobedience, impairment, and incapacity. BT persists to reinforce the unworthiness of failed and problematic groups as less capable than more successful social groups of consciousness, cognition, and self-determination.

Effectiveness

Contrary to the field's promoters, the effectiveness of behavioral therapy has not been established through rigorous clinical tests. Indeed, the noncognitive behavior therapy research is customarily too weak to emerge in the field's stronger journals covering psychotherapy.[2] The typical BT research is impaired by a variety of self-serving pitfalls. Following the example of animal research, behavioral research has regressed methodologically to embrace single subject designs—methods that lack nontreatment or placebo controls and instead compare the patient's own baseline of behavior (that is, prior to therapy) against the patient's behavior after therapy.

Randomized controls, when they exist in BT research, are customarily compromised, while standard treatment controls often do as well as the experimental BT conditions. Most problematically, the theoretical considerations of the interventions—reasons to expect their effectiveness or the precise conditioning pathways of therapy—are rarely specified. Indeed, many have recognized that both the methodological failures of BT research as well as its inconsistent findings raise serious questions about the effectiveness of BT. These doubts have sped the movement away from pure BT interventions and toward cognitive-behavioral therapy (CBT).

Rather than provide evidence for the effectiveness of various behavioral self-control training programs including bibliotherapy for problem drinkers, Skutle and Berg (1987) demonstrated only that people motivated to reduce their drinking may do so. Their self-selected group of "early-stage problem drinkers" were recruited through local media by advertising for those who wanted to drink less. Severe alcoholics were excluded from the study. Results indicated that weekly drinking was reduced by more than 50%, from about 35 drinks to about 15 drinks. Improvement was apparently maintained for one year after treatment. However, "the drop in consumption from the intake values had already taken place by the week after treatment started" (p. 498). Thus it appears likely that the patients' own motivation rather than any condition of therapy accounted for the change. Moreover, consumption of alcohol was measured only by self-report. No nontreatment control was employed.

In fact, the sample seems to include few problem drinkers. Moreover, the only behavioral characteristic of the interventions lies in their potential for being objectively measured, although in this case it is not clear that the critical measurement—actual alcohol consumption—was either objective or reliable.

Foy, Nunn, and Rychtarik (1984) randomly assigned problem drinkers to "broad-spectrum behavioral treatment including controlled drinking skills training or the same broad-spectrum treatment package without training in controlled drinking skills" (p. 220). The broad-spectrum behavioral treatments included "alcohol education, group therapy, individual therapy, self-management training, job seeking and interpersonal-skills training, drink-refusal-skills training, and relaxation training" during four weeks of hospitalization and eleven aftercare visits during the year after hospitalization (p. 218). The authors reported that in the six months after treatment the group trained in controlled drinking reported significantly less drinking, although more incarceration, than the group not trained in controlled drinking—about 25% more days abstinent and less alcohol consumption. None of the differences were significant one year after treatment. Both groups reported significant reductions in heavy drinking days and job-related problems after treatment. However, no significant improvements in either group were reported in social adjustment outcomes, for example, personal relationships.

However, the research, lacking a nontreatment control for broad-spectrum behavioral intervention, cannot separate the modest improvements from the motivation of patients or the degree to which their reports were influenced by the demand characteristics of the research situation. It is also notable that about half the sample volunteered to take Antabuse during the first three months after treatment. Thus the significant positive reductions in drinking may more logically be attributed to the Antabuse (perhaps as further evidence of patient motivation) than to the behavioral treatment.

It is curious that the authors only acknowledged the use of Antabuse as an aside, largely ignoring its likely contribution to their outcomes. It is even more telling that the *Journal of Consulting and Clinical Psychology* obviously failed to insist on a more forthcoming discussion of the authors' findings. In short, if in fact the patients' outcomes improved during the course of the study, the least likely explanation rests with the package of behavioral interventions and the more likely causes rest with their own motivation, family pressure, and Antabuse.

In the treatment of post-traumatic stress disorder, Tarrier, Pilgrim, Sommerfield, Faragher, Reynolds et al. (1999) claimed that "either imaginal exposure (flooding) or a challenge to cognition can result in symptom reduction, although neither resulted in complete improvement" (p. 13). However, their design lacks a nontreatment control, with the result that maturation, accustomization, and patient motivation seem more likely explanations for their modest findings. Nevertheless, on the basis of similarly flawed research, Gauthier (1999), reflecting the bravado of the field, insisted that "across each of the anxiety disorders, effective cognitive-behavioural approaches have been developed and empirically validated" (p. 4).

Klesges, Haddock, and Lando (1999) reported that a forced smoking cessation program—a smoking ban for all basic-training troops in the military "24 hours a day, 7 days a week, for 6 weeks together with brief health lectures"—during basic training for the United States Air Force produced an improvement. However, improvement was the same in both the treatment group and the nontreatment control. Moreover, smoking initiation rates appeared to be very high. Yet, given the strong obvious preference of the military to discourage smoking and the reliance of the research on self-report, it is questionable whether the modest reported findings are reliable. After all, the acknowledgment of smoking was a confession of breaking a military order.

Apparently the Air Force is unconstrained by either experimental logic or informed consent, although the rates of noncompliance among enlisted personnel might itself be a cause for some concern.

Dumas and Albin (1986) marveled at the fact that behavioral treatments—usually parent skills training—for noncompliant, aggressive children failed as "adverse social and material conditions increased" for their families. The suggestion is that treatment succeeds for relatively less beleaguered families, but the design characteristics of the study also lead to a contradictory possibility: behavioral treatments for aggressive children are not needed in skilled, motivated families. In other words, parental skills training does not provide parental skills sufficient to treat any notable behavioral problem in children.

In reporting gains for a number of behavioral treatments for anxiety, Butler and Anastasiades (1988), Butler, Cullington, Hibbert, Klines, and Gelder (1987), and Butler, Gelder, Hibbert, Cullington, and Klimes (1987) share similar pitfalls. All relied on patient self-reports in situations that probably encouraged exaggerated reports of progress. All lacked true nontreatment controls, relying usually upon wait-listing that may encourage the maintenance of symptoms. All recruited amenable, motivated patients whose symptoms might have frequently subsided by themselves and whose initial report of symptoms may have been exaggerated so that they could become eligible or maintain eligibility for treatment. All of the studies were conducted by researchers with an apparent stake in the behavioral interventions they were evaluating.

Perri, Nezu, Patti, and McCann (1989) treated obesity with behavioral techniques—self-monitoring, stimulus control, self-reinforcement, cognitive modification, problem solving, and programmed aerobic exercise—comparing the effectiveness of 20 sessions against 40 sessions. The 48 patients, recruited from newspaper advertisements, were between 25% and 100% overweight (averaging about 72 pounds) and were randomized to the two conditions. One-third dropped out. After one year of treatment, the remaining patients in the extended treatment group lost about 20 pounds and the shorter treatment group lost about 10 pounds, a significant difference. However, the modest weight reduction was achieved by unusually motivated patients, and the results were not adjusted for the substantial number of patients who dropped out and presumably failed to lose weight.

While the extended treatment group lost more weight than the shorter treatment group, they were also heavier by about 10 pounds to begin with. The very modest findings for extended treatment also need to be considered in light of the researchers' probable expectancy biases and the long-term ability of the patients to maintain weight loss. Both groups were beginning to gain back substantial weight after treatment, replicating the common pattern of failure. Moreover, the long-term gains of the extended treatment group were measured only 32 weeks after the intensive surveillance of treatment but 52 weeks later for the shorter treatment group. Rather than boast about the curative ability of extended treatment, it seems likely, especially in consideration of the pitfalls of the research, that all of the modest weight loss would be gradually regained. Apparently self-restraint for the chronically obese is a constant problem even when it is redefined as a problem of conditioning.

In perhaps the most thorough current review of BT for adults, Krijn, Emmelkamp, and Olafsson (2004) largely ignored the problems of the research to cobble together an advertisement. Unfortunately, it is about as credible as a television doctor pushing an herbal cure for anxiety, constipation, obesity, and age spots. Krijn et al. summarized research in the previous decade that hardly improves on earlier studies. Much of the evidence continues to be provided through single case testimonials and analogue studies, which might be acceptable if psychotherapy had an underlying theory of emotional and mental functioning that was as powerful as physiology and pathology are for medicine. Yet it does not; conditioning theory is challenged to predict accurately in humans.

With hardly an exception, the controlled primary studies in Krijn et al. (2004) are impaired by self-selected patients, patient self-reports, short-term follow-ups, unrepresentative samples, inappropriate and imperfect controls, and committed researchers—in short, the very same problems that beset earlier studies by allowing for serious bias and, thus, substantial grounds for skepticism. Notably too, the findings are frequently contradictory or ambiguous—for example, imaginal versus in vivo treatment, BT versus CBT versus drug therapy versus even nontreatment, controlled drinking versus abstinence, and many others. Indeed, Krijn et al. cite evidence that BT for generalized anxiety disorder is only slightly superior to drug therapy. Yet the research offers a suspicious symmetry between the clinical orientation of the researchers and the findings they provide. Indeed, in less professionally loyal hands, the same review might have called attention to confirmational response bias in the field, that is, the ability of researchers to concoct compatible findings.

If anything, the suspicion remains strong that remission of clinical symptoms is a tribute more to initial patient motivation than to any value added by BT. Indeed, patient self-selection and maturation may be the critical elements in reported improvements; the therapist may simply be providing a ceremony of remission that could be conferred by a less pretentious and expensive source. The cultivation of patient expectancies as the substance of

BT recalls Christian Science and mind cures rather than the promises of psychotherapy. In this case, psychotherapy may be the only publicly supported service appropriate for complete conversion from state to church auspices.

There is little theoretical consistency in Krijn et al. (2004). They offer very few comments on the jumble of poorly sustained clinical generalizations that explain clinical outcomes, only a final aside that "relatively little attention has been devoted to the therapeutic process" (p. 431). Thus Krijn et al.'s state-of-the-art study is a collection of ad hoc treatments with separate and distinct references to underlying causal propositions. The laboratory success of conditioning simple behaviors in animals and the treatment of humans for complex behavioral dysfunctions are worlds apart, related metaphorically but not through scientifically established behavioral theory. Their conclusion that "research on behavioral-based treatments for anxiety disorders has clearly and consistently shown the positive effects of interventions" is more heroic and fanciful than analytic or careful (p. 430).

More troubling, the growing consensus that "evaluating the outcome of behavioral techniques whose effects have already been established for the 'average' patient are not likely to produce new knowledge" encourages research that probes the processes of healing before healing itself is properly established (p. 431). The methodological problems of the primary research undercut any conclusion except ineffectiveness. Permission to proceed into studies of internal mechanisms is a political gambit to get past the field's faulty research and assume BT's clinical powers. The acceptance of the new research agenda says much about social preferences and the symbolic standing of psychotherapy, the utility of BT as a metaphor of radical self-reliance and a punishment for populations that cannot or do not seem to be adequately independent.

Krijn et al. (2004) applauded recent "innovations" in BT for phobia that rely on self-help manuals for home remedies. Apparently, in proselytizing the heroic folklore of self-invention, the field is going so far as to eliminate the in vivo therapist and the necessity of the therapeutic relationship in favor of decentralized mail-order business with on-line and phone backup. BT-at-home is more reminiscent of buying a computer from Gateway or Dell than seeking cure from a healer. Alternative medicine has customarily had a greater genius for adaptations to changing consumer styles than any demonstrable ability to cure, prevent, or rehabilitate.

Rather than a noble reach for neutral, well-considered, and careful scientific knowledge, the tactful might conclude that these studies and their ponderous reviews are triumphs of heart over intellect or, with less tolerance, wasted resources . . . assuming for the moment that the research is actually funded to provide objective, neutral knowledge. Yet the previously discussed

examples and Krijn et al.'s (2004) base of studies are among the more prominent and stronger studies culled from the near endless chapters and summary
arguments for the effectiveness of BT. Just as these studies fall far short of scientific credibility, so it is with the rest of the evidence for BT's effectiveness.
The body of research is a premature attempt to measure outcomes; the field
is ill equipped to test its effects objectively or to apply a tough communal
standard of skepticism. Indeed, the failure of the BT research, as of psychotherapy generally, begins to mark the divide between a true scientific enterprise, even in its early stages, and alternative science—the flummery of lab
coats, statistical designs, and professed high purpose but devoid of rigorous
methods and communal dedication.

The Therapeutic Exchange:
Appropriating Science for Metaphor

The language and process of behavioral therapy are ineffective in achieving
clinical goals. BT's success lies in the reinforcement of social values. On the
one hand, BT promotes heroic individualism by insistence on self-reliance.
On the other hand, in the sense that incarceration celebrates liberty by
depriving prisoners of freedom, BT stigmatizes numerous groups by denying
assumptions of their capacity for self-direction and imposing stringent operant conditions, usually punishments, to modify their behavior. Yet BT has not
changed the humaneness of maintaining order in near total institutions.
Adorning prisons, state hospitals, reform schools, orphanages, domestic violence shelters, homeless shelters, and other congregate settings with the terms
of BT obscures their coercive, intrusive, and sometimes violent nature and
their failure to treat defiance, mental or emotional incapacity, physical impairment, and other problems. In fact, total institutions rarely succeed at more
than incapacitation, that is, restricting harmful behaviors through involuntary commitment of one sort or another. BT as some form of token economy
is applied without the delicacy of informed consent, often as the punishment
for undisciplined, impulsive, and bizarre behaviors that are interpreted as
rebellions against personal responsibility.

Still, outside of rare applications to severely incapacitated patients, BT
must rely on obviously cognitive processes. BT for most patients customarily
employs dialogue through a therapeutic relationship as pivotal tools of communication. Not only does the therapeutic relationship provide direction
and encouragement for patients, but the authority of the therapist is also the
source for reinforcing the patient's appropriate behaviors.

In its narrow sense, that is, without great reliance on cognitive processes,

BT reconditions the patient through the therapeutic situation, including the therapeutic relationship. Either through classical or operant conditioning, the therapist controls the unconditioned stimuli and the reinforcers to elicit remedies for the patient's behavioral complaints. Theoretically, patients play the same roles in therapy that dogs played for Pavlov and pigeons for Skinner. Yet the therapeutic situation remains an open field, a very imperfect Skinner box, the antithesis of controlled laboratory conditions.

Wolpe (1973) has made much of "assertive training" in overcoming phobia. "With a reasonable amount of pressure and encouragement, most patients begin to be able to assert themselves in a matter of days, or a week or two" (p. 87). He has provided an example of a "typical assertion-instigating conversation:

THERAPIST: Let us talk about your mother-in-law.
MRS. A: She is a bully, says a lot of things and does a lot of things to me that I sit back and take. I really should open my mouth and not be big about it. . . . She steps over me and I let it boil up inside.
T: Now what would happen if you let it out on your mother-in-law— which is what you really want to do, isn't it? . . .
A: My in-laws don't like the way I behave, by the way . . . Suppose my husband starts up with me, "You shouldn't talk like that to my mother. You are not cementing relationships; you are putting them farther apart." How do I handle that situation?
T: You have to say, "If your mother makes unjust remarks I have to tell her and I will tell her. If your mother makes reasonable criticisms, I will be very interested in what she has to say. But she is always at me, and she has gotten into the habit of it because I have been allowing her to say whatever she likes. I am not going to have it any more." (pp. 87–88)

The learning dynamic of reciprocal inhibition in this exchange assumes that assertiveness can be classically conditioned to substitute for phobia so long as the assertive act produces a response that is preferable to fear. The pleasurable response (at least the absence of fear, although hopefully some positive result of the assertive behavior) will operantly reinforce assertiveness. Wolpe cautioned: "*never instigate an assertive act that is likely to have punishing consequences*" (p. 87).

But there is no compelling evidence that this "instigation" of assertion logically follows through to assertion itself. That is, the implicit "encouragement" in the therapist's statement is not necessarily sufficient to elicit the desired response. The fact of the patient's pursuit of therapy, by itself an assertive act, may well be the necessary precursor of assertive behavior. In this sense, therapy becomes a ritual of the patient's activity, although a ritual that requires an authority to certify the behavior.

There is a seeming contradiction inherent in both encouraging individual assertion and increasing the authority of the therapist in order to provide a sufficient reinforcement for the behavior. Indeed, it is at least theoretically possible that the patient will become perversely conditioned to rely on authority for personal motivation in handling phobia; it is not clear which is worse, especially as phobic patients may generalize their reliance on the clinical authority of the therapist to social authority generally, in direct contradiction of personal autonomy and self-determination. This is still speculative, since BT has not demonstrated credible clinical success. However, it brackets the metaphoric meaning of BT as a ritual of social bonding that underscores the dogma of personal reliance even while the therapy itself may undermine individual autonomy.

Systematic desensitization repeats the ambiguity of therapy. The conditioning logic of systematic desensitization employs relaxation or some other pleasurable, unconditioned stimulus to substitute for fear in the face of the fear-producing stimulus. The expectation is that the fear-producing stimulus will become paired with (conditioned to) relaxation. In the following example, Wolpe asks the patient to elicit the phobic stimulus cognitively, that is in the patient's imagination, after having been relaxed.

> THERAPIST: I am now going to ask you to imagine a number of scenes. You will imagine them clearly and they will generally interfere little, if at all, with your state of relaxation. . . . As soon as a scene is clear in your mind, indicate it by raising your left index finger about one inch . . .
>
> After a few seconds the patient raises her left index finger. The therapist pauses for five seconds.
>
> T: Stop imagining that scene. By how much did it raise your anxiety level while you imagined it?
>
> MISS C: Not at all.
>
> T: Now give your attention once again to relaxing.
>
> There is again a pause of 20–30 seconds.
>
> T: Now imagine that you are home studying in the evening. It is the 20th May, exactly a month before your examination.
>
> After about 15 seconds Miss C. raises her finger. Again she is left with the scene for 5 seconds. (p. 123)

And so the therapy continues, with progressively more fearful scenes being elicited and paired with relaxation, ultimately graduating into successful in vivo exposure. Yet a number of concerns diminish the credibility of the procedure. There is little demonstration of the superiority of systematic desensitization over appropriate controls, that is, control conditions that the patient believes to be therapeutic but are not. The control is particularly important to handle the claim that the supposedly scientific techniques of systematic desensitization are improvements over simple, naive encouragement. People have typically learned to handle their irrational fears by confronting them and taking wisdom from the absence of the feared consequences. The clinical problem of proof for BT is to demonstrate that it achieves more favorable outcomes, more often, than the accumulated folklore of history, that is, the unplanned, received wisdom of almost all human civilizations.

Further, the process of systematic desensitization is essentially cognitive rather than behavioral. Patients who can elicit emotions simply through imagination and recall without the presence of initial stimuli are probably amenable to some form of rational induction without the adjuncts of conditioning theory. Yet systematic desensitization is behavioral only in the more recent sense of explicitness. In fact, the imaginal content and the reliance on patient report defies the core tenets of behaviorism that were elaborated in conditioning theory. Moreover, Wolpe's detailed patient case histories, with their implicit theory of psychosocial development, elide the critical differences between behavioral therapies—for example, assertive training and systematic desensitization—and the psychodynamic therapies. They both erect a superstructure of untestable theory and unobservable intrapsychic events.

The patient's expectancies of cure are recruited through a gnomic process of belief. The patient is made amenable to BT through faith in the curative powers of the therapist. Much has been made of placebo effects, but they do not require an expensively trained clinician. Shamanistic healing converts science into a totem, in turn reinforcing a belief in magic rather than autonomous thought toughened by reality. But the process of systematic desensitization and BT for voluntary patients emphasizes their responsibility to handle their own problems, subtly burdening them with guilt and shame for any failure to heal.

The large cognitive component is notable in this exchange. But the cognitive processes of desensitization and BT generally are not equivalent to conditioning a rat to run a maze or a pigeon to peck at a key in a cage. The learning dynamics of BT are extremely ambiguous. It is not clear what stimuli the patient is responding to—cognitive or behavioral, internal or related to the therapeutic exchange—or whether the therapist's verbal encouragement in

184 Psychotherapy as Religion

assertive training or desensitization has the same predictability as classical pairing or operant reinforcement with animals. Thus the terms of conditioning in BT are metaphoric, appropriating the authority of laboratory conditioning for the ceremonial affirmation of social values.

Ritualism seems to be a logical explanation for much of the BT dialogue, notably in the absence of credible proof of BT's effectiveness. In the following exchange, a child is being taught the conditions of "systematic exclusion" under which his "bizarre behavior" will result in his being sent home from school.

> THERAPIST: In order to help you, J.F., we have made three rules for you. You are to follow these rules whenever you are in class. The rules are: One, no talking. This means talking out in class, with neighbors, laughing, or making any noise with your voice or mouth. How do you get permission to say something?
> J.F.: Raise my hand.
> T: Good. Do you understand this rule?
> J.F.: Yes.
> T: Very good. Do you have any questions about this rule?
> J.F.: No.
> [And so on for rules two and three.]
> T: Now, J.F., will you tell us these three rules? [J.F. names them.] Now, we all know that boys your age forget rules. To help you remember, each time you forget your teacher will give you one of these. [J.F. was shown a half sheet of paper that had blanks for date and time and the statement, "To the office: Please call Mrs. F. and tell her that J.F. is on his way home."] This means that, when you forget, to help you remember, you will go home for the rest of the day. You will come back the next morning and try again. When you go home, you are to stay at home until the usual time you get home from school. When you come back to school the next morning, we start fresh. We don't worry or talk about what happened yesterday. This is being done to help you remember the rules. Do you understand what I've been saying?
> J.F.: Yes.
> T: Why might you be sent home?
> J.F.: When I forget a rule. (Shier, 1969, pp. 119–120)

The dialogue continues, with similar repetitions of the rules and consequences by J.F. No punishments other than systematic exclusion from the school are applied by the school staff or the boy's parents. As it turns out, J.F.'s behavior does not change much until a neurologist prescribes Dexedrine. But the bizarre behaviors, similar to ADHD, return the next school year when J.F. is taken off of the Dexedrine. Shier concludes that systematic exclusion was effective—"drug therapy in addition to systematic exclusion resulted in total behavior modification"—but wonders whether drug therapy need be continued with BT (p. 123).

Aside from the fact that Shier's own data suggest that BT was not necessary for J.F.'s improvements, systematic exclusion seems to be staged for the rest of the school population, underscoring the necessity of obedience. It really does not matter much whether J.F. changes but rather that the school be orderly. J.F. provides the opportunity to affirm institutional order. It is intriguing that the focus of the failed therapy is on J.F.'s self-control, the ability of the child to modify his own behavior, even after the neurologist concludes that J.F. has "an organic problem with attention span," which itself may be a specious excuse for the recourse to sedation (p. 123). Even in the face of medication for an organic source of J.F.'s problems, BT is continued for ritualistic purposes to emphasize personal responsibility . . . that J.F. and all other students must abide by the rules. "Help" for J.F. is contrived within the distorted theatrics of institutional control and personal responsibility. Yet J.F. is still accorded some respect for his capacity for reflection and self-control, even while both are undercut in the actual treatment. Currently, disruptive behavior is "treated" to plastic obedience by a promiscuity of drugs—the prison in a pill—for the convenience of understaffed schools, overwhelmed parents, and neglectful, indifferent communities.

In a transcript of therapy with an anxious patient, Goldstein (1972) explains BT's assumptions about anxiety. It is notable that conditioning does not inform this description of treatment, which asks the patient to rely upon a largely gnomic, mystical explanation for his disorder: "something" happened.

> DR. GOLDSTEIN: . . . Through the kinds of experiences that we have in life we end up responding to particular situations in particular ways and the hardest job for us is finding out what situations trigger uncomfortable feelings when there is no objective danger. Once we have done that, things become much more simple to deal with because there are ways we can change the kind of automatic anxiety response that occurs. . . .
>
> I think some of the confusion you are experiencing is that you are trying to put this into a rational context when in fact these kinds of feelings are not at all rational in that they are not appropriate to the

reality of the situation. They are logical in the sense that they tend to be consistent—certain events or people will trigger it. But they are not rational in terms of the kind of analysis that you make of a situation. And that tends to confuse you if you are looking for some reason. The reason simply is that because of some past experience with this particular set of personality traits, or something about that person, or something about that particular event, has taken on the capacity to elicit an anxiety response, a response of being uncomfortable. There is consistency, I am sure, and in that sense it is logical. (pp. 224–225)

The nature of the dialogue and especially the BT that entails imaginal techniques bears a strong resemblance to psychodynamic therapy. Backgrounds are explored for important events that are accorded standing as conditioners for behavioral therapists and traumatic experiences for the psychodynamically oriented. The discovery of an early event of importance by itself enhances treatment, for there are similarly large cognitive and emotional components in both treatments. The purely behavioral commitments of BT are contrived, superficial, and linguistic rather than truly analogous to the science of animal conditioning.

Institutional Behavior Modification:
Token Economies in Mental Hospitals, Orphanages, and So Forth

Gambrill (1977) argues that BT does not dehumanize people. Yet its application as behavior modification of one sort or another in a variety of congregate-care institutions for involuntary patients often flies in the face of Gambrill's insistence that BT should recognize "the roles of thoughts and feelings . . . offering the client skills that will enable greater influence over his environment" (p. 15). In fact, BT has taken on a very different role in many institutions, appropriating a language of helping in order to mask its frank use to preserve order. Despite the repeated incorporation of more cognitive components, the fundamental assumption of behaviorism, largely carried into forms of BT intended for the involuntary patient, is that environmental reinforcements and cues determine the behavior of organisms. The recent attempts in CBT to soften this tenet mystifies the actual role of BT in understaffed, under-funded, and frequently neglected residential programs for a public that wishes to confuse coercion as philanthropy.

BT may be useful for some severely debilitated patients. Yet even for these groups, its success is questionable. Still, the generalization of BT methods from the back wards to more functional populations tends to justify the broader use of restriction. Indeed, it constitutes a form of coercion without adjudication, treating troubled people as if they were criminals and justifying the very neglect that BT was initially developed to confront. The use of a solution as a symbol that actually perpetuates a problem is not all that unique. For example, Stein and Test (1980) demonstrated the possibility of maintaining long-staying psychiatric patients in community settings with appropriate support services; however, the cost of community care *exceeded* the cost of hospital care. The Stein and Test demonstration was routinely cited by the federal and state governments to justify the deinstitutionalization of the mentally ill, but perversely, in order to *decrease* allocations for their care.

Treatment for psychiatric patients customarily requires drug therapy; BT is adjunctive. BT for the psychiatric patient reflects the assumption that "abnormal behavior, even that stemming from biological disturbances, can be favorably influenced by therapeutic arrangements of an individual's inter-action with his or her environment . . . [because] instrumental and interpersonal behaviors are more readily changed than cognitive and affective levels of behavior" (Corrigan and Liberman, 1994, p. 3). BT assumes that cognitive and affective changes will follow behavioral adaptations. Thus the typical BT for the psychiatric patient applies a pattern of rewards and punishments to the patient in order to elicit desired behaviors.

BT in the psychiatric hospital entails token economies and skills-training methods "to enable patients to acquire and perform behaviors that help them cope with interpersonal stressors" (Corrigan and Liberman, 1994, p. 15). BT involves attempts to establish an environment that prevents patient violence and promotes "prosocial behaviors" through social learning theory. Token economies reinforce adaptive patient behaviors that have already been learned with tokens that can be exchanged for a variety of desired items. The following example of a token-economy program is drawn from the Camarillo State Hospital.

> THERAPIST: So, how did you do washing your face? I would like you to look in the mirror and tell me if your face is clean.
> PATIENT (*examining face in mirror*): It's OK.
> T: Any soap still on it?
> P: No, looks clean to me.
> T: I agree. You did an excellent job washing your face. How many tokens do you earn for that?
> P: Two.
> T: OK, what's next? (Corrigan and Liberman, 1994, p. 48)

Importantly, the reinforcement effects of the tokens cannot be separated from the reinforcement effects of the therapist's commendation. Indeed, no token-economy experiment has provided adequate controls to learn whether the tokens or the environment of therapy itself, including the relationship between staff and patient, accounts for behavioral changes. All of the nine examples of BT that Corrigan and Liberman (1994) describe rely upon single subject designs that substitute baseline comparisons for randomized non-treatment controls. It is notable that all of the baseline measures are taken in the absence of staff/patient relationships comparable to those that existed during the experimental BT procedures. Thus it remains quite likely that the tokens are only metaphors of the necessary ingredients for successful therapy. Rather than an advance in treatment, they are a symbol that cheapens the actual warmth and caring that may produce behavioral change in severely disabled patients. However, as metaphor, the reduction of the disabled to automatons only capable of mechanistic responses is apparently preferable to pressing their capacity for human emotions and their rights to humane care.

The other important component of BT for psychiatric patients, social-skills training, teaches adaptive behaviors that have not previously been learned or have been forgotten. These skills include "interpersonal communication, coping, and problem-solving abilities . . . including self-care, conversation, assertion, job seeking, dating and friendship, and symptom and medication self-management" (Corrigan and Liberman, 1994, p. 1920). A variety of tech-niques are intended to assist patients in transferring these skills to less super-vised situations outside of the hospital, hopefully enabling them to rejoin families. These extended applications of behavioral principles include train-ing families to care for their severely disabled relative and vocational rehabil-itation for the patient. The community services are remarkably similar to Stein and Test's (1980) program.

Yet the literature of BT for the psychiatric patient has diverted attention away from the probable sources of patient improvements, assuming they have occurred. Rather than the "scientific" nature of the BT interventions or the specificity of techniques, the compassion and effort of the staff in the demon-stration hospitals probably explains any therapeutic outcome. The culture of psychiatry in particular undercuts less lofty and possibly more effective care for the mentally ill. In fact, in all of the studies that testify to the benefits of BT in mental hospitals, the staffs were enormously motivated both personally and professionally to prove the effectiveness of their techniques. They were advocates, if not actually zealots, of BT for the mentally ill, hardly dispassion-ate scientists. Many patients probably responded to human kindness and con-cern more than to the game of tokens.

At the same time, the basic research that adapted BT for the psychiatric hospital was compromised by a host of likely biases and methodological pitfalls, not least of all, by the absence of adequate controls. Even the few randomized experiments suffer a large number of problems in isolating the cause of their outcomes as well as establishing the outcomes themselves. Paul and Lentz (1977) reported impressive gains for milieu therapy and especially for social-learning therapy over customary in-patient care during more than five years of in-hospital and community treatment. The treatment groups evidenced more adaptive patient behaviors, much less use of psychotropic drugs, higher community placement rates, and better and longer adaptation to community settings.

However, the demonstration was conducted in a chaotic political and funding situation, with the project being terminated prematurely and unexpectedly. Indeed, the threats to its continuation encouraged the staff to exaggerate in-patient improvement, to increase community placements of treated patients, and to maintain those placements. The potential biases were facilitated by the measurement procedures and the lack of blinding; staff conducted all patient assessments while aware of the patients' assignment to milieu therapy, social-learning therapy, and control conditions. In addition, treatment staff were responsible for decisions to place patients in community settings and to readmit them to the hospital. Yet because of the extremely impaired condition of the patients whom the experiment ended up treating, the study sample had "a zero probability of release to relatively independent functioning" (Paul and Lentz, 1977, p. 16). Rather than relative independence, the goal of the community placements changed to "significant release" and conditions in the community placements that appear to have replicated many of the restrictive conditions of hospitalization.

The problem of compromised neutrality, reactive assessments, and biased placement decisions in the Paul and Lentz experiment recalls the California Youth Authority's community placement program for delinquents in the 1960s (Palmer, 1974). That experiment's positive results were notoriously concocted through the administrative decisions of staff to "re-incarcerate" failed delinquents within the community setting and, therefore, boost at least the perception of its success in keeping them out of prison (Lerman, 1975). Similarly, Paul and Lentz's (1977) administrative and assessment procedures seem to have created the possibility that the impressive reported gains of BT with very disabled psychiatric patients were largely a tribute to impaired objectivity and a demonstration effect created by the unusually motivated staff. In fact, the staff's reluctance to terminate community placements is suggested by Paul and Lentz's observation that "about one fifth of all releases [disproportionately including the BT patients] had declined in functioning after community placement to levels that were lower than those that existed when they were previously rejected for community placement" (p. 411).

Thus, through the subtle manipulations of complex social and clinical experiments, BT and community placement persist as unsubstantiated treatments but, more importantly, as metaphors for heroic individualism—the insistence that self-reliance is possible for even extremely debilitated psychiatric patients. Even in this case, self-reliance implies diminished public responsibility. Perhaps the production of socially useful metaphors resolves the paradox of many social-service experiments that experimental staff with obvious personal and professional stakes in the success of their programs are permitted to evaluate the outcomes of those programs.

The evaluative research of BT for psychiatric patients reduces to the mundane likelihood that any actual gains are the result of common decency, surveillance, and surrogate care—the decision to treat disabled people well—rather than to any elegance or insight of care. Getting beyond the verbiage of conditioning and the grandiosity of BT, Corrigan and Liberman's (1994) experiments simply provided a number of practical and humane services for psychiatric patients: close surveillance in the hospital and during aftercare, opportunities and encouragement for patients to perform at their level of capacity, and surrogate care for what they cannot do themselves. The therapeutic value is debatable, but the practical value of creating a supportive environment to handle chronic afflictions is obvious.

Following the Stein and Test (1980) experience, BT for the psychiatric patient appears to be expensive and staff intensive. Cost rather than caring explains the observation that "despite three decades of empirically documented success in psychiatric hospitals, clinically applied behavioral technology has a poor sales record" (Corrigan and Liberman, 1994, p. 221). Corrigan and Liberman attributed the resistance to differences in treatment approaches, ignorance, and a lack of resources. The more telling point, a derivative of their observations, is that most psychiatric hospitals may not be particularly concerned about the welfare of their patients. The positive effects in the demonstration hospitals cannot be replicated in others that simply try to apply the enumerated techniques of BT to lessen costs. The replications require the attention, compassion, and motivations of the demonstrations. Indeed, that may be all that is necessary to achieve the modest effects of the literature. The history of care for severely handicapped people, especially poor ones, continues as a sorry commentary on American life.

BT in psychiatric settings did not translate to other institutions as simple decency but rather as a scientific endorsement of sternness and regimentation, perhaps even serving to endorse neglect of the severely disabled. In orphanages such as Boys Town and in other residential settings for youths, notably the typical reform school, BT, with its unremitting emphasis on "consequences," has trained up a generation of youth that curse the regimentation—"the [expletive] rules." They are treated like feral animals that need to be broken. The luckiest go on to military careers; the others disappear quickly into the Willow World of American society. Indeed, it is unusual for researchers to reach even 20% of foster children two years after they are "emancipated" at the age of eighteen from the court supervision of foster care. But the appalling neglect of congregate residences for youth is given the cachet of "treatment" by the invocation of BT theory. Punishment is made necessary and noble by reference to animal studies of avoidance behavior; rewards are narrow and institutionally sterile, and again, made desirable by reinforcement theory. Good staff frequently have the sense to employ the language of BT in their reports to board and funding authorities but display a far more discretionary affection for the children themselves.

However, the possibility of greater freedom, more specialized and personalized care, middle-class opportunities for education and cultural development, staff with the capacity to develop warm relationships, and an assurance of relative permanence in placement have been pushed aside by social acceptance of the correctness of BT for troubled youth. It is also telling that the severity of public foster care seems largely reserved for the children of poor and lower-status parents. The environment of encouragement at residential schools for wealthy children is very different. In fact, the harsh emotional environment for children in public congregate care enacts the nation's bare-knuckles attitude toward poor and lower-status groups—the witlessly intemperate and brutishly impulsive—rather than its generosity, patience, and affection for more prosperous citizens.

BT for the profoundly mentally retarded is implemented to teach rudimentary behaviors, but frequently the learned behaviors appear to have little more than ritualistic meaning.

Three profoundly mentally retarded nonverbal institutionalized men were identified as subjects for an experimental study to determine whether behavioral techniques could enhance their participation in a service of worship. A series of nine gestures were trained which were a physical expression of a simplified confession of faith. Intervention with quiet verbal prompts by observer-trainers during recitation of the gestural confession of faith by a congregation of worshipers tripled the number of gestures performed by the subjects. It was concluded that behavioral techniques can enhance participation in religious events by profoundly mentally retarded nonverbal people. (Henricksen and Mahr, 1987, p. 151)

"Participation" in this case takes on a Brave New World meaning. Institutional adaptation is obviously important, but the issue of enforced ceremonial obedience to social norms, such as religiosity, does not appear to have any semblance of therapeutic value or even meaning as free choice.

Conclusion

BT is only metaphorically related to behaviorism and conditioning, both of which reject hypothetical constructs as causes of behavior and dispute the experimental utility of subjective states of consciousness. Yet except in the rarest situation—perhaps token economies with severely handicapped patients—BT is still talk therapy, depending largely on cognition and other inner states that mediate between environmental stimuli and behavioral responses. Self-control, self-reliance, self-motivation, self-monitoring, self-reinforcement, indeed the stagy self-invention at the core of behavioral techniques for the needy who seek assistance, are not effective. Rather, BT underscores moral improvidence, that is, the incapacity for self-restraint, particularly among the institutionalized. Behavioral techniques that are imposed on reluctant, recalcitrant, rebarbative, or otherwise noncompliant, deviant, and maladaptive patients are pointless clinical interventions. Instead, they make sense ritualistically, as metaphors that condemn the lack of self-restraint as sin, debase patients for their deficits, and justify the deprivation of needed care.

9: Cognitive-Behavioral Therapy as Christian Science

Cognitive-behavioral therapy (CBT)—initially developed by Aaron Beck as cognitive therapy in the early 1960s but also variously called rational-emotive therapy, cognitive-behavioral modification, multimodal therapy, and other names depending on the theorist—emerged from a rejection of both psychodynamic therapy, notably psychoanalysis, as well as behavioral therapy. It added a largely volitional definition of cognition to each one, in return accepting some notions of unconscious motivation and conditioning. Its core assumption is that the individual is capable of changing personal behavior through conscious thought, that is, cognition. At least theoretically, cognitive assumptions differ from psychodynamic ones, emphasizing prior socialization, particularly within the family, and behavioral modes of learning, notably conditioning and Bandura's adaptations in social-learning theory.

The psychotherapeutic treatments inspired by psychotherapy, even the behavioral treatments, emphasize the patient's ability to modify personal behavior while they suggest different metaphors of personal responsibility. Perhaps the declining interest in behavioral therapies reflects a general preference for individual self-invention more than its inability to provide successful outcomes. That is, compared with CBT and the psychodynamic interventions, the basic tenets of behavioral therapy—environmental conditioning and mechanistic learning—were not adequately heroic in their assumptions of personal responsibility. Yet even the behavioral therapies made great demands on the individual; after all, the willingness to proceed through the successive approximations of systematic desensitization reflected on the patient's character.

Since all of the psychotherapeutic theories usually defy direct tests of their accuracy except through the therapies they inspire, the universal failure of clinical experiments to provide scientifically credible evidence of effective outcomes suggests that psychotherapy's major contribution is metaphoric. Rather than as a successful clinical form, psychotherapy as a cognitive process, that is, CBT, provides a socially cherished symbol—individual thought, cognition—that explains its popularity. In fact, CBT appears to be the favored contemporary choice of psychotherapy, eclipsing psychodynamic and behavioral treatments as American society intensifies its preference for personal responsibility over social responsibility, exaggerating an already exaggerated heroic individualism.

Yet CBT, like all of psychotherapy, is more akin to the mysticism of mind cure and faith healing than to clinical science. Its tenets, demands on patients, and metaphysical texts, except for its contemporary style, recall Christian Science. Both make much of patient expectancies, true belief, faith in healing, and the curious proposition of mind over matter. While the literary styles of their founding texts differ dramatically (although neither in beauty nor in clarity), their social roles are remarkably alike. Both dramatize dominant social values; both emphasize heroic individualism. And, not to miss the point, both fail to provide predictable clinical cures. While modern medicine has made a mockery of Mary Baker Eddy's teachings, there is no similar rational threat to the continuation of CBT. As long as its central metaphor of individual cognition implies individual responsibility, and barring the unlikely rebellion of the field against itself on grounds of ineffectiveness, CBT will endure as a cherished social religion. CBT and Christian Science are two kindred fables of heroic individualism, scripted for different times but for similar audiences.

The Theory of CBT

The energetic entrepreneur who founded the Beck Institute for Cognitive Therapy, Aaron Beck is one of the earliest exponents of CBT and continues to publish voluminously. Beck claims that the cognitive model—its basic assertions about psychopathology—and it application to clinical practice rest on sound empirical evidence of effectiveness. He proposes twelve theoretical propositions that undergird treatment. One, people form cognitive representations of the environment. Two, they process information at different levels of consciousness in promoting efficiency and adaptability. Three, reality is personally constructed. Four, information serves as "a guiding principle for the emotional, behavioral, and physiological components of human experience," which means that cognition is not simply expressive but importantly causative, perhaps even determinative of human behavior (Clark and Beck, 1999, p. 62). Five, cognition consists of interaction between stimulus-driven behavioral processes and "higher-order" semantic processes, that is, conscious thought (ibid., p. 63). Yet six, cognitive constructions only approximate experience, distorted by "egocentric" motives that "filter" reality. Seven, meaning is imposed on experience by the interaction of environment with "innate rudimentary schemas" (ibid., p. 65). Eight, meaning is hierarchical: broader concepts encompass more specific concepts. Nine, different meaning processes are activated at different thresholds. Ten, the information processing is geared to two types of activities ("goals"): primary survival activities of cognitive, behavioral, affective, motivational, and physiological schemas operate largely at the "preconscious" level; the second level of activities pursues "personal goals and aspirations . . . as well as the norms and guiding principles of society" (ibid., p. 68). Eleven, psychological problems emerge because meaning, "the schemas," is either overactivated or underactivated. The assumption is that the misactivation distorts reality. Twelve, therefore, therapy focuses on changing the misactivated schemas by bringing cognition into better alignment with objective reality.[1]

Thus people are depressed because they have learned preconsciously to react automatically to stimuli in a depressed way. That is, their distorted depressive schemas, "their negative automatic thoughts," are activated by a variety of situations: "Certain cognitive patterns could be responsible for the patients' tendency to make negatively biased judgments of themselves, their environment, and their future" (ibid., p. 49). These distortions ("the cognitive errors") include arbitrary inference, selective abstraction, overgeneralization, magnification/minimization, and others.

Yet none of these negative judgments are compared to the reality of the patients' situations but only contrasted with the patients' own assessments of the consistency of their behaviors. Cognitive research, in the manner of most psychological research, is impaired in assessing any internal function except by means of associated behaviors that in the context of treatment are named through patient self-report. However, the items under study, for example, depression and anxiety, are invariably internal states—moods, dispositions, attitudes, and so forth. In treatment, the only behavior that is under investigation in most of the clinical research is the patients' language, that is, their self-reports. Still, the necessity for accurate description that lies at the heart of any true science may be sidestepped for practical ends if, in fact, the theory produces credible evidence of patient improvement despite the conceptual imprecision and lack of rigorous specification.

Further, the distinction between schemas and modes that Beck makes much of exists only as an interpretive device. Like Freud's three components of the psyche—id, ego, and superego—schemas and modes have no relationship to physical functions or anatomical locations. It is not even clear that the reported behaviors, emotions, and beliefs that are customarily used to define the clinical conditions do, in fact, constitute adequate definitions of the clinical problems.

Clark and Beck (1999) concluded on the basis of "considerable empirical support" that, as two examples among many that sustain their cognitive model, "negative cognitive organization plays an important role in shaping the depressive experience" (p. 172) and depressive thinking exists even in those who are not yet depressed (p. 290). Yet this base of research has even more problems of specificity than the outcome research. It invariably employs abstractions of the clinical problem—for example, "depressogenic" events—and thought processes that are only patient self-reports, lacking any objective standing except as language with uncertain meaning. Thus explorations of these phenomena that attempt to pinpoint the order of their occurrence (for example, whether automatic thoughts precede depression or whether modes are presets of emotional reactions) and, therefore, attempt to pinpoint their causal roles are again greatly hampered by the problem of specification and the absence of neutral, physical (objective) assessment. Preconscious learning, schemas, personal construction of reality, cognitive constructions, basic purposes, and the rest are all elusive notions—hypothetical constructs. Indeed, Beck's theory is reminiscent of ex post facto attempts to impose motive on a consistency of behavior, with the result that motive often exists more in the observer than the observed, raising the issue of the intentions of research itself.

It is notable that Beck's theory appears in many regards to recast the form and occasionally even the substance of Freud, for example, distortions instead of defense mechanisms, automatic activation and electrical charges (A. Beck, in Salkovskis, 1996) rather than pneumatic processes, including unconscious motives. While Beck insists that the theory has been impressively validated by research, the validating research is even more tenuous than the clinical tests of effectiveness. Aside from the constant problem of researchers evaluating their own theories without maintaining distance from the love of their own hypotheses, nearly all of the critical information about the patient's or subject's internal states is self-reported. Accordingly, there remains a serious problem of accuracy in the self-report and a serious inability to measure psychological states objectively. But even more debilitating, none of the twelve principles are easily specified for testing. They remain hypothetical constructs, states of mind, rather than specified, objective entities.

Most problematic, the central notion of causal direction, that cognition rules emotion, behavior, and perhaps even physiology, has not been adequately proven by any test. Indeed, alternative assumptions—for example, that the environment or primitive emotion determines behavior and that cognition is usually expressive post hoc representation—remain equally plausible. Notably in relation to cause but also in many other portions of the theory, Beck and others are evasive.

> Because it was proposed [by Beck himself in earlier works] that schemas take a primary role in directing the dysfunctional information processing that characterizes depression, other writers assumed that the cognitive model asserts that the activation of maladaptive schemas causes

depression. However, cognitive theory is quite clear in stating that a combination of factors may cause depression including biological, genetic, stress, and personality variables. . . . Thus the theory restricts the conceptualization of schema activation to that of a hypothetical explanation for the development of depression. . . . From this perspective, then, negative self-referent schemas constitute a hypothesized feature of depression that can be tested at the descriptive level without invoking any notion of causality. (Clark and Beck, 1999, p. 217)

Yet if not as an important point for clinical intervention, that is, as a cause of depression, what is the point of simply describing schema activation? The central position of schema activation in CBT is precisely what has led many to conclude that it is proposed as an important sustaining (if not original) cause of depression and therefore a focus for clinical intervention. A. Beck (in Salkovskis, 1996) has insisted that his theory has matured over thirty years to abandoning "simple schematic processing" in favor of modal processing, presumably now amplifying cognition with affect, behavior, physiology, genetics, and motivation. Yet cognition—distorted automatic thoughts—still retains central billing as a *cause* for emotional problems, and therefore cognition is maintained as the strategic target of interventions. In particular, while Beck has recognized that environmental cues trigger problematic reactions, his theory only attends to the individual's responses to those conditions and clearly not to the conditions themselves.

After all, the individual, the captain and master of personal destiny and fate, is presumed to own his or her emotions. Otherwise, CBT would not make any sense at all. This is no small point, since CBT and psychotherapy generally intervene with individuals and not with the environment. However, the strategic choices of CBT are not made rationally (although they may be cognitive) in consideration of interventions that may make the most sense for patients (that is, changing their environment) but as a result of convenience and social preference, predicated on the assumption of self-determining individual action and therefore individual responsibility—heroic free will leading to extreme personal responsibility. Moreover, it needs to be emphasized that the subtle relationship between the individual and the environment has not been worked out, or there would exist little dispute between personal and social responsibility.

In fact, the cognitive model, that is, CBT theory, becomes dissociated from CBT practice if the activation of depressive schemas or the later identification of modes fails as a cause for depression. However, because the literature cannot sustain a causal relationship, Clark and Beck (1999) fell back on the explanation that they were simply describing depression rather than defining its etiology. A theory built upon a series of hypothetical constructs can retreat quickly from any conflict with empirical evidence by claiming that it is simply descriptive, that it does not predict other events, or that the wrong predictions were derived.

Yet even in his revised format, A. Beck (1996, in Salkovskis) was quite clear that dysfunctional modes are impediments to cure and that the favored strategic interventions are cognitive.

> There are three major approaches to "treating" the dysfunctional modes: first, deactivating them, second, modifying their structure and content, and third, priming or "constructing" more adaptive modes to neutralize them. In actual practice, the first and third procedures are carried out simultaneously, for example, demonstrating that a particular belief is wrong or dysfunctional and that another belief is more accurate and adaptive. . . . If [patients] recognize that their interpretation of "danger" was wrong, or when they determine the danger has passed, the primal mode is deactivated. . . . Corrective information from an acknowledged authority not only contradicts the content . . . embodied in the mode but also activates a "safety mode," incorporating a more realistic belief. (pp. 15–16)

In a curious way, the creation of an "acknowledged authority" cuts against a cognitive faith in reason, recalling psychodynamic forces and even perhaps psychoanalytic assumptions about transference as the essential element of successful therapy. With an unfortunate kinship to Freudian psychoanalysis, CBT seems to defy testing in that it explains both confirmatory and disconfirmatory information, failing to specify the conditions under which it can be falsified. For example, if the patient reports automatic thoughts, well and good, but if the patient does not, then he or she is unaware of them due to preconscious or subconscious hypothesized processes, which are difficult to specify and measure. Thus cognitive theory becomes sealed off from empirical tests of its tenets. As a result, it collapses from scientific theory to a metaphysics disguised by the elaborate jargon of social-science research and by a large number of periphrastic relationships between uncertain entities. In fact, CBT has been variously criticized within the field for many of these defects (Blaney, 1977; Coyne and Gotlib, 1983; Teasdale and Bernard, 1993). Yet its popularity seems to make it impervious to criticism.

Despite the enormous amount of research cited to sustain the different propositions of the cognitive model and thus CBT, the theory has a contrived, ad hoc quality. It retreats from disconfirming evidence, proposing the unmeasurable to explain inconvenient findings. It relies on very uncertain discordant research that only allows box-score summaries of "many studies" or of "most research" or of "most evidence," or of seemingly "reasonable conclusions" or of "our review" or of some "evidence [that] was found." Like the rest of psychotherapy, CBT's clinical evidence is constructed almost entirely through patient self-reports, ignoring the demand characteristics of the research. Moreover, Clark and Beck (1999) as well as the rest of the field have suffered a partisan blindness toward research that challenges their views and a patriot's passion for confirmatory studies: disconfirmatory studies are closely critiqued, while supportive evidence is readily accepted. In short, cognitive evidence fails to sustain the causal propositions of the cognitive model.

Indeed, cause is often arbitrary in the sense that any behavior can be traced back infinitely to a variety of precursors. In this sense, the cognitive model and CBT exist as theories of the middle range, following Robert Merton. CBT does not purport to explain original or comprehensive factors but rather identifies the functional elements of positive clinical treatment. As a theory of the middle range, the sustaining causes of clinical problems identified by cognitive theory and, by implication, the usefulness of cognitive theory itself are assessed by the success of CBT in relieving those problems. Thus empty forms of clinical practice that are sustained in spite of their failure to cure, prevent, or rehabilitate beg for interpretation as rituals and ceremonies of social value.

The Practice of CBT

The assumptions of the cognitive model dictate the strategies, tactics, and techniques of CBT. Judith Beck (1995) has summarized her father's cognitive model in ten principles. One, the patient's problems are defined in cognitive terms: current thinking, precipitating factors, and enduring patterns of interpretation. Two, CBT requires "a sound therapeutic alliance" with the patient that, three, emphasizes collaboration and active participation in order to be, four, goal oriented and problem focused. Five, CBT initially emphasizes the present. Six, it is educative, emphasizing self-therapy and relapse prevention. Seven, it is time limited and, eight, structured. Nine and most central, CBT "teaches patients to identify, evaluate and respond to their dysfunctional thoughts and beliefs." The acknowledged ambiguity of these principles naturally leads to the tenth principle: CBT "uses a variety of techniques to change thinking, mood, and behavior" (J. S. Beck, 1995, pp. 5–9). The treatment assumptions probably boil down to a single theoretical assumption: "when a client argues against an irrational thought, and does so repeatedly, the irrational thought becomes progressively weaker" and rational behaviors become proportionately more likely (McMullin, 1986, p. 3).

In the foreword to his daughter's book, Aaron Beck has enthusiastically endorsed Judith's efforts as representative of "a new generation of therapists/ researchers/teachers" who have successfully applied CBT to "a broad spectrum of psychiatric disorders" (J. S. Beck, 1995, p. x).

> The applications of cognitive therapy to a host of psychological and medical disorders extended far beyond anything I could have imagined when I treated my first few cases of depression and anxiety with cognitive therapy. On the basis of outcome trials, investigators throughout the world, but particularly the United States, have established that cognitive therapy is effective in conditions as diverse as posttraumatic stress disorder, obsessive-compulsive disorder, phobias of all kinds, and eating disorders. Often in combination with medication it has been helpful in the treatment of bipolar affective disorder and schizophrenia. Cognitive therapy has also been found to be beneficial in a wide variety of chronic medical disorders such as low back pain, colitis, hypertension, and chronic fatigue syndrome. (Ibid.)

Judith Beck's (1995) session-by-session description of practice detailed the application of the cognitive model to CBT. It also provided a narrative of therapy that is amenable to a different interpretation than one based on the centrality of the patient's problems.

The first session of treatment is designed to orient the patient and set expectations for therapy. It entails "establishing trust and rapport, socializing the patient into cognitive therapy, educating the patient about her disorder, about the cognitive model, and about the process of therapy, normalizing the patient's difficulties and instilling hope, eliciting (and correcting, if necessary) the patient's expectations for therapy, gathering additional information, using this information to develop a goal list" (J. S. Beck, 1995, p. 26). These objectives are structured into specific tasks such as "doing a mood check," "identifying problems and setting goals," and so forth. These tasks are worked out through enumerated procedures. Throughout, Judith Beck has illustrated treatment by quoting from the session transcripts of a depressed patient she treated. The patient was apparently an undergraduate student.

In order to assess the patient's mood at the first session, the therapist has the patient rate her mood prior to the session and then goes over the ratings with her during the session, graphing the responses to demonstrate progress over the subsequent sessions. A variety of instruments to measure mood are apparently appropriate, each one repeated at each session.

> THERAPIST (T): Okay, next. How about if we start with how you've been doing this week. Can I see the forms you filled out? (*Looks them over.*) It seems as if you're still pretty depressed and anxious; these scores haven't changed much since the evaluation (*Presumably the intake evaluation*). Does that seem right?
> PATIENT (P): Yes I guess I'm still feeling pretty much the same.
> T: (*Giving rationale.*) If it's okay with you, I'd like you to come to every session a few minutes early so you can fill out these three forms. They help give me a quick idea of how you've been feeling in the past week, although I always want you to describe how you've been doing in your own words, too. Is that okay with you?
> P: Sure. (J. S. Beck, 1995, pp. 29–30)

Similarly, the agenda items for each session are worked out through prescribed dialogue and content. Rapport is established and constantly refreshed by the therapist, whose

> implicit and sometimes explicit messages are that he cares about and values the patient; that he is confident they can work together; that he believes he can help her and that she can learn to help herself; that he really wants to understand what she's experiencing and what it's like "to walk in her shoes"; that he's not overwhelmed by her problems, even though *she* might be; that he has seen and helped other patients much like her; and that he believes cognitive therapy is the appropriate treatment for her and that she will get better. (Emphasis in original; ibid., p. 27)

The therapist seems oblivious to the likelihood that the patient's repeated self-assessments on the same instruments create practice effects and distortions that emerge from the established "rapport," the therapeutic alliance between therapist and patient. The therapist *expects* the patient to improve session by session. Without much attention to accuracy, concrete measurement—the essential behavioral component of CBT—itself becomes a ritual of participation.

Inappropriate thoughts are the defining characteristic of CBT. "The cognitive model states that the interpretation of a situation (rather than the situation itself), often expressed in automatic thoughts, influences one's subsequent emotion, behavior, and physiological response" (J. S. Beck, 1995, p. 75).

During the first session and then throughout each subsequent session, the therapist has corrected the patient's negative thoughts under the assumption that thoughts lead to feelings and behavior rather than the reverse, that is, that emotions lead to thoughts and behaviors or that pleasurable behaviors induce cognitive justifications.

> P: I was afraid you'd think I was crazy.
> T: Not at all, you have a fairly common illness or problem called depression, and it sounds as though you have a lot of the same problems as most of our patients here. But again, that's a good automatic thought, "You'll think I'm crazy." How do you feel now that you've found out it isn't true?
> P: Relieved.
> T: So correcting your thinking *did* help. If you have any more thoughts like that, would you write them down for homework so we can evaluate them at our next session?
> P: Sure.
> T: This kind of very negative thinking is one symptom of your depression. Depression affects how you see yourself, your world, and your future. For most people who are depressed, it's as if they're seeing themselves and their worlds through eyeglasses covered with black paint. Everything looks black and hopeless. Part of what we'll do in therapy is to scrape off the black paint and help you see things more realistically . . . Does that analogy make sense to you?
> P: Yeah. I understand. (Emphasis in original; J. S. Beck, 1995, pp. 38–39)

At the end of each session the patient is assigned homework to reinforce the lessons of therapy and provide continuing involvement with the content of the sessions. All of the subsequent sessions are structured in the same way: checking on mood and updating concerns, bridging from the prior session, setting the agenda, reviewing homework, discussing and handling progress, summary, and feedback—but always with an eye to correcting distorted cognitions, that is, inappropriate automatic thoughts and more fundamental distorted beliefs, as demonstrated in a subsequent session:

> T: . . . What emotion were you feeling: sad? anxious? angry?
> P: Sad.
> T: What was going through your mind?
> P: I was looking at these other students, talking or playing frisbee, hanging out on the lawn.
> T: What was going through your mind when you saw them?

p: I'll never be like them.

t: Okay. You just identified what we call an *automatic thought.* Everyone has them. They're thoughts that just seem to pop into our heads. We're not deliberately trying to think about them; that's why we call them automatic. Most of the time, they're real quick and we're much more aware of the emotion—in this case, sadness—than we are of the thoughts. Lots of times the thoughts are distorted in some way. But we react *as if* they're true. (Emphasis in original; J. S. Beck, 1995, p. 78)

In order to handle automatic thoughts, the therapist must have the skills to elicit them during sessions. A variety of techniques are suggested for this end, for example, asking the basic question, "What was going through your mind just then?" and then following up with a series of questions to probe the response, for example, "What did the situation mean to you?" role playing, and others. Freeman and Dattilio (1992) provide an extended list of these techniques: downward arrow, idiosyncratic meaning, labeling of distortions, questioning the evidence, examining options and alternatives, reattribution, decatastrophizing, exaggeration, turning adversity to advantage, replacement imagery, cognitive rehearsal, behavioral techiques, assertivenss training, behavioral rehearsal, graded task assignments, bibliotherapy, relaxation and meditation, social skills training, schema attacking exercises, and, always, homework (p. 7).

The basic assumption pervades CBT that even when the patient is unaware of them, automatic thoughts cause problematic emotions and must be handled. Thus much time is spent encouraging the patient to identify automatic thoughts, differentiating between automatic thoughts and interpretations, between those that are useful and less useful, and even between thoughts and emotions. After all, if the inappropriate cognitions cannot be identified, there is nothing for CBT to focus on.

There are a great variety of cognitive distortions corrected by the therapist: all-or-nothing thinking, catastrophizing, disqualifying the positive, and so forth. Indeed they appear to be quite similar to Freud's identification of defense mechanisms such as rationalization, projection, and sublimation.

t: When people predict the worst, we call it fortune telling or catastrophizing—believing that a catastrophe might happen. Are you aware of catastrophizing much?

p: I think I probably do.

t: How about if you try this week to catch yourself catastrophizing? When you write down an automatic thought, see if that's what you're doing, and if so, write "catastrophizing" next to it. (J. S. Beck, 1995, p. 120)

Cognitive distortions are customarily handled through a presumably rational process of testing the patient's thoughts against the reality of the patient's environment. Yet it should be noted that the rational content is always filtered through the patient's perceptions and reports. There are no independent assessments of the patient's situation.

> T: How much do you believe that the professor won't think you're wasting his time or, if he does, that that's what he's being paid for anyway?
>
> P: I do believe it, but—
>
> T: But?
>
> P: But I still think I should work it out myself.
>
> T: Well, that's another possibility, maybe you should. Should we look rationally at whether you're better off working it out yourself or going to him for help? (J. S. Beck, 1995, p. 124)

Patients are encouraged to keep "automatic thought records" and refer back to them during their homework. Automatic thought records constitute a graphic reminder of therapy and the patient's responses that Beck claims may be helpful in preventing relapse. Together with the overall structure of CBT— an emphasis on cognitions and rationality, the therapist as teacher, enumerated sessions, notebooks and homework, lesson plans, follow-up, and so forth—CBT looks like an adaptation of schooling. It is not surprising, therefore, that Beck chose a university student as the case example. But schooling is as much a social institution with defined social roles as it is a specific method of achieving educational goals. Indeed, the ritual of CBT seems modeled after the ritual of schooling. However, deprived of credible evidence of effectiveness, the schooling ritual of CBT raises issues about its use of a common, trusted social authority (the teacher) to undermine the natural skepticism of patients.

CBT also modifies inappropriate intermediate beliefs, "the deeper, often unarticulated ideas or understandings that patients have about themselves, others, and their personal worlds which give rise to specific automatic thoughts" (J. S. Beck, 1995, p. 137). Again, by invoking a variety of amorphous, unconscious levels of thought, CBT parallels psychodynamic therapy in retreat from a commitment to rigorous objectivity. The therapist is directed to draw a "cognitive conceptualization diagram" (copyrighted in 1993 by J. S. Beck) to relate intermediate thoughts to the patient's automatic thoughts.

Intermediate thoughts are elicited during therapy especially in order to overcome a variety of patient blockages. The therapist identifies intermediate beliefs by recognizing when a belief is expressed as an automatic thought, providing the first part of an assumption, using the downward arrow and other techniques. Beck illustrates the downward arrow technique:

> T: . . . what would that mean to you?
> P: I didn't do a very good job in class.
> T: Okay, if it's true that you didn't do a very good job in class, what would that mean?
> P: I'm a lousy student.
> T: . . . what does that mean about you?
> P: I'm not good enough. [I am inadequate] [*core belief*] (J. S. Beck, 1995, p. 145)

The admission of inadequacy is central to the beliefs of the therapist, the notion that as an intermediate belief it gives coherence to depression. Yet feelings of inadequacy, along with the other characteristics of depression, may be related to more global and central experiences and not directly amenable to therapeutic resolution. Indeed, bad feelings may be the results of inappropriate environmental influences that typically defy modification by discussion. But here and throughout the therapeutic exchange, it is not clear whether the patient is handling her own reality or simply conforming to the therapist's coherence in becoming a psychological equivalent of the "rice Christian." Especially when the therapist fancies herself as a teacher of a very specific theory, the therapeutic relationship may be the vehicle for achieving the patient's conformity with the therapist's demands for agreement. The therapist rewards the patient for identifying, at long last, what the therapist expects to hear, and the patient enjoys a brief moment of approval. However, continuing problems may persist even while the therapeutic environment creates obvious incentives, indeed, instructions, for the patient to misrepresent improvement and maintain, at least symbolically, the therapist's continued loyalty and warm regard.

Educating patients about beliefs is important. But the education is not grounded in the prowess of the cognitive model to rationally establish the causal therapeutic relationships of the cognitive mode.

> T: Well, the bad news is that you currently have a set of beliefs which aren't bringing you much satisfaction, right? The good news is that since you *learned* this current set of beliefs, you can unlearn them and learn others. . . . How does that sound? (Emphasis in original; J. S. Beck, 1995, p. 149)

This is precisely the promise of organizations seeking members, churches seeking converts, and spiritual movements seeking believers: your current behavior is wrong, self-defeating, and unsatisfying; we can teach you better ways of living. The recruitment becomes cultish to the extent that coercive forms of persuasion are employed in substitution for objective proof and to the extent that the proffered doctrine occupies the personality and constrains the free will of the potential recruit. CBT is constantly pressing, chiding, encouraging, and inveighing the patient, through the demands of the therapeutic relationship, to believe, believe, believe in the curative ability of treatment and the authority of the therapist. Moreover, CBT, with all of its occupying techniques, can easily transcend the bounded concerns of specific emotional problems and become a philosophy and a prescriptive regimen of adaptation and adjustment to social norms.

The issue of norms—the advantages and disadvantages of beliefs—is central to treatment and frequently implies accepting the customary social virtues. One example:

T: What are the *advantages* of believing if you don't do your best then you're a failure?

P: Well, it might make me work harder.

T: I'd be interested to see if you actually *need* such an extreme belief to keep you working hard. . . . *Disadvantages?* . . .

P: I feel miserable when I don't do well on an exam. . . .

T: . . . Okay so on one hand, it may or may not actually be true that this belief is the only thing that makes you work hard. On the other hand, this belief about having to live up to your potential makes you feel miserable when you don't do great, makes you more nervous than you have to be before presentations, cuts into your enjoyment of your work, and stops you from doing other things you like. Is that right?

P: Yes.

T: Is this an idea, then, that you'd like to change? (Emphasis in original; J. S. Beck, 1995, pp. 149–150)

There are a number of expressions of heroic individualism in this exchange: first, that hard work is important and that living up to one's personal potential, a national resource, verges on a moral obligation, but second and more important, that through a largely introspective process, the patient can by herself, through her own will, achieve personal change. The idea of a heroic overcoming is constantly conveyed through therapy, and with CBT, largely short-term therapy—that within a few months the patient can overcome environment and autobiography largely through the heroic will to achieve personal goals. Not coincidentally, these are also the promises of cults and sects—that true belief, in its methods and faith, will activate hidden powers.

CBT designs a variety of presumably objective behavioral tests for the patient to take to evaluate her automatic thoughts and beliefs. Thus the therapist encourages a patient who believes that she will be belittled when she asks others for help to check out her beliefs by asking for help.

T: . . . It would be useful to find out if other people, in general, are more like me or not [that is, supportive and helpful]. How could you find out?

P: Ask other people for help, I guess.

T: . . . How about if we make a list of some of the possibilities? . . . After we have a list, you can decide whom you'd like to test these ideas with.

P: Okay.

T: Could you ask your roommate?

P: Yeah, actually I already do. And I could ask my resident advisor for help with something. (J. S. Beck, 1995, p. 155)

Yet both the patient's resistence as well as her subsequent effort are known only through the patient's self-reports. Indeed, it is never clear what the patient actually suffers from nor what she actually does. More problematically, the research has not clarified what the patient would do in the absence of CBT. In fact, it seems likely from the large placebo effects reported in the outcome literature that patients would routinely attempt to test their beliefs drawing encouragement from those around them. Thus this exchange with the therapist could be reinterpreted as a form of dependency, teaching the patient to rely upon an authority figure to gain motivation for simple tasks rather than to explore her own environment independently. Particularly in the present situation of a young student living in a college dorm, it seems likely that beliefs about her environment will be tested in the scheme of things through the usual social opportunities of her college experience. It is never clear whether the behavioral tests, along with the other obvious and simplistic techniques of CBT, are integral contributions to psychic relief or merely a series of rituals that bind the patient to the therapist and to conventional social authority for the performance of basic tasks.

Following the Becks, CBT posits only two types of negative core beliefs: inadequacy and unlovability, "the most central ideas about the self" that persist in the "mind." They are fundamental motivations that are formed in childhood. Again reminiscent of psychodynamic therapies, CBT's core beliefs are not fully

articulated until the therapist peels back the layers [of the mind] by continuing to ask for the meaning of the patient's thoughts. . . . The therapist begins to formulate a conceptualization (including core beliefs)
from the beginning of therapy. He does so mentally at first or privately
on paper. At some point in therapy he shares his conceptualization with
the patient, presenting it as a hypothesis and asking if it "rings true" to
her. (J. S. Beck, 1995, pp. 166–67)[2]

Yet the dualism of mind and body has still not been resolved; mind remains
an amorphous place, and its structures are hypothetical constructs, not locations in the brain. Still, clinical psychology recognizes, at least formally, the
experimental psychologist's distinction between the testable and the stubbornly metaphysical. "It is important to note that the new explanations proposed by learning theorists still relate directly to physical events and physiological processes. Researchers in clinical psychology seem less likely to anchor
their explanations in such events and processes, and we would caution that
when theorizing relies too heavily on indefinite terminology and analogous
reasoning, it loses explanatory power" (McMullin and Giles, 1981, p. 13). In
this way, automatic, intermediate, and core beliefs, lacking manifest anchors,
have a value only to the extent to which their use predicts important outcomes of CBT. This has not occurred; the outcomes of CBT are uncertain.
Instead, the jumble of CBT verbiage mystifies the patient's motivation and
emotional distress without demonstrating an ability to cure, prevent, or rehabilitate. The appearance of objectivity, for example in CBT's behavioral tests,
actually serves to further subjectify personal experience. It offers a new language of experience to patients as a totem of belief, an apotropaic charm, for
their recovery. The CBT process again looks like an induction ceremony into
a cult more than a serious attempt to describe emotional processes—a metaphysic of therapy rather than a clinically useful anatomy of emotions.

Furthermore, negative feelings may not be as dysfunctional as CBT con-
tends but rather formed by the secondary rewards of people performing their
roles, rejecting in a profound way more socially acceptable or desirable behaviors. In all probability, the patient has already failed to find motivation from
naturally occurring behavioral tests or has resisted their lessons or simply does
not find that the rewards of change outweigh the pleasures and attentions of
continued dysfunctionality. Rather, the patient continues to subjectivize reality in support of her negative feelings. Following both Zilbergeld (1983) and
Becker (1973), perhaps the patient needs to accept herself as a negative, unmo-
tivated person, opposed to the dominant American demand for optimism,
uplift, and self-help—a contribution to the diversity of American society.

The rejection of the dysfunctional core beliefs also implies an acceptance of the American ethos of heroic striving. It is difficult to bid against the economy of happy feelings, and CBT quite clearly proselytizes American buoyancy and hope. Still, reality for the downcast, the sad, the inattentive, the uncooperative, the violent, the oblivious, the depressed, and even the psychotic may, in fact, contain a sad social environment that needs correction before a greater incidence of happiness can be realized. Many people have earned their sorrow.

It is improbable that a person who has learned sadness over many years, and perhaps through the benefits of a long face, will change fundamental orientations during a few weeks of discussions with a therapist. This skepticism is sustained by the outcome literature's uniform failure to certify the curative ability of CBT. Moreover, the typical therapeutic exchange in the less systematic case material would not constitute credible theater, let alone credible treatment.

> T: Sally, we've been talking about this core belief, "I'm inadequate." What do you rationally think a more accurate belief might be?
> P: I am adequate?
> T: That's good. Or we could work on a new belief that might be easier for you to adopt, say, "I'm adequate in most ways, but I'm only human, too." Which sounds better?
> P: The second. (J. Beck, 1995)

Yet this exchange displays little that is rational, only the therapist's assurance that arriving at this conclusion is somehow superior, that is, rational. While the new belief seems reasonable, it is offered only as a first approximation of change. If the patient has not come to this modest conclusion in all her years, it seems improbable that she will now reach an epiphany in the temporary shelter of her therapist's office. In fact, if she does arrive at this conclusion, it is more likely the result of life changes rather than the product of a banal dialogue with a therapist.

The logic of successive approximation may appear to be rational, with modest change postulated as the antecedent of greater progress. But, in fact, this has not been empirically endorsed by the research. Instead, the process of little steps for little feet dramatizes cultural belief in individual change. It ritualizes the heroic credo of the United States. It is Franklinesque, a tenet of *Poor Richard's Almanac,* one of the culture's core beliefs, a command performance of institutional patriotism.

CBT has caused the proliferation of an enormous number of concrete techniques and strategies as well as a demand for detailed record keeping of specific behaviors. Each session is charted; moods are assessed; behaviors are recorded in detail; alternatives are weighed in behavioral terms; outcomes are measured. Yet just like the more complex outcome protocols, these little exercises in objectivity are neither reliable nor free of bias, failing on many points of actual and persistent subjectivity to handle the ambiguities of patient self-report. Moreover, the appearance of progress in therapy can simply be attributed to patient selection (that is, therapists treat patients who are motivated to seek therapy and might well have recovered from their complaints in any event) or patient expectancies, which can be as powerfully formed without the rare skills of the therapist, their long and expensive training, or the conditions of specific therapies. Thus CBT, with its trappings of science cultivated within a society entranced with its own pretentious rationality, is shamanistic and ritualistic but not specialized, truly coherent, or clinically productive.

More rational attention might revert to American society's failure to nurture citizen expectancies through greater conditions of economic and social parity rather than constantly hovering over self-invention and personal motivation through institutions such as psychotherapy. But in this way, by emphasizing the individual over the social, CBT and psychotherapy in general deflect attention away from the material deprivations of the society in favor of a disembodied insistence on individual responsibility.

CBT conveys a distinct preference for a client type despite its repeated insistence on near universal relevance. It is typical that Judith Beck's case example is a student and that the common recipient of CBT is a professional and relatively wealthy. As McMullin (1986) observed, "the typical profile for [the cognitive restructuring] client was that he or she was from an upper middle-class background, well-educated, and a very high achiever" (p. 3). Of the 32 case examples presented in Freeman and Dattilio (1992), 23 fit McMullin's description. The cases of the schizophrenic patient, the drug addict, and the child abuser were among the few that involved poor patients. Others are even more direct in acknowledging that CBT, with its emphasis on reasoning and logic, is intended for the highly verbal and productive. Indeed, the central metaphor of CBT as thought conveys a snobbery of intellect and class. Apparently the mute forms of behavior therapy, with their emphasis on punishment, are reserved for the lower orders, while psychodynamic therapy is affordable only by the truly wealthy embarked on a voyage of self-discovery and insight. Yet it is rare for any case example to present poor people in treatment for depression, anxiety, and phobia; the uninsured are apparently the residue of child molesters, psychotics, and addicts. In this subtle way, CBT endorses the distorted social schemas (stereotypes) that justify America's class divisions.

Additionally, the cultural patriotism of CBT reduces to the commonsensical and common injunction, folklore, to check personal belief against objective reality. CBT, however, has not demonstrated a systematic ability to encourage the unwilling to become more concrete, reasonable, or grounded. It seems rather to have fritzed up the process with unacknowledged parallels to existing social institutions—for example, schooling, optimism, guided self-help—and an endless number of contrived techniques channeled through the therapist to foster heroic individualism through an obsession with the concrete.

The romance of cognition and self-determination are obedient expressions of heroic overcoming and self-invention. CBT insists that the patient is sufficient, indeed, must be sufficient, to change his or her own thoughts and thus gain control of emotions and behavior but also that the patient carries a moral and ethical obligation to correct his or her distorted notions and dysfunctional behaviors. Thinking right, feeling right, and doing right compose the mantra of CBT, paeons to heroic and responsible self-control. Yet inevitably, control is exercised to transmit social norms that curiously tame the inflamed heroic imagination.

Heroic individualism, gnomic knowing, and a cultural loyalty with a strong sense of individual chosenness constitute a CBT of recruitment, cultish in its reliance on the patient's self-report and the therapist's manipulations. The therapist inspires and mediates the patient's reality checks, assisting the patient at all points to identify emotions, perceptions, thoughts, and feelings. The process leads the susceptible to conclusions that are convenient for the therapist, not necessarily the patient. After all, it is not really known what is in the true interest of the patient. Perhaps changing his or her environment is basic to any cure and should be the first line of attack. Yet the constant stress on individual adaptation to social institutions contradicts the ethereal promises of heroic overcoming.

Ad hoc theory has produced ad hoc therapy, simplistic and commonsensical in every way except for its complicated obedience to social mores. While jury-rigged and piecemeal, neither theory nor practice is accidental, unplanned, or critical of the American ethos. On the contrary, theory and practice have distorted science in scripting heroic fables of personal responsibility. The ad hoc simplicity of CBT comes along with the same superstitions as faith-based religion and the same demands for belief. Both American religion and CBT take on a particular cultural form. They are both popular because of their irrationality and their endorsement of the culture's core beliefs. The parallel between CBT and Christian Science is uncanny: heroic individualism expressed as faith in mind over matter, expectancy effects, and spiritual causation. Christian Science works through God, CBT through the self-positing mind, but both emphasize personal responsibility over any sense of social compulsion. Indeed, implicit in both is a rejection of the environment as fate: the will is supreme; nineteenth-century Romanticism triumphs over Enlightenment rationality.

Christian Science and CBT

Christian Science is the revelation, invention, or hysterical insight of Mary Baker Eddy, its founder and prophet. Eddy wrote the sect's basic text, *Science and Health with a Key to the Scriptures,* in 1875, and it has had constant revisions since then—432 clarifying editions according to Caroline Fraser (1999). The practice of Christian Science is predicated on the notion that purity of mind creates purity of body. The body is immortal and nonmaterial but suffers physical disease as a manifestation of a diseased soul in the manner of Dorian Gray's portrait. Physical disease is cured through spiritual cleansing. Mental conditions trump physical reality. The key to personal transformation lies in the ability of mind to transcend the limitations of matter. Man, made in God's image, is also immortal. As a result, early Christian Science adamantly rejected medical cures; all disease could be cured and prevented through the pure life of the soul. Eddy presented the techniques and procedures of soul cleansing to a suffering world.

However, the logic and the protection against falsification of its principles allies Christian Science with psychotherapy, notably CBT. While Christian Science's pretenses to bodily cures have been discredited by the success of modern medicine, its claims to healing mental and emotion problems are about on a footing with CBT. Both rely on the supremacy of the will and the power of cognition to alter mood. Both offer proofs that are largely anecdotal. And most notably, both consciously confuse patient expectancies and placebo effects with professional interventions.

For Christian Science, human life is Spirit. Disease is a condition of the Spirit, not the body. Sin is the cause of physical and mental suffering; disease is the penalty for wrongdoing, not just wrong thinking. Both mental and physical diseases are corrected through mind cures. "It is error to suffer for aught but your own sins. Christ, or Truth, will destroy all other supposed suffering, and real suffering for your own sins will cease in proportion as the sin ceases" (Eddy, 1994, p. 404). "Healing the sick and reforming the sinner are one and the same thing in Christian Science" (ibid., p. 404).

Contrast this with CBT's claim that emotional and mental problems are the results of distorted cognitions. These problems are not the result of environmental insults but cognitive "errors" in processing cues from the environment. Sin for CBT lies in self-blame and the list of cognitive distortions, all evidence of inappropriate thoughts, leading to dysfunctional behaviors. Healing requires true perceptions of reality. While Christian Science engages in the "spiritualization of thought," CBT subjectivizes it through the perceptions of the therapist.

"Sin [is] a form of insanity . . . which mistakes fable for fact. . . . Those unfortunate people who are committed to insane asylums are only so many distinctly defined instances of the baneful effects of illusion on mortal minds and bodies" (ibid., pp. 407–408). Substitute depression, panic, and so forth for sin and cognitive distortion for illusion in order to arrive at the basic tenets of CBT. Eddy's description of successful Christian Science practice works well for CBT; the notion of bringing sin to the surface recalls the value of the subconscious for CBT: "What I term *chemicalization* is the upheaval produced when immortal Truth is destroying erroneous mortal belief. Mental chemicalization brings sin and sickness to the surface, forcing impurities to pass away, as is the case with a fermenting fluid" (emphasis in original; ibid., p. 401).

Each theory insulates itself from falsification. "Expose the body to certain temperatures, and belief says that you may catch cold and have catarrh; but no such result occurs without mind to demand it and produce it" (ibid., p. 386). If one freezes to death in the cold, then it means that the mind, soul, and spirit were not pure. If one persists, then they were pure. Thus those who get sick are sinful, and those who do not are pure: the proposition and its effects are tests of each other. In its turn, CBT's distorted beliefs function in largely the same way: when dysfunctional behaviors occur, by metaphysical assumption, cognitive distortions have preceded them. There are no independent predictions for the causal relation between thoughts and either emotional disease or dysfunctional behaviors; distorted thoughts are *defined* as causative and defy independent testing.

Eddy constantly presented edifying examples of the prowess of Christian Science healing. Dr Judith Beck's (1999) book is a prolonged anecdote. Neither provides independent verification of her healing, let alone controlled objective tests of her theories. Indeed, the systematic outcome literature is largely a statistical summary of anecdotes. In conferences such as "The Evolution of Psychotherapy," practitioners sell their psychic wares through compelling anecdotes.

The cures for Christian Science and CBT rely on the same processes of patient expectation: "Avoid talking illness to the patient. . . . the refutation of the testimony of material sense is not a difficult task in view of the conceded falsity of this testimony. . . . *At the right time explain to the sick the power which their beliefs exercise over their bodies*. Give them divine and wholesome understanding, with which to combat their erroneous sense, and so efface the images of sickness from mortal mind" (emphasis added; Eddy, 1994, p. 414).

Patient expectancies dominate Christian Science: "Homeopathic remedies, sometimes not containing a particle of medicine, are known to relieve the symptoms of disease. What produces the change? It is the *faith* of the doctor and the patient, which reduces self-inflicted sufferings and produces a new effect upon the body" (emphasis added; ibid., p. 398). The distortions for Christian Science also work through "automatic mechanisms": "If Mind is the only actor, how can mechanism be automatic? Mortal mind perpetuates its own thought. It constructs a machine, manages it, and then calls it material" (ibid., p. 399).

Both are focused on the receptivity of the patient and the educative relationship between therapist and healer:

> The treatment of insanity is especially interesting. However obstinate the case, it yields more readily than do most diseases to the salutary action of truth, which counteracts error. The arguments to be used in curing insanity are the same as in other diseases: namely, the impossibility that matter, brain, can control or derange the mind, can suffer or cause suffering; also the fact that truth and love will establish a healthy state, guide and govern mortal mind or the thought of the patient, and destroy all error, whether it is called dementia, hatred, or any other discord.
>
> To fix steadfastly in your patients' thought, explain Christian Science to them, but not too soon—not until your patients are prepared for the explanation—lest you array the sick against their own interests by troubling and perplexing their thought. (Ibid., p. 414)
>
> [For example] Palsy is a belief that matter governs mortals, and can paralyze the body, making certain portions of it motionless. Destroy the belief, show mortal mind that muscles have no power to be lost, for Mind is supreme, and you cure the palsy. (Ibid., p. 375)

CBT substitutes accurate beliefs for Eddy's truth, behavior or environment for matter (brain), therapy for love, and depression for palsy. Both sets of concepts are hypothetical constructs, that is, metaphysics, not physical entities amenable to objectification.

> Because the so-called body [CBT's behavior] is a mental concept [beliefs and thoughts] and governed by mortal mind, it manifests only what that so-called mind expresses. Therefore the efficient remedy is to

destroy the patient's false belief by both silently and audibly arguing the true facts in regard to harmonious being—representing man as healthy instead of diseased, and showing that it is impossible for matter to suffer, to feel pain or heat, to be thirsty or sick. Destroy fear, and you end fever. Some people, mistaught as to Mind-science, inquire when it will be safe to check a fever. Know that in Science you cannot check a fever after admitting that it must have its course. To fear and admit the power of disease, is to paralyze mental and scientific demonstration. (Eddy, 1995, p. 376)

Eddy's euphuisms mirror much of the textbook verbosity of CBT. In both forms of mind cure, "science" is arrogated and given a special meaning devoid of science. However, Christian Science has the virtue of clearly equating "science" with metaphysics. The following juxtaposition of a few Christian Science notions [with the CBT equivalent] highlights their spiritual propinquity, suggesting the essential ways Eddy anticipated the Becks:

The moral and spiritual facts of health, whispered into thought, produce very direct and marked effects on the body [inappropriate schemas cause depression]. A physical diagnosis of disease—since mortal mind must be the cause of disease—tends to induce disease. (Ibid., p. 370)

The prophylactic and therapeutic (that is, the preventive and curative) arts belong emphatically to Christian Science, as would be readily seen, if psychology, of the Science of Spirit, God, was understood. Unscientific methods [psychodynamic and behavioral therapies] are finding their dead level. Limited to matter by their own law, what have they of the advantages of Mind and immortality? (Ibid., p. 369)

Once let the mental physician believe in the reality of matter [behavioral causes] . . . [and] he is unfitted for the successful treatment of disease. (Ibid., pp. 368–369)

If the Scientist reaches his patient through divine Love [the therapeutic relationship], the healing work will be accomplished at one visit [short-term CBT], and the disease will vanish into its native nothingness like dew before the morning sunshine. If the Scientist has enough Christly affection [clinical skill and imagination] to win his own pardon, and such commendation as the Magdalen gained from Jesus, then he is Christian enough to practice scientifically and deal with his patients compassionately [by establishing a therapeutic alliance]; and the result will correspond with the spiritual intent. (Ibid., p. 365)

The author never knew a patient who did not recover when the belief of the disease [distorted cognitions] had gone. (Ibid., p. 377)

Both CBT and Christian Science are successful forms of naive spirituality, sharing the ability to marshal belief past skepticism, faith over reason, in sustaining dominant social values. In both cases, faith in mind over matter is nurtured through anecdotes of personal testimony and appeals to the authority of scientific proof—a primitive form at the turn of the nineteenth century and a sophisticated form at the turn of the twentieth but in both cases lacking the substance of scientific proof. Both CBT and Christian Science purvey social fables of personal responsibility, initially through their anecdotes and later, for CBT, through charades of supposedly definitive clinical trials. The dogma, central to both but equally without credible proof, that individuals have the capacity to change their behavior in spite of social conditions presses the culture's preference for personal over social responsibility. Personal responsibility and personal effort to pursue cure remain an issue of character for both forms of treatment: salvation for one, emotional health for the other, but perhaps the same in the end.

> We say that one human mind can influence another and in this way affect the body, but we rarely remember that we govern our own bodies. The error, mesmerism—or hypnotism, to use the recent term— illustrates the fact just stated. The operator would make his subjects believe that they cannot act voluntarily and handle themselves as they should do. If they yield to this influence, it is because their belief is not better instructed by spiritual understanding. (Eddy, 1994, p. 402)

Eddy parallels CBT's insistence that rational behavior is possible, that patients are capable of analyzing their beliefs and thus changing their behaviors. She was competing with a variety of mind cures and spiritualist claims— hypnosis, phrenology, seances to chat with the dead, nutritional schemes, hydrotherapy, and so on. The nineteenth century's many quacks, crackpots, and superstitions are refreshed today by the different psychotherapies and also with diet cures, past-life therapy, aroma therapy, sleep learning, biofeedback, and the host of alternative medical treatments. Rather than having any distinction of rational content or proof, Eddy's Christian Science competing with CBT simply represents the clerical competing against the secular for market share.

Christian Sceince and CBT pose belief itself as a personal responsibility in overcoming resistance to treatment, but in both cases the credulity of a defenseless faith is created by stripping away skepticism through the pressures of authority. Heroic responsibility for personal change ironically leads in each case to cultish conformity, to the submission of the individual to God, "the immortal Mind," or the truths of CBT and the authority of the therapist. "The author [Mary Baker Eddy] has raised up the dying, partly because they were willing to be restored" suggests that personal responsibility follows the corpse into the grave (Eddy, 1995, p. 373). But it is no less grandiose than A. T. Beck's earlier claim that CBT succeeded with the full range of emotional disorders because patients were willing to correct their erroneous thoughts.

The parallel between CBT and Christian Science may be explained by the fact that both are elaborated expressions of the common ethos rather than scientific truths, that is, they follow the logic of cultural tastes rather than objective clinical outcomes. Since the normative preferences of the nation have been astonishingly consistent throughout the years of the nation, it is not surprising that CBT and Christian Science promote the same social values. Both express the same cultural preferences for metaphysical certainty and individual responsibility, assuring congregants and patients of a sense of chosenness. Both are empirical in so far as they rely upon the same forms of testimony: case testimonials that largely rely on placebo effects rather than true cures. However, both sustain themselves on response falsification, choosing the benefits of subjectivity over the trials of objective proof. Aside from predictable placebo benefits, both are equally uncertain but equally committed to manipulating expectancies through disingenuous alliances with the patient that subvert prudent doubt.

Christian Science faded as its antagonism toward medicine and public health became mindless denial of their obvious benefits. But Christian Science did not fail in its central conformity with American preferences for a gnomic, personal style. Similarly, CBT persists in spite of its tenuous clinical value, hiding behind a stewardship of American values. CBT is less confrontational toward obvious truths and tends to avoid claims for physical cures that can be easily tested; indeed, it has adapted science to its own form. Both are metaphysical, but the churchly style of Christian Science, with its hysterical depreciation of the material, has given way to the secular style of CBT, which ritualizes science but eludes its substance.

Cognitive theory, for all its deficiencies, has not inspired effective clinical practice. As noted in earlier chapters, the best research offers no credible evidence of any successful psychotherapy for any condition. In just this way, both the theory and the practice of CBT are social languages, that is, "schemas" of social meaning, a Wittgenstein language-game, a universe of discourse. Failing as science, cognitive theory and cognitive-behavioral treatments become interesting as social phenomena of belief—it is fascinating to speculate why contemporary culture accepts the metaphysics of CBT rather than BT or psychodynamic therapy, or for that matter Christian Science, colonic irrigation, or phrenology.

In rejecting the mentalism of psychodynamic therapy, CBT has proliferated behavioral evidence. Yet the constant recording of CBT itself is predicated on hypothetical constructs (for example, automatic, intermediate, and core beliefs, preconscious processes) that lack physical reality. It is as mystical as Christian Science and as barren of credible evidence to support its efficacy. Its mysticism is one of the concrete, like an actor dressing in a lab coat to sell aspirins, but its core processes are gnomic and spiritual. It is a secular Christian Science relying on patient expectations, that is, placebo effects, for mind-over-matter cures that testify to the judicious wisdom of heroic individualism and, therefore, epic personal responsibility.

The death of Mary Baker Eddy should have refuted the immortality of the pure human being, just as the failure of its evaluative enterprise should have signaled the demise of CBT. Yet both thrived past their rational denouement. Just as Christian Science was sustained to the limits of its social use, so too is CBT sustained as a ceremony of American values. The meaning of both lies in their social message, not their ability to cure, their ceremonial functions, not their clinical abilities. "Mary Baker Eddy's child, her Church, is dying. But unlike the Church's own lost children, who have not been resurrected, Christian Science may well be. It may wear a different face or call itself by a different name, but in American life, extreme self-reliance is here to stay" (Fraser, 1999, p. 400).

The extravagant promises of mind cures, the primacy of human consciousness, are heroicly individual yet ironically promote group conformity—freedom through unquestioning belief. For America's religions, the churchly as well as the secular, heroic individualism is not a programmatic goal, a tangible achievement, but rather a doctrinaire romanticism of American culture. Two values are pressed: the formal, explicit tenets of heroic individualism, which, except with the rarest patients, are unobtainable, and the informal but decisive reality of its fables, which bind citizens to their culture through identification with existing social institutions: Mary Baker Eddy and Aaron Beck, two styles, one author.

Hope without Faith

Psychotherapy offers little if any proof that consciously planned interventions can modify human behaviors. There is even less evidence that the unwilling can be moved to become less self-destructive or less troublesome. In fact, the constant perfectionism of American society may actually abet personal problems as millenarianism and liberal markets, the demand for constant improvement and the mechanism to quickly unseat tradition, create profound dissatisfaction with life as it is, a rejection of necessarily imperfect humans. Heroic individualism is an impossible ideal and probably even a harmful one. The more that American culture insists on personal invention and extreme individual responsibility, the more that many will retreat inward in self-protection, rejecting sociability and civility and, in the end, undercutting the possibility of true heroism. Narcissism supplants sacrifice for others, the essence of heroism, as a personal strategy and a social goal. Read as fable, psychotherapy is more than simply complicit with American culture; it is one of its important institutions.

Psychotherapy is a shopkeeper of American manners, retailing the social etiquette of individual responsibility to loyal customers. Psychotherapy is one of the symbols of heroic individualism in the same way that the peace pipe had significance beyond its function. Its ceremonial role is all the more profound since there does not appear to be any clinical role that the field can credibly demonstrate. The persistent failure of its treatments and the field's success in thwarting credible evaluation beg for explanation in terms of society's stake in its rituals rather than in any sign of emerging clinical prowess.

At best, the outcomes of psychotherapy are indeterminate. Yet even the very best of the recent research, appearing in the most highly regarded and selective journals, has failed to apply rigorous tests to psychotherapy. It is a stunning commentary that after so many decades during which sophisticated techniques of clinical research—randomized controlled trials—were available to the inquisitive researcher, the probative tests of psychotherapy's outcomes are still deeply flawed. Even when randomized controlled trials are employed, random assignment is frequently breached, random selection of subjects rarely takes place, samples are small, attrition and censoring are high, measurement is compromised by a lack of neutrality, measurement instruments themselves are typically unreliable and questionable, measures are soft and subjective, usually relying on patient self-report and therapist evaluation, and so forth. In fact, there has never been a scientifically credible study that attests to the effectiveness of any form of psychotherapy for any mental or emotional problem under any condition of treatment.

Still, the obvious and deep biases of the research, consistently exaggerating if not actually creating positive findings, have only produced modest estimates of the field's effectiveness. Yet those positive outcomes are nearly wiped out by adjustments for placebo effects—empathic care or, for Wittgenstein, old women nursing the sick. Dawes (1994) and many others have made far too much of the field's distorted estimates. Taking into account the research's multitude of biases generated by committed researchers, patient expectancies, patient self-reports, and the other demand characteristics of the research situation, psychotherapy emerges as routinely ineffective. In consideration of the enormous amount of positive outcomes that are accounted for by biases and placebo effects, psychotherapy may even be harmful for many patients.

Furthermore, the estimates of psychotherapy's effectiveness are usually derived from university research, in which presumably superior practitioners are closely monitored. The typical community setting is very different, avoiding scrutiny and tolerating a far greater number of marginal therapists. Thus even under optimal conditions of treatment, psychotherapy fails; in more customary situations, as Masson (1988), Gross (1978), and Zilbergeld (1983) have observed, it is often destructive.

In short, psychotherapy lacks both a clinical function in cure, prevention, or rehabilitation and a community of scholars and practitioners dedicated to the canons of science. Certainly, few people are aware of the weakness of the field's research or even its routine clinical ineffectiveness, and perhaps the argument could be pressed that the society tolerates psychotherapy out of ignorance. Yet few people have expert knowledge in any area of social activity. It is more to the point that psychotherapy has not been held to credible scientific standards of clinical proof because the society is not terribly concerned with its clinical role. Rather, psychotherapy persists as a civil religion, a purely ceremonial social role.

Psychotherapy affirms broadly shared social values through the vehicle of faith. Rather than the paladin of revolutions in human consciousness, the field acts much to the contrary, molding adaptation to cultural norms. Those norms—the tenets of civic virtue in the United States—press heroic individualism through highly subjective and emotional mechanisms on a population convinced of its chosenness and the exceptionalism of the American destiny. Rather than a form of social responsibility, psychotherapy promulgates the extreme self-reliance and extreme personal responsibility that results from a belief in self-invention, in people creating themselves. In loyalty to nineteenth-century Romanticism, heroic individualism disputes the force of social imperatives on development and the structural influences of family, community, and society.

The American ethos of patriotism, spirituality, chosenness, and individualism is expressed in the general American religion, both the churchly and the civic. The truths of the American religion's core experiences—an immediate apprehension of the divine and individual transcendence—are spiritual, ineffable, and knowable only through sublime faculties. Embracing the basic beliefs and even the forms of America's standard god-centered religions in rejection of a communal or organic logic, psychotherapy is also an America religion. While it customarily lacks a specific place for a god, its commitment to essentially nonempirical methods of proof, although usually dressed up as science, still acts through gnomic processes of faith to subvert rationality, objectivity, and coherent proofs of the senses.

Psychotherapy's heroic individualism consistently promises to release hidden talents in pursuit of the patient's unique creativity, offering each patient a heroic role and the therapist the heroism of psychic healer. However, the psychotherapist, like the shaman, is only associated intermittently, not causally, with a patient's healing if it occurs at all. Frank (1974) might have profitably reversed his comparison. It is not the shaman who acts as a psychotherapist, but the therapist who performs the rituals of a shaman. Yet the intermittent coincidences of psychotherapy with apparent cure are not the point. The face toward the culture, that is, psychotherapy's affirmation of core social values, determines the success of the field.

While psychotherapy shares the basic form and function of mainstream American religions, it frequently also acts with the fervor and cunning of American cults and superstitions—Christian Science, Madame Blavatsky's Spiritualism, Scientology, and others. Indeed, psychotherapy is a pseudoscientific enterprise not simply in its marginal forms or because it deals with psychic phenomena but also in its most accepted practices: psychodynamic psychotherapy, behavioral therapy, and cognitive-behavioral therapy.

Yet heroic individualism is an oxymoron, actually mock-heroic in the grand tradition of Swift, Pope, and Dryden. Heroism implies sacrifice for others, but psychotherapeutic treatment is self-centered, even narcissistic in a literary sense. It focuses more on celebrity and fame than on service to others. Indeed, prominent practitioners have become celebrities who appear on television, promote their books, and are covered as topics of great general interest and gossip in the tabloids. Poor Frodo, after returning to America from Mordor, would be booked for celebrity tours and endorsements, eventually succumbing to pious obliteration in Las Vegas, greeting casino guests and signing cards, hats, and keno sheets: the Joe Louis of mythic has-beens and American unconcern.

Heroic individualism is a form of pernicious liberalism, a blind faith in personal reinvention and the salvation of social adaptation rather than in the provision of greater institutional and material equality. True heroism requires self-sacrifice, courage under duress, perseverance, and leadership on behalf of others, notably those in need. In contrast, heroic individualism mocks the notion of personal sacrifice with its monomania of attention to individual ambition. Heroic individualism cheapens the recurring and deep problems of American society, requiring only shallow right thinking rather than the repair of failed social institutions. Psychotherapy is the quintessential expression of social efficiency—that any program to cure, prevent, or rehabilitate must be compatible with cultural preferences for minimal provisions. Indeed, psychotherapy is one of the principal cultural devices by which American society patrols the boundaries of its individualistic values. It is not simply ironic that individual identity is diminished in the cult of the heroic. Rather, the loss of individualism may be the sustaining purpose of rabid participation in the binding delusions of mass appeal. Uniformity rather than tolerance or diversity proceeds from common myths. Patients and therapists reveal a dull sameness even as they prattle on endlessly about their imagined uniqueness.

C. M. Hall's (1998) exposition of the heroic self was tortured by the contradiction between the myopically self-serving psychotherapy patient and the broader heroism of self-sacrifice and service to others. Yet "living the larger life" is not a demonstrable outcome of psychotherapy, and Hall only presented a few questionable case studies. Instead, the pursuit of the heroic appears to rest on the vain assumption that "choosing to be heroic selves, and thereby choosing to live the larger life, inevitably benefits others" (C. M. Hall, 1998, p. 125). In good Adam Smith fashion, personal interest presumably graduates into social benefit, transforming psychotherapy's creed of individualism into an act for the general good. Approaching the fervor of a sacrament, the assumption that individual benefit extends to others frees psychotherapy from any obligation to evaluate its actual outcomes. Psychotherapy becomes increasingly unmoored from objective discipline, reality reduced to mood, with assumptions that the patient is freed "seeing self as hero rather than as sinner or victim" (ibid., p. 105). Thus victimization becomes the victim's choice and unwanted behaviors become personal sins—a refusal to control matter with mind, a faulty will, and a malingering "learned helplessness"—in denial of economic and political barriers, lack of opportunities, and grossly unequal investments in family and community.

The hospitality of both psychotherapy and the American people to notions of extreme self-invention and spiritual proofs have maintained a near blind credulity for ever-replenished absurdities of belief and treatment. Moody's *Life after Life* (1975) purported to provide evidence of an afterlife through interviews with those having returned from the dead. By 2001, it had sold *13 million* copies. A charming psychiatrist with a Ph.D. in philosophy, Moody never claimed that his book was science, only that it was "an entertainment," defusing any potential criticism of its faulty evidence and methods. Nevertheless, some years later he did rise above entertainment to insist that belief in the afterlife, again based on the evidence of near-death experiences but now also invoking a "special death sense," was psychotherapeutic and, of course, profitable (Moody, 2001). Some years later, perhaps in recognition of monumental sales, he titled his new book *The Last Laugh* (Moody, 1999).

Absent a rigorous application of science, only style separates mainstream psychotherapy from the fringes of its own practitioners and of American enthusiasms for the spectacularly surreal—space abduction, unexplained pregnancies, Rapture, Adepts, teleportion, sleep learning, transmigrations of the soul and reincarnation, visitations from the Virgin Mary. Still, the relationship between American faith in the supernatural and psychotherapy is too profound to be threatened by the rigors of objectivity and coherence.

Authentic clinical practices can be distinguished from the ridiculous, improbable, and false only by the quality of their proofs. There is little that separates Moody's little entertainments from psychotherapy's mawkish sincerity. Both have failed to place their interventions and beliefs under tough scrutiny, defying accountability. Put another way, psychotherapy is more akin to Moody's profitable sense of humor than to clinical medicine. Christian Science, Theosophy, and psychotherapy are in competition for the same shriveled souls. Psychotherapy in its many materializations keeps tradition alive for subsequent generations that need magical reinvention and emotional seances to maintain regard for their existential heroism: victory without effort, peace without struggle, immortality without immortal works, and, of course, illusion without psychosis.

Blavatsky, Eddy, Freud, and the field of psychotherapy are united in their disdain for objective proof, although the good Madame had the decency to respect Theosophy without grasping for the legitimacy of science, at least not too often. In contrast, Freud endures with greater regard than Blavatsky, probably because he limited his inventive spirit to the fantastic, avoiding the specificity that allows for the falsification of testable assertions. Alas, Blavatsky's materializations did not materialize without the assistance of stuffed sleeves and hidden cords; no distance was ever discerned between the floor and her levitated body; and, the drama of speaking to the dead was cheapened by proxy actors. Even the staunchest true belief in the ability of the faithful to pass through solid walls is eventually dispelled by the reality of nosebleeds and bruised shins.

Madame Blavatsky's Theosophy is too bohemian and out of touch with contemporary demands for a Second Coming, Rapture, alien abductions, or scientific clinical practice like Moody's. In the end, Blavatsky transmigrated the soul of Theosophy to the place where Mehitabel the cat is perpetually reincarnated as Cleopatra. However, Freud's sincerity, medical degree, and grand pen were just right, inspiring revisions of refreshed faith: Oedipus morphed into developmental stages; infantile sexuality into age-specific demands; ten years of treatment collapsed into two years, then a few months. Emotionality became the vanity of thoughtful cognition, and nonmedical practitioners were let into the club of treatment.

Heroic individualism accompanies America's devotion to classical liberalism, with particular affection for Smith's proposition that the individual's pursuit of self-interest confers general benefits—the "spontaneous orders" of productive markets and social cohesion. Ever greater economic prosperity in the United States is endorsed by social values: "Our suspicions fade that the quality of life may not be a synonym for the standard of living" (Rieff, 1966, p. 243). The national ethos has traveled from the community and the ethnic group to the extended family, then to the nuclear family, and finally to the individual. Psychotherapy has been one of the mythmakers in this change, reconciling the individual to the goodness of a culture increasingly devoid of communal protections and pleasures. Indeed, psychotherapy itself is a product of the changing culture and hardly the autonomous philosophy or practice it flatters itself to be. The myth of heroic individualism justifies the desirability, if not actually the inevitability, of extreme self-attention—taking care of each "self-positing ego" by reducing anxiety and guilt over self-absorption and justifying self-interest as heroic. However, the true hero, recanting pleasure and advantage, intentionally submerges the self in sacrifice for the community. The therapeutic has triumphed with its "gospel of self-fulfillment" (ibid., p. 252).

Rieff emphasized that the "doctrine of the therapeutic" is in fact a language of morality, a "moral demand system" (ibid., pp. 251, 247). However, he may have been optimistic in predicting a self-limiting therapeutic morality. "A full transition to a post communal culture may never be achieved. It is a persuasive argument, still, that maintains there are safeguards, built into both human nature and culture, limiting the freedom of men to atomize themselves" (ibid., p. 11).

Yet contrary to Rieff (1966), the therapeutic ethos is the individual empty of communal obligations—the citizen without civility. Heroic individualism imposes the stringency of a near-ascetic imperative to care only for oneself. The psychotherapeutic discourse is devoid of any injunction for the patient to be socially or morally responsible. Rieff's nostalgia for community, like Marx's, and his faith in self-correcting social mechanisms lack historical veracity. Still, the isolation of individualism and the constant little tyrannies of communalism defy easy comparison or evaluation. Nevertheless, with the encouragement of American society, psychotherapy has become an advocate of heroic individualism and, consequently, an apologist for the lost spirit of community, in the process eroding the safeguards of community, if they ever existed.

Becker (1973) offered no promise of cure, prevention, or rehabilitation for psychological counseling. He seemed to suggest that all citizens should have access to a wise person at different times in life to review their personal experiences, to explore the meaning of existence, and to reevaluate ethical and moral choices. As a social institution, broad access to wise counseling may be universally desirable as a humane way of maintaining ethical standards. It is only a hope that wise counsel will modify human behavior, in the same way that it is a hope that participation in other American institutions will produce a nurturing culture. Becker has found no evidence in the experience of psychotherapy that this will be so, and his sense of the personally heroic does not resolve the problem. He is not advocating a clinical form but rather a discussion of ethics in existing social institutions. There is no coercion; opportunities for guided self-reflection are simply to be created by common consent as a structure of civilized America, perhaps as an adjunct to public education. Yet Becker's noble therapy may be possible only in a noble society.

In practice, psychotherapy turns its back on egalitarian, universal rights to participate in basic social institutions. Even the interminable treatments of psychoanalysis seem to have failed to do more than ingratiate a privileged class and indulge its outsized vanity. Psychotherapy is often mandated through the courts, schools, and business for miscreants—criminals, drunks, unruly children, drug users, spouse beaters, the insane, the raucous, the inattentive, and so forth. In contrast, through the essentially market-based, fee-for-service organization of psychotherapy, the voluntary patient is largely in control of the nature of the therapeutic exchange. Therapists have convinced themselves that maintaining the therapeutic relationship is essential for treatment—except, of course, when the analyst declares the process a success after the patient terminates treatment out of boredom or is terminated because the insurance lapses.

Patient satisfaction, feeding off of patient self-absorption rather than behavioral change or the creation of a more sociable citizen, is the desideratum of successful treatment. But self-deception is the worst kind of deception, and psychotherapists, enthralled by their heroic role in psychic healing, reinvent their own market stakes as noble service in which sales become a beneficence, the charity of self-interest. The free market fosters a pleasing contract between buyer and seller—therapist and patient—but contrary to faith in the spontaneous orders of free markets, psychotherapy creates external diseconomies, that is, broader prices that society may pay in narcissism and antisocial individualism. As Freedheim (1992) has observed, we hire the therapist "to act as a guide to our success and happiness." Rarely does one speak of duty to one's society; "almost everyone undergoing therapy is concerned with individual gain, and the psychotherapist is hired to assist in this endeavor" (p. xxv).

Bellah, Madsen, Sullivan, Swidler, and Tipton's (1985) treatment of American individualism is derived more from a reading of the ceremonial, idealized texts of America than from its operating ethos. Their four notions of biblical, civic, utilitarian, and expressive individualism are praised as sacred rights of citizenship. But in practice individualism has been shorn of social obligation and the self becomes "the main form of reality" (p. 143). Individualism is consistently challenged to define itself in a positive fashion and not simply as the absence of inhumane coercion. The appropriate trade-off between the individual's rights to personal development and the obligations for social duty and sacrifice is neither obvious nor simple but perhaps "a profound impasse." Heroic or "modern individualism seems to be producing a way of life that is neither individually nor socially viable, yet a return to traditional forms would be to return to intolerable discrimination and oppression" (p. 144). The operative form of individualism, the heroic, has emerged as a grand consensus from the enduring negotiation among the components of American society, including its traditions. The heroic form is a tectonic plate of America's social geology.

By promoting a false heroism based upon self-absorption rather than sacrifice, psychotherapy and the culture that sustains it are encouraging the very behaviors that civic ideals and psychotherapy profess to handle. The cure becomes the cause of the disease. Similarly, selfishness confused with virtue or even seen as a necessary motive nurtures an isolating narcissism that threatens community itself. Wealth is achieved at an awful price.

The notion of the therapeutic is characteristically American and is repeated with almost eidetic precision in both psychotherapy and the nation's different churches: extreme personal responsibility paired with nearly perpetual opportunities for salvation through self-correction. However, the opportunities for salvation through psychotherapy are rarely paired with the resources that might facilitate personal adaptation. For example, there are few jobs for exconvicts; the conditions of foster children are deplorable; the destitute have few opportunities to make a living. Indeed, therapeutic sessions are morality skits that reaffirm broader social values without offering the resources for a better life.

The patient's recognition of social sin, acceptance of personal responsibility, and then at least a voiced commitment to personal change provide the cathartic spectacles of justice triumphant and the rectitude of cherished social values. The refusal to change, especially after the enlightenment of psychotherapy, condones punishment, which once again reinforces cultural values. Personal problems only become a general concern when they aggregate with political and social force. A few gang members are morally instructive as bad examples that vindicate the persistence of America's ghettos, but an interminable underground subverting common institutions and the general peace threatens social stability.

To take responsibility for oneself is the epiphany of America's formal religions, the manner in which they handle sin. It is also the manner in which psychotherapy handles deviance: the patient must take responsibility for his or her own actions. People who fail in therapy refuse to take responsibility for themselves and, thus, disqualify themselves from the community's generosity. In the puritanical eye, wayward patients demonstrate their lack of grace, their sinfulness, their ineligibility for salvation (Erickson, 1966).

The therapeutic exchange, irrespective of type, is a narrative of American social values, demanding loyalty to the communal values of heroic individualism, the vaunted independence, and self-creation embedded in American folklore, popular culture, and regnant intellectual life. Citizens are largely expected to fend for themselves despite the obvious consequences of unequal investments in families, schools, communities, and so forth. It appears to be a consistent sociological truth (that is, more true than not true or customarily true or apparently true or seemingly plausible or culturally coherent or some other middling compromise with reality) that those who succeed have enjoyed greater benefits of schooling and family than those who do not succeed. Yet psychotherapy, in the manner of the Latter-day Saints, assumes that each person, regardless of environment, has the capacity to make good choices. "If a person were tied up in a dungeon all his life he would still have moral choice. He could think good thoughts or bad. He could be kind or mean. Like Victor Frankl taught, he could choose how to respond. No one can take away agency. But we can lose agency through sin. An immoral personal may reach the point where he cannot control his thoughts."[1]

Thus bad choices are signs of bad character or one of the cataloged disorders listed in the American Psychiatric Association's *Diagnostic and Statisti-*

cal Manual, and in fact may be the same thing. Psychotherapy insists through a process of introspection (conscience) that patients consider their evil ways and reform. Reform is largely expected without any bribe to conformity—the provision of greater equality through a more generous social welfare. Rather, wealth and social standing are the consequences of righteousness, not the reasons for it. Perhaps subtle in their labeling but profound in their effects, the ministrations of psychotherapy are little different from the preacher's calling attention to sin and thus invoking awesome communal pressures to coerce obedience or, failing this, to isolate the sinner from the communion of the righteous.

The social role of psychotherapy as a civil religion of heroic individualism also has political implications. It collaborates with minimalist social-welfare provisions in the United States by exaggerating individual self-invention and personal responsibility. Psychotherapy is a form of libertarian neglect rather than communal support and offers one explanation for the inadequacies of the American welfare state in comparison with other modern industrialized nations. The minimalism of the American social-welfare system is an even greater marvel in light of the nation's spectacular wealth, which is greater than it has ever been and greater than that of any other society. The commitment to the creed of psychotherapy, so central to an enormous number of social-welfare programs, blocks even experimentation with greater equality.

Psychotherapy is American's core strategy in many social-welfare programs that attempt to change problematic personal behaviors, including crime, poverty, and mental and social disorders. The psychotherapeutic strategy substitutes moral suasion for material sustenance or direct investments in social institutions such as families, schools, and communities. The therapeutic rather than the communal inspired the 1996 welfare reforms that replaced Aid to Families with Dependent Children with Temporary Assistance to Needy Families (TANF). Among other restrictions in benefits and eligibility, TANF terminated welfare as a right, placing each recipient under the discretion of a personal case manager as if poverty were proof of moral inadequacy.

A very experienced and intelligent therapist has argued that empathic listening is inherently confirmation of the other person's dignity and thus enhances self-esteem. "I also believe that the lack of empathic understanding of children (and in later stages of life) is a major contributor to violent behavior."[2] Thus therapy has value. However, an intuition of cause, no matter how valuable as a moral precept, is not by itself adequate foundation for professional practice; propositions about clinical treatment require testing. Empathic listening, in contrast with the listening ear, suggests a professional, systematic, refined ability to engineer outcomes.

Almost all human activities profess goodness: it is good to build strong buildings; it is good to play baseball well; it is good to design safe cars. Similarly, it is good to be sympathetic, understanding, kind, attentive, thoughtful, decent, and truthful. However, the issue lies with the clinical effectiveness of psychotherapy's achievement of goodness. Aside from the theory that is implicit in the claim for empathic listening (for example, its salubrious effects on self-esteem and positive outcomes), does empathic listening reduce the problems to which it is applied? The related but still speculative idea of prior deprivation also needs specific empirical testing: does, in fact, the lack of empathic understanding produce violent behavior in later life? Will empathic listening compensate for the deprivation?

The humanistic content in human relations is very important; indeed, empathic listening, along with the other virtues, should be taught within the culture as modes of decent human interaction. But the issue of the humanistic content in psychotherapy is ancillary to the issue of its effectiveness. Well-meaning failures are still failures, although as symbols they have a separate social significance. Unfortunately, the symbolic significance of psychotherapy is not all that humanistic but rather consistently affirmative of some of the cruelest tendencies in American culture.

For a variety of practical and technical reasons psychotherapy may not be testable, and given the field's self-protection, it may not even be researchable. The best that can be said for the current literature is that it is presumptive and premature. However, it will remain this way until reliable measures are developed and neutral researchers are in charge of the research. Less apologetically, the field actually frustrates good research, knowingly and with the society's encouragement. It even appears that the prestige of research auspices—medical schools and hospitals affiliated with Columbia, Yale, Stanford, the University of Pittsburgh, and so forth—and the academic achievements of practitioners are offered in lieu of scientifically credible research: faith and style over science and substance.

Furthermore, the outcomes of psychotherapy do not compel the society, or failed patients would be clamoring for effective cures and the complacency of practitioners, their smug assurances of being able to treat psychic ailments, would be disturbed by a hostile public. The tacit social stake is in the mythology the field promotes, not in the facts of cure, prevention, and rehabilitation. Investigations of the field have been given over to the field. Clinical meaning has shrunk into patient satisfaction even when there are ostensible behaviors that all participants wish to change (for example, addiction, anxiety, obesity).

A field that employs alternative science is not scientific but something else. This is not necessarily bad, just outside of scientific understanding, and only the fastidious would press the issue of truth and accuracy. Yet psychotherapy as pseudoscience implies science distorted as social invention; the logic of discovery mimicked as the campaign for belief; acultural fact surrendering to the ineluctable, undeniable, irrepressible forces of socialization, adaptation, and social integration.

The practice of science persists as a distinct logic despite its many enigmas and ambiguities. Even as an acceptable social institution, it is differentiated from all other social forms by its rigorous skepticism and its communal discipline. Yet precisely because psychotherapy functions outside of science's precincts as a civil religion, it loses the cachet of science. The difficulties of accurately assessing the outcomes of psychotherapy do not provide a warrant for its practice. The best information available may not be good enough, with the result that social satisfaction rather than its clinical outcomes explains the field's acceptance.

Freud (1961) concluded his own investigations with a concession to modesty: "Our enquiry concerning happiness has not so far taught us much that is not already common knowledge. And even if we proceed from it to the problem of why it is so hard for men to be happy, there seems no greater prospect of learning anything new" (p. 33).

If Freud had taken counsel from his own comment in *Civilization and its Discontents,* the world would have enjoyed a very honest and wise man although quite a silent one. In fact, the literature of psychotherapy subsequent to Freud has borne out his observation; there is no credible clinical practice of the heart or mind that is effective. However, Freud muttered on throughout a lifetime of publication, disrespectful both of science and of the possibility of learning anything new about the human psyche. His insights have been unmasked as both culturally and temporally bound, not the hardwired universal truths of his intuitions; at best they have provided coherence to literary fiction, while Freudian psychoanalysis has maintained a cult fervor stoked by the obscure, egocentric revelations of true belief.

The principal lesson of psychotherapy is that it has failed. The routine failure of therapy, together with the fact that 75% of psychotherapists have themselves been in therapy, suggest that very troubled people may have been placed in the troubled hands of therapists so committed to their own biographies that they are unwilling or incapable of participating in those of others (Norcross, Karpiak, and Santoro, unpublished). The ambitious youths who endure years of graduate training in becoming psychotherapists may have been diverted from more substantive occupations such as engineering, farming, and physical therapy into psychotherapy by virtue of their intense civic spirituality, that is, their own pretensions to psychic healing and mind cures, their fantasies of themselves as avatars of the heroic. The diversion, however, like the mute, blind, and inadvertent logic of Darwinian selection, has little to do with their consciousness of the actual role of psychotherapy or their ability "to restoreth the soul" but rather with an impenetrable and possibly harmful process by which society makes gnomic choices to sustain itself. Psychotherapists may be chosen by fate and culture for their weaknesses, not their strengths.

The universal failure of psychotherapy implies that failed social institutions may be expensive to revive. Socially efficient interventions do not compensate for the deprivations that attend problematic human behaviors. Indeed, psychotherapy may even sustain those deprivations as it promotes the heroic self-invention and extreme personal responsibility that are enacted by American social-welfare programs in denial of greater social responsibility. The heroic human will by itself is a loathsome, antisocial impulse, even infantile and narcissistic in its insistence on being treated subjectively as a cultural form immunized from science.

There is greater peril in society's convincing itself of the necessity, the chosenness of its institutions than in recognizing that they exist without any moral, scientific, or divine sanction. If the remission of psychic pain and mental disorder is the goal, then the search needs to continue. Yet the soul's ease may not be the social function of psychotherapy. Rather, psychotherapy abides the social imperative to affirm America's institutionalized ethos.

Zilbergeld and Becker each advised greater psychic acceptance of individual limitations and variations from social ideals, although this would seem to require the concurrence of a society that does the same thing. However, American civilization has structured its ethos around heroic individualism, celebrating its callousness to personal shortcomings as compassion and refusing to extend its wealth and open its institutions to all of its citizens.

Myth is a collective enterprise that expresses itself without cunning or coaching. It is not speech writing or occasional entertainment or even art, but an informal, symbolic, and compromised negotiation between a society's aspirations and reality. Psychotherapy as myth expresses American society's sense of itself, its faith narrated as a series of analects, morality tales, injunctions, definitions, characterizations. Heroic individualism, and therefore psychotherapy, may be little more than America's cruel optimism that truth has arrived despite graphic evidence that it has not. In spite of countless sessions with Dr. Pangloss, psychotherapy mocks enlightenment. The search for remedies might proceed under the banner of hope without faith.

NOTES

DEDICATION

A riff on Mother Goose:

I do not like thee, Doctor Fell,
The reason why I cannot tell;
But this I know, and know full well,
I do not like thee, Doctor Fell.

INTRODUCTION

1. The contemporary logic of falsification is accepted: scientific theory can only be falsified, not verified. However, maintaining this logic makes for stilted prose. Thus throughout the book, the concept of proof implies the absence of disconfirming evidence consequent to tests conducted in conformity with rigorous science, discussed below. This latter point addresses the logic of means—the differences between means of experimental and control groups—rather than Popper's insistence on the probative value of single instances.

2. Smith, Glass, and Miller (1980) seem to confuse standard error-type measures and standard deviations, with the result that their estimates of the variances of therapeutic outcomes grossly underestimate true variation. The implication is that the actual outcomes are not tightly wound around means but suggest a Wild West of therapy. For detailed discussion, see Epstein 1984a and 1984b.

3. The "shift" is *not* Kuhnian. Psychotherapy has not experienced the grandeur of a paradigm shift; there is no accumulation of any evidence to justify a new way of looking at things. Rather than leaps in human betterment or even the slow but sure march of progress, psychotherapy's adaptations are the weak and frequently mindless adjustments that constitute routine organizational and institutional adaptation. There is little in psychotherapy that is profound, powerful, transformative, or even heroic.

3: THE ADDICTIONS

1. Portions of this analysis of Winters, Fals-Stewart, O'Farrell, Birchler, and Kelley (2002) and a few additional sentences that appear later in the chapter are drawn from Epstein (2005).

6: MAGIC, BIAS, AND SOCIAL ROLE

1. This sense of religion plays a variation on Harold Bloom's notion of the American religion (Bloom, 1992).

2. Madanes (1995; Zeig, 1997) has not been censured for her use of humiliation in therapy. Indeed, she prods violent patients to change through enforced acts of humiliation, which in turn seem to reflect a cultural acceptance, even vicarious sadism, of humiliation as a tool of socialization.

7: PSYCHODYNAMIC PSYCHOTHERAPY

1. Throughout, distinctions between psychoanalysis and psychodynamic psycho-therapy are drawn only when pertinent. As employed here, PP encompasses both unless specifically qualified. Psychoanalysis is the intervention developed by Freud and elaborated by his disciples and their organizations. While its goals are ambiguous, expressive and supportive psychodynamic psychotherapy—although relying largely on psychoanalytic theory—are clearly clinical forms, intended from the outset to change behavior if not character itself.

2. The psychoanalytic literature exceeds by multiples the capacity of any single human being to read through in a lifetime. With the key word *psychoanalysis,* the Library of Congress identifies about 10,000 books; the Social Sciences Citation Index comes up with 6,800 articles since only 1980 in its limited base of journals; Psych-INFO lists more than 38,000 articles. An extraordinarily well-read adult will rarely cover even 5,000 books in a lifetime (100 per year for 50 years). It is a terrible comment on culture's obdurate self-deception that PP is pointless as clinical science. Indeed, its fecklessness and futility as treatment commands attention to its social symbolism. Some of the psychoanalytic literature is "breathtakingly unreadable," but much of it is lucid and convincing in the sense of a novel or play although not in any sense of scientific credibility. How then is it possible to write about psychoanalysis and avoid the charge of being unaware of its nuances and insensitive to its debates? The problem is handled by focusing on its claims: first, by addressing its clinical role and, therefore, the implicit promise to be effective even while acknowledging its disingenuous claim to only provide insight; second, by holding it to its endlessly repeated assertion that it is scientific and, thus, to the criteria of theoretical coherence, procedural rigor, objectivity, and sequential logic; third, by focusing on its communal attributes, notably as it fails the tests of effective clinical practice and science and appears to persist as a secular church of the Eternal American Hero.

3. Norcross, Karg, and Prochaska (1997); Norcross, Karpiak, and Lister (unpublished); and Norcross, Karpiak, and Santoro (unpublished) report that psychodynamic psychotherapy is the principal orientation of 15% of the members of the American Psychological Association's (APA's) Division of Clinical Psychology. This is the most popular orientation after cognitive therapy (28%) and eclectic/integrative approaches. Still, psychodynamic theory remains a strong component of cognitive therapies and an important component of eclectic treatments. Indeed, more than 45% of those with an eclectic/integrative orientation came from a psychodynamic orientation. It seems quite likely that the increasing preference for cognitive approaches is more stylistic than real; therapists continue to maintain faith in primitive metaphysics and simply redecorate their beliefs within current fashions. Moreover, Norcross esti-

mates in a separate communication with the author that the psychodynamic orientation is probably much more popular in other clinical divisions of APA.

4. Perhaps, too, Eddy was inspired by Blavatsky or, as Randi argues, the other way around, since *Isis Unveiled* was shown to have "been copied from previous works of other authors" (1997, p. 33). Then again, maybe both drew inspiration from the nineteenth-century German idealists, notably Fichte and Hegel, and from the spirit of the second Great Awakening in the United States. The similarity of phrasing and often of structure is striking between Eddy's *Science and Health* and Blavatsky's *Isis Unveiled*. While Eddy originally published her volume in 1875, it went through an enormous number of substantial revisions before reaching its final form. *Isis Unveiled* first appeared in 1877.

8: BEHAVIORAL THERAPY—THE OWL AND THE MULE

1. The authors acknowledge that BT is usually ineffective but then go on to recommend it strongly in the next section, seemingly oblivious to their prior comment. In the manner of most textbooks, this is probably considered the balanced treatment that inspires the demand for creationism to be given equal standing with evolution in biology courses. Further, the authors define behavioral techniques as products of classical and operant conditioning but then go on to describe eleven forms of BT without any reference to conditioning. They frequently fail to cite research in support of their comments, and when they do, their interpretation is frequently inaccurate. They acknowledge the customary ineffectiveness of pure behavioral forms but then go on in the very next section to recommend them for treating the problems of marginal, lower-class populations. Publishers like Allyn and Bacon—and there are many—make a living from feeding the seemingly insatiable appetite of undergraduate education for simplistic, redacted, and colorized cartoons of ideas, in this case, treatments of complex social and intellectual phenomena. Students naturally go on to become citizens who insist upon encapsulated testimonial dogma in public discourse that discards complexity for the soothing flatteries of ideology. While it seems that James and Gilliland are typical of the field, there are still occasional voices of greater intellectual strength, but they have had hardly any influence on the clinical fascination with BT.

2. Specific attention to BT outcomes here is necessitated by the routine absence of studies of pure behavioral interventions that emerged in the initial search strategy, that is, from the three major journals screened for the initial chapters. The absence is occasioned first, by the enchantment of BT with single-subject designs, and second, by serious methodological lapses in the studies that did employ randomization. The studies discussed in this and subsequent sections are representative of the most relevant research that was cited by a leading state-of-the-art analysis of psychotherapy (Emmelkamp, in Lambert, 2004), a prominent annual review of behavior therapy (Franks, Wilson, Kendall, and Foreyt, 1990), a representative textbook now in its fourth edition (James and Gilliland, 2003), and others.

9: COGNITIVE-BEHAVIORAL THERAPY AS CHRISTIAN SCIENCE

1. Aaron Beck's cognitive theory and the case material presented by his daughter Judith Beck are representative of the enormous amount of material on this subject. Rather than an area of vital investigation and discussion, CBT is an area of near hypnotic monotony, with casebooks largely repeating the same techniques on patients who share similar problems and social class (for example, J. S. Beck, 1995; J. Scott, Williams, and Beck, 1989; Stern and Drummond, 1991; Freeman and Dattilio, 1992). Theoretically, the distinctions between the avalanche of repetitive writers are not worth a small essay, let alone the small library that has emerged from the field's hypergraphia (for example, A. T. Beck, 1967; Meichenbaum, 1977; Ellis, 1962; Lazarus, 1989). Leahy (1996) would probably dispute the conformity and uniformity of the field, arguing that there are many CBTs and not just Beck's cognitive theory. However, all the others—Rehm, Meichenbaum, Ellis, Mahoney, and so forth—share a few common assumptions: (1) the causal centrality of thought in determining behavior and emotion; (2) patient will: the ability of the patient to alter his or her own thoughts through encouragement and the techniques of therapy; (3) therapy as structured and seemingly explicit, amenable to behavioral measures; and (4) the importance of the treatment alliance. The integrative books are apparently cranked out for the inexhaustible college textbook market, requiring ever greater simplification and visualization in charts, graphs, and cartoons (for example, Leahy, 1996; Person, Davidson, and Tompkins, 2001; Salkovskis, 1996; Dobson, 2001; Dobson and Craig, 1996). It is as though CBT was mounting a campaign for conversion based on the weight of its published testimonials.

2. The curious use of male gender for the therapist and female gender for the patient is entirely Judith Beck's choice and perhaps again with the approval of her father, Aaron.

HOPE WITHOUT FAITH

1. The extract is from a letter by Steve Fotheringham, Las Vegas Nevada Institute of Religion, Church Educational System, Church of Jesus Christ of the Latter-day Saints (Mormons), October 23, 2002, to the author in response to a query regarding the Church's position on free agency. Bloom in *The American Religion* argued that Mormonism is the quintessential American religion.

2. Personal communication.

REFERENCES

Ablon, S. J., & Jones, E. E. (2002). Validity of controlled trials of psychotherapy findings from the NIMH treatment of depression collaborative research program. *American Journal of Psychiatry, 159(5),* 775–783.

Agras, W. S., Walsh, B. T., Fairburn, C. G., Wilson, G. T., & Kraemer, H. C. (2000). A multi-center comparison of cognitive-behavioral therapy and interpersonal psychotherapy for bulimia nervosa. *Archives of General Psychiatry, 57,* 459–466.

Andersen, H. C. (1987). *Andersen's fairy tales.* New York: Signet.

Anderson, D. A., & Williamson, D. A. (2002). Outcome measurement in eating disorders. In W. W. IsHak, T. Burt, & L. I. Sederer (Eds.), *Outcome measurement in psychiatry: A critical review* (pp. 289–301). Washington, DC: American Psychiatric Publishing.

Anderson, E. M., & Lambert, M. J. (1995). Short-term dynamically oriented psychotherapy: A review and meta-analysis. *Clinical Psychology Review, 15,* 503–514.

Antoni, M. H., August, S., Bagget, L., Klimas, N., Fletcher, M., & Schneiderman, N. (1991). Cognitive-behavioral stress management intervention buffers distress responses and immunologic changes following notification of HIV-II seropositivity. *Journal of Consulting and Clinical Psychology, 59 (6),* 906–915.

Appiah, K. A. (2003). Into the woods. *New York Review of Books, December 18,* 46–51.

Atkeson, B. M., Calhoun, K. S., & Resick, P. A. (1982). Victims of rape: Repeated assessment of depressive symptoms. *Journal of Consulting and Clinical Psychology, 50(1),* 96–102.

August, G. J., Realmuto, G. M., Hektner, J. M., & Bloomquist, M. L. (2001). An integrated components preventive intervention for aggressive elementary school children: The early risers program. *Journal of Consulting and Clinical Psychology, 69(4),* 614–626.

Bachrach, H. H., Weber, J. J., & Solomon, M. (1985). Factors associated with the outcome of psychoanalysis (clinical and methodological considerations): Report of the Columbia Psychoanalytic Center Research Project (IV). *International Review of Psychoanalysis, 12,* 379–388.

Bankart, C. P. (1997). *Talking cures: A history of western and eastern psychotherapies.* New York: Brooks/Cole.

Barber, J. P., & Crits-Christoph, P. (Eds.). (1995). *Dynamic therapies for psychiatric disorders (Axis 1).* New York: Basic Books.

Barber, J. P., & Muenz, L. R. (1996). The role of avoidance and obsessiveness in matching patients to cognitive and interpersonal psychotherapy: Empirical findings from the treatment for depression collaborative research program. *Journal of Consulting and Clinical Psychology, 64(5),* 951–958.

Barkham, M., Rees, A., Stiles, W. B., Shapiro, D. A., Hardy, G. E., & Reynolds,

S. (1996). Dose-effect relations in time-limited psychotherapy for depression. *Journal of Consulting and Clinical Psychology, 64(5),* 927–935.

Barkley, R. A., Guevremont, D. C., Anastopoulis, A. D., & Fletcher, K. E. (1992). A comparison of three family therapy programs for treating family conflicts in adolescents with attention-deficit hyperactivity disorder. *Journal of Consulting and Clinical Psychology, 60(3),* 450–462.

Barrett, P. M., Dadds, M. R., & Rapee, R. M. (1996). Family treatment of childhood anxiety: A controlled trial. *Journal of Consulting and Clinical Psychology, 64(5),* 333–342.

Barrowclough, C., Haddock, G., Tarrier, N., Lewis, S. W., Moring, J., O'Brien, R., Schofield, N., et al. (2001). Randomized controlled trial of motivational interviewing, cognitive intervention for patients with comorbid schizophrenia and substance use disorders, behavior therapy, and family. *American Journal of Psychiatry, 10(158),* 1706–1713.

Barrowclough, C., King, P., Colville, J., Russell, E., Burns, A., & Tarrier, N. (2001). A randomized trial of the effectiveness of cognitive-behavioral therapy and supportive counseling for anxiety symptoms in older adults. *Journal of Consulting and Clinical Psychology, 69(5),* 756–762.

Basen-Engquist, K., Edmundson, E. W., & Parcel, G. S. (1996). Structure of health risk behavior among high school students. *Journal of Consulting and Clinical Psychology, 64(4),* 764–775.

Beck, A. T. (1967). *Depression: Causes and treatment.* Philadelphia: University of Pennsylvania Press.

Beck, A. T., Brown, G. K., & Steer, R. A. (1997). Psychometric characteristics of the scale for suicide ideation with psychiatric outpatients. *Behavior Research and Therapy, 35(11),* 1039–1046.

Beck, A. T., Steer, R. A., & Garbin, M. G. (1988). Psychometric properties of the Beck Depression Inventory: Twenty-five years of evaluation. *Clinical Psychology Review, 8(1),* 77–100.

Beck, A. T., Ward, C. H., & Mendelson, M. (1961). An inventory for measuring depression. *Archives of General Psychiatry, 4,* 561–571.

Beck, J. S. (1995). *Cognitive therapy: Basics and beyond.* New York: Guilford Press.

Beck, J. S., Stanley, M. A., Baldwin, L. E., Deagle, E. A., & Averill, P. M. (1994). Comparison of cognitive therapy and relaxation training for panic disorder. *Journal of Consulting and Clinical Psychology, 62(4),* 818–826.

Becker, E. (1973). *The denial of death.* New York: Free Press.

Bellack, A. S., Hersen, M., & Kazdin, A. E. (Eds.). (1982). *International handbook of behavior modification and therapy.* New York: Plenum Press.

Bellah, R. N., Madsen, R., Sullivan, W. M., Swidler, A., & Tipton, S. M. (1985). *Habits of the heart: Individualism and commitment in American life.* Berkeley, CA: University of California Press.

Beretvas, S. N., & Pastor, D. A. (2003). Using mixed-effects models in reliability generalization studies. *Educational and Psychological Measurement, 63(1),* 75–95.

Bergin and Garfield's handbook of psychotherapy and behavior change (5th ed). (2004). M. J. Lambert (Ed.). New York: Wiley.

Beutler, L. E., Engle, D., Mohr, D., Daldrup, R. J., Bergan, J., Meredith, K., & Merry, W. (1991). Predictors of differential response to cognitive, experiential, and self-directed psychotherapeutic procedures. *Journal of Consulting and Clinical Psychology, (59)2,* 333–340.

Beutler, L. E., Scogin, F., Kirkish, P., Schretlen, D., Corbishley, A., Hamblin, D., Meredith, K., et al. (1987). Group cognitive therapy and alprazolam in the treatment of depression in older adults. *Journal of Consulting and Clinical Psychology, 55(4),* 550–556.

Birmaher, B., Brent, D. A., Kolko, D., Baugher, M., Bridge, J., Holder, D., Iyengar, S., et al. (2000). Clinical outcome after shorter-term psychotherapy for adolescents with major depressive disorder. *Archives of General Psychiatry, 57,* 29–36.

Blaney, P. H. (1977). Contemporary theories of depression: Critique and comparison. *Journal of Abnormal Psychology, 86(3),* 203–223.

Blatt, S. J., Zuroff, D. C., Quinlan, D. M., & Pilkonis, P. A. (1996). Interpersonal factors in brief treatment of depression: Further analyses of the National Institute of Mental Health treatment of depression collaborative research program. *Journal of Consulting and Clinical Psychology, 64(1),* 162–171.

Blavatsky, H. P. (1877). *Isis unveiled.* Wheaton, IL: Theosophical Press.

———. (1972). *Dynamics of the psychic world.* Wheaton, IL: Theosophical Publishing House.

Blomberg, J., Lazar, A., & Sandell, R. (2001). Long-term outcome of long-term psychoanalytically oriented therapies: First findings of the Stockholm outcome of psychotherapy and psychoanalysis study. *Psychotherapy Research 11,* 361–382.

Bloom, H. (1992). *The American religion: Emergence of the post-Christian nation.* New York: Simon & Schuster.

Boney-McCoy, S., & Finkelhor, D. (1995). Psychological squeal of violent victimization in a national youth sample. *Journal of Consulting and Psychology, 63(5),* 726–736.

Bornstein, R. F., & Masling, J. M. (1998). *Empirical Studies of the Therapeutic Hour.* Washington, DC: American Psychological Association.

Boscarino, J. A. (1996). Posttraumatic stress disorder, exposure to combat, and lower plasma cortisol among Vietnam veterans: Findings and clinical implications. *Journal of Consulting and Clinical Psychology, 64(1),* 191–201.

Brent, D. A., Holder, D., & Kolko, D. (1997). A clinical psychotherapy trial for adolescent depression comparing cognitive, family, and supportive therapy. *Archives of General Psychiatry, 54(9),* 877–885.

Brown, C., Shulberg, H. C., Madonia, M. J., Shear, M. K., & Houck, P. R. (1996). Treatment outcomes for primary care patients with major depression and lifetime anxiety disorders. *American Journal of Psychiatry, 153,* 1293–1300.

Buckley, T. C., Parker, J. D., & Heggie, J. (2001). A psychometric evaluation of the

BDI-II in treatment-seeking substance abusers. *Journal of Substance Abuse Treatment, 20(3),* 197–204.

Burish, T. G., Snyder, S. L., & Jenkins, R. A. (1991). Preparing patients for cancer chemotherapy: Effect of coping preparation and relaxation interventions. *Journal of Consulting and Clinical Psychology, (59)4,* 518–525.

Butler, G., & Anastasiades, P. (1988). Predicting response to anxiety management in patients with generalised anxiety disorders. *Behavior Research and Therapy, 26,* 531–534.

Butler, G., Cullington, A., Hibbert, G., Klines, I., & Gelder, M. (1987). Anxiety management for persistent generalised anxiety disorder. *British Journal of Psychiatry, 151,* 535–542.

Butler, G., Fennell, M., Robson, P., & Gelder, M. (1991). Comparison of behavior therapy and cognitive behavior therapy in the treatment of generalized anxiety disorder. *Journal of Consulting and Clinical Psychology, 59(1),* 167–175.

Butler, G., Gelder, M., Hibbert, G., Cullington, A., & Klimes, I. (1987). Anxiety management: Developing effective strategies. *Behavior Research and Therapy, 25,* 517–522.

Byerly, F. C., & Carlson, W. A. (1982). Comparison among inpatients, outpatients, and normals on three self-report depression inventories. *Journal of Consulting and Clinical Psychology, 38(4),* 797–804.

Carroll, K. M., Ball, S. A., Nich, C., O'Connor, P. G., Eagan, D. A., Frankforter, T. L., Triffleman, E. G., et al. (2001). Targeting behavioral therapies to enhance naltrexone treatment of opioid dependence. *Archives of General Psychiatry, 58,* 755–761.

Casacalenda, N., Perry, J. C., & Looper, K. (2002). Remission in major depressive disorder: A comparison of pharmacotherapy, psychotherapy, and control conditions. *American Journal of Psychiatry, 159(8),* 1354–1360.

Celio, A. A., Winzelberg, A. J., Wilfley, D. E., Eppstien-Herald, D., Springer, E. A., Dev, P., & Taylor, C. B. (2000). Reducing risk factors for eating disorders: Comparison of an Internet and a classroom-delivered psycho-educational program. *Journal of Consulting and Clinical Psychology, 68(4),* 650–657.

Chemtob, C. M., Novaco, R. W., Hamada, R. S., & Gross, D. M. (1997). Cognitive-behavioral treatment for severe anger in posttraumatic stress disorder. *Journal of Consulting and Clinical Psychology, 65(1),* 184–189.

Chen, X., Rubin, K. H., & Li, B-S. (1995). Depressed mood in Chinese children: Relations with school performance and family environment. *Journal of Consulting and Clinical Psychology, 63(6),* 938–947.

Chessick, R. D. (1996). *Dialogue concerning contemporary psychodynamic theory.* Northvale, NJ: Jason Aronson.

Clapp, J. D. (1999). *The community/collegiate AOD prevention partnership: Project CAPP.* U.S. Department of Education, Application #S184H990014.

———. (2000). *Alcohol & other drug prevention models on college campuses.* U.S. Department of Education, Application #S184 N010020.

———. (2001). *High risk drinking/violent behavior among college sudents.* U.S. Department of Education, Application #s184H010044.

Clapp, J. D., Lange, J. E., Russell, C., Shillingon, A., & Boas, R. B. (2003). A failed norms social marketing campaign. *Journal of Studies on Alcohol, May,* 409–414.

Clark, D. A., Beck, A. T., & Alford, B. A. (1999). *Scientific foundations of cognitive theory and therapy of depression.* New York: John Wiley & Sons.

Clarke, G. N., Hornbrook, M., Lynch, F., Polen, M., Gale, J., Beardslee, W., O'Connor, E., et al. (2001). A randomized trial of a group cognitive intervention for preventing depression in adolescent offspring of depressed parents. *Achives of General Psychiatry, 58,* 1127–1134.

Classen, C., Butler, L. D., Koopman, C., Miller, E., Dimicelli, S., Giese-Davis, J., Fobair, P., et al. (2001). Supportive-expressive group therapy and distress in patients with metastic breast cancer. *Archives of General Psychiatry, 58,* 494–501.

Cobham, V. E., Dadds, M. R., & Spence, S. H. (1998). The role of parental anxiety in the treatment of childhood anxiety. *Journal of Consulting and Clinical Psychology, 66(6),* 893–905.

Connors, G. J., Carroll, K. M., DiClemente, C. C., Longabaugh, R., & Donovan, D. M. (1997). The therapeutic alliance and its relationship to alcoholism treatment participation and outcome. *Journal of Consulting and Clinical Psychology, 65(4),* 588–598.

Cooper, Z., Cooper, P. J., & Christopher, G. (1989). The validity of the Eating Disorder Examination and its subscales. *British Journal of Psychiatry, 154,* 807–812.

Corrigan, P. W. (2001). Getting ahead of the data: A threat to some behavior therapies. *The Behavior Therapist, October,* 189–193.

Corrigan, P. W., & Liberman, R. P. (1994). *Behavior therapy in psychiatric hospitals.* New York: Springer Publishing.

Coyne, J. C., & Gotlib, I. H. (1983). The role of cognition in depression: A critical appraisal. *Psychological Bulletin, 94(3),* 472–505.

Crews, F. (1993). The unknown Freud. *New York Review, 30(19),* 55–66.

Crits-Christoph, P., Crits-Christoph, K., Wolf-Palacio, D., Fichter, M., & Rudick, D. (1995). Brief supportive-expressive psychodynamic therapy for generalized anxiety disorder. In J. P. Barber & P. Crits-Christoph (Eds.), *Dynamic therapies for psychiatric disorders (Axis 1)* (pp. 43–83). New York: Basic Books.

Curran, P. J., Stice, E., & Chassin, L. (1997). The relationship between adolescent alcohol use and peer alcohol use: A longitudinal random coefficients model. *Journal of Consulting and Clinical Psychology, 65(1),* 130–140.

Curry, S. J., McBride, C., Grothaus, L. C., Louie, D., & Wagner, E. H. (1995). A randomized trial of self-help materials, personalized feedback, and telephone counseling with non-volunteer smokers. *Journal of Consulting and Clinical Psychology, 63(6),* 1005–1014.

Dadds, M. R., & Mchugh, T. A. (1992). Social support and treatment outcome in behavioral family therapy for child conduct problems. *Journal of Consulting and Clinical Psychology, (60) 2,* 252–259.

Dawes, R. M. (1994). *House of cards: Psychology and psychotherapy built on myth.* New York: Free Press.

Deale, A., Chalder, T., Marks, I., & Wessely, S. (1997). Cognitive behavior therapy for chronic fatigue syndrome: A randomized controlled trail. *American Journal of Psychiatry, 154 (3),* 408–414.

Devilly, G. J. (2001a). The influence of distraction during exposure and research allegiance during outcome trials. *The Behavior Therapist, 24,* 18–21.

———. (2001b). Effect size and methodological rigor in EDMR: A reply to Lipke's (2001) comment. *The Behavior Therapist, October,* 195.

Diguisto, E., & Bird, K. D. (1995). Matching smokers to treatment: Self-control versus social support. *Journal of Consulting and Clinical Psychology, 63(2),* 290–295.

DiMaggio, P., Evans, J., & Bryson, B. (1996). Have Americans' social attitudes become more polarized? *American Journal of Sociology, 102(3),* 690–755.

DiMascio, A., Weissman, M. M., Prusoff, B. A., Neu, C., Zwilling, M., & Klerman, G. L. (1979). Differential symptom reduction by drugs and psychotherapy in acute depression. *Archives of General Psychiatry, 36,* 1450–1456.

Dineen, T. (1996). *Manufacturing victims.* Montreal: Robert Davies Publishing.

Dishion, T. J., & Andrews, D. W. (1995). Preventing escalating in problem behaviors with high-risk young adolescents: Immediate and 1-year outcomes. *Journal of Consulting and Clinical Psychology, 63(4),* 538–548.

Dobson, K. S. (1989). A meta-analysis of the efficacy of cognitive therapy for depression. *Journal of Consulting and Clinical Psychology, 57,* 414–419.

———. (2001). *Handbook of cognitive-behavioral therapies.* New York: Guilford Press.

Dobson, K. S., & Breiter, H. J. (1983). Cognitive assessment of depression: reliability and validity of three measures. *Journal of Abnormal Psychology, 92(1),* 107–109.

Dobson, K. S., & Craig, K. D. (1996). *Advances in cognitive-behavioral therapy.* Thousand Oaks, CA: Sage.

Drake, R. E., McHugo, G. J., Becker, D. R., Anthony, W. A., & Clark, R. E. (1996). The New Hampshire study of supported employment for people with severe mental illness. *Journal of Consulting and Clinical Psychology, 64 (2),* 391–399.

Dryden, W. (1996). *Developments in psychotherapy: Historical perspective.* London: Sage.

Dryden, W., & Feltham, C. (1992). *Psychotherapy and its discontents.* Buckingham: Open University Press.

Dufresne, T. (2000). *Tales from the Freudian crypt.* Stanford, CA: Stanford University Press.

———. (2003). *Killing Freud.* London: Continuum.

Dumas, J. E. (1986). Parental perception and treatment outcome in families of aggressive children: A causal model. *Behavior Therapy, 17,* 420–432.

Dumas, J. E., & Albin, J. B. (1986). Parent training outcome: Does active parental involvement matter? *Behavior Research and Therapy, 24,* 227–230.

Eddy, M. B. (1994). *Science and health with key to the Scriptures.* Boston, MA: Christian Science Board of Directors.

Ehlers, A., Stangier, U., & Gieler, U. (1995). Treatment of atopic dermatitis: A comparison of psychological and dermatological approaches to relapse prevention. *Journal of Consulting and Clinical Psychology, 63(4),* 624–635.

Eisner, D. A. (2000). *The death of psychotherapy.* Westport, CT: Praeger.

Elkin, I., Gibbons, R. D., Shea, M. T., Sotsky, S. M., Watkins, J. T., & Pilkonis, P. A. (1995). Initial severity and differential treatment outcome in the National Institute of Mental Health Treatment of Depression Collaborative Research Program. *Journal of Consulting and Clinical Psychology, 63(5),* 841–847.

Elkin, I., Shea, M. T., Watkins, J. T., Imber, S. D., Sotsky, S. M., Collins, J. F., Glass, D. R., et al. (1989). National Institute of Mental Health Treatment of Depression Collaborative Research Program: General effectiveness of treatments. *Archives of General Psychiatry, 46(11),* 971–982.

Ellis, A. (1962). *Reason and emotion in psychotherapy.* Secaucus, NJ: Lyle Stuart.

Endicott, J., Spitzer, R. L., Fleiss, J. L., & Cohen, J. (1976). The Global Assessment Scale: A procedure for measuring the overall severity of psychiatric disturbance. *Archives of General Psychiatry, 33,* 766–771.

Epstein, W. M. (1984a). Technology and social work, part 1: The effectiveness of psychotherapy. *Journal of Applied Social Sciences, 8(2),* 155–175.

———. (1984b). Technology and social work, part 2: Psychotherapy, family therapy and implications for practice. *Journal of Applied Social Sciences, 8(2),* 175–87.

———. (2005). The problem of psychotherapy in social work. In S. Kirk (Ed.), *Mental disorders in the social environment.* New York: Columbia University Press.

———. (in press). Response bias in opinion polls and American social welfare. *Social Science Journal, 43(3).*

Erikson, K. T. (1966). *Wayward Puritans.* New York: John Wiley.

Erle, J. B. (1979). An approach to the study of analyzability and analysis: The course of forty consecutive cases selected for supervised analysis. *Psychoanalytic Quarterly, 48,* 198–228.

Eysenck, H. F. (1965). The effects of psychotherapy. *International Journal of Psychiatry, 1,* 97.

Fals-Stewart, W., Birchler, G. R., & O'Farrel, T. J. (1996). Behavioral couple therapy for male substance-abusing patients: Effects on relationship adjustment and drug-using behavior. *Journal of Consulting and Clinical Psychology, 64(5),* 959–972.

Fava, F. A., Rafanelli, C., Grandi, S., Conti, S., & Belluardo, P. (1998). Prevention of recurrent depression with cognitive behavioral therapy. *Archives of General Psychiatry, 55,* 816–820.

Foa, E. B., Rothbaum, B. O., Riggs, D. S., & Murdock, T. B. (1991). Treatment of posttraumatic stress disorder in rape victims: A comparison between cognitive behavioral procedures and counseling. *Journal of Consulting and Clinical Psychology, 59(5),* 715–723.

Foy, D. W., Nunn, L. B., & Rychtarik, R. G. (1984). Broad-spectrum behavioral treatment for chronic alcoholics: Effects of training controlled drinking skills. *Journal of Consulting and Clinical Psychology, 52*, 218–230.

Frank, E., Shear, K. M., Rucci, P., Cyranowski, J. M., Endicott, J., Fagniolini, A., Grochocinski, V. J., et al. (2000). Influence of panic-agoraphobic spectrum symptoms on treatment response in patients with recurrent major depression. *American Journal of Psychiatry, 157(7)*, 1101–1107.

Frank, J. D. (1974). *Persuasion and healing.* Baltimore, MD: Johns Hopkins University Press.

Franklin, M. E., Abramowitz, J. S., Kozak, M. J., Levitt, J. T., & Foa, E. B. (2000). Effectiveness of exposure and ritual prevention for obsessive-compulsive disorder: Randomized compared with nonrandomized samples. *Journal of Consulting and Clinical Psychology, 68(4)*, 594–602.

Franks, C. M., Wilson, G. T., Kendall, P. C., & Foreyt, J. P. (1990). Review of behavior therapy: Theory and practice. (Vol. 12). New York: Guilford Publications.

Fraser, C. (1999). *God's perfect child: Living and dying in the Christian Science Church.* New York: Henry Holt.

Freedheim, D. K. (1992). *History of psychotherapy: A century of change.* Washington, DC: American Psychological Association.

Freedman, S. R., & Enright, R. D. (1996). Forgiveness as an intervention goal with incest survivors. *Journal of Consulting and Clinical Psychology, 64(5)*, 983–992.

Freeman, A., & Dattilio, F. M. (1992). *Comprehensive casebook of cognitive therapy.* New York: Plenum Press.

Freeston, M. H., Ladouceur, R., Giagnon, F., Thibodeau, N., Rhéaume, J., Letarte, H., & Bujold, A. (1997). Cognitive-behavioral treatment of obsessive thoughts: A contolled study. *Journal of Consulting and Clincial Psychology, 65(3)*, 405–413.

Freud, S. (1961). *Civilization and its discontents.* New York: W. W. Norton.

Gaffan, E. A., Tsaousis, I., & Kemp-Wheeler, S. M. (1995). Researcher alliance and meta-analysis: The case of cognitive therapy for depression. *Journal of Consulting and Clinical Psychology, 63*, 966–980.

Gallagher-Thompson, D., & Steffen, A. M. (1994). Comparative effects of cognitive-behavioral and brief psychodynamic psychotherapies for depressed family caregivers. *Journal of Consulting and Clinical Psychology, (62)3*, 543–549.

Gambrill, E. D. (1977). *Behavior modification: Handbook of assessment, intervention, and evaluation.* San Francisco: Jossey-Bass.

Gardner, M. (1952). *In the name of sciences.* New York: Putnam.

Gauthier, J. G. (1999). Bridging the gap between biological and psychological perspectives in the treatment of anxiety disorders. *Canadian Psychology, 40*, 1–11.

Gayle, J. B., Stanley, M. A., Baldwin, L. E., Deagle, III, E. A., & Averill, P. M. (1994). Comparison of cognitive therapy and relaxation training for panic disorder. *Journal of Consulting and Clinical Psychology, 62(4)*, 818–826.

Giambra, L. M. (1977–1978). Adult male daydreaming across the life span: A replication, further analyses and tentative norms based upon retrospective reports. *International Journal of Aging and Human Development, 8(3)*, 197–228.

Gittell, R., & Vidal, A. (1998). *Community organizing: Building social capital as a development strategy.* Thousand Oaks, CA: Sage.

Glueckauf, R. L., & Quittner, A. L. (1992). Assertiveness training for disabled adults in wheelchairs: Self-report, role-play, and activity pattern outcomes. *Journal of Consulting and Clinical Psychology, 60(3),* 419–425.

Goldman, A., & Greenberg, L. (1992). Comparison of integrated systemic and emotionally focused approaches to couples therapy. *Journal of Consulting and Clinical Psychology, 60(6),* 962–969.

Goldstein, A. (1972). Behavior therapy. In R. Corsini (Ed.), *Current psychotherapies.* Itasca, IL: Peacock.

Goodkin, K., Blaney, N. T., Feaster, D. J., Baldewicz, T., Burkhalter, J. E., & Leeds, B. (1999). A randomized controlled clinical trial of a bereavement support group intervention in human immunodeficiency virus type 1-seropositive and -seronegative homosexual men. *Archives of General Psychiatry, 56(1),* 52–59.

Gordon, L. (1992). Social insurance and public assistance: The influence of gender in welfare thought in the United States, 1890–1930. *American Historical Review,* February, 19–54.

Greene, B., & Blanchard, E. B. (1994). Cognitive therapy for irritable bowel syndrome. *Journal of Consulting and Clinical Psychology, 62(3),* 576–582.

Gross, M. L. (1978). *The psychological society.* New York: Random House.

Grunbaum, A. (1984). *The foundations of psychoanalysis.* Berkeley, CA: University of California Press.

———. (1993). *Validation in the clinical theory of psychoanalysis.* Madison, CT: International Universities Press.

Guthrie, E., Moorey, J., Margison, F., Barker, H., Palmer, S., McGrath, G., Tomenson, B., et. al. (1999). Cost-effectiveness of brief psychodynamic-interpersonal therapy in high utilizers of psychiatric services. *Archives of General Psychiatry, 56,* 519–526.

Hall, C. M. (1998). *Heroic self: Sociological dimensions of clinical practice.* Springfield, IL: Charles C. Thomas.

Hall, S. M., Muñoz, R. F., & Reus, V. I. (1994). Cognitive-behavioral intervention increases abstinence rates for depressive-history smokers. *Journal of Consulting and Clinical Psychology, 62(1),* 141–146.

Hamilton, K. E., & Dobson, K. S. (2002). Cognitive therapy of depression: Pretreatment patient predictors of outcome. *Clinical Psychology Review, 22(6),* 875–894.

Hamilton, M. (1960). A rating scale for depression. *Journal of Neurology, Neurosurgery and Psychiatry, 23,* 56–61.

———. (1967). Development of a rating scale for primary depressive illness. *British Journal of Social and Clinical Psychology, 6(4),* 278–296.

Hammen, C. L. (1980). Depression in college students: Beyond the Beck Depression Inventory. *Journal of Consulting and Clinical Psychology, 48(1),* 126–128.

Harcum, E. R., & Rosen, E. F. (1993). *The gatekeepers of psychology: Evaluation of peer review by case history.* Westport, CT: Praeger.

Hardy, G. E., Barkham, M., Shapiro, D. A., Stiles, W. B., Rees, A., & Reynolds, S. (1995). Impact of cluster c personality disorders on outcomes of contrasting brief psychotherapies for depression. *Journal of Consulting and Clinical Psychology, 63(6),* 997–1004.

Heatherton, T. F., Kozlowski, L. T., & Frecker, R. C. (1991). The Fagerström Test for Nicotine Dependence: A revision of the Fagerström Tolerance Questionnaire. *British Journal of Addiction, 86(9),* 1119–1127.

Heimberg, R. G., Liebowitz, M. R., Hope, D. A., Schneier, F. R., Holt, C. S., Welkowitz, L. A., Juster, H. R., et al. (1998). Cognitive behavioral group therapy vs phenelzine therapy of social phobia. *Archives of General Psychiatry, 55,* 1133–1141.

Heineman, M. B. (1981). The obsolete scientific imperative in social work. *Social Service Review, 55(3),* 371–397.

Henggeler, S. W., Melton, G. B., Brondino, M. J., Scherer, D. G., & Hanley, J. H. (1997). Multisystemic therapy with violent and chronic juvenile offenders and their families: The role of treatment fidelity in successful dissemination. *Journal of Consulting and Clinical Psychology, 65(5),* 821–833.

Henggeler, S. W., Melton, G. B., Brondino, & Smith, L. A. (1992). Family preservation using multistyemic therapy: An effective alternative to incarcerating serious juvenile offenders. *Journal of Consulting and Clinical Psychology, 60(6),* 953–961.

Henricksen, G. I., & Mahr, J. M. (1987). A behavioral approach to enhanced participation of mentally retarded people in the religious experience. In J. A. Mulick & R. F. Antonak (Eds.), *Transitions in Mental Retardation* (pp. 150–166). Norwood, NJ: Ablex.

Herceg-Baron, R. L., Prusoff, B. A., Weissman, M. M., DiMascio, A., Neu, C., & Kerman, G. L. (1979). Pharmacotherapy and psychotherapy in acutely depressed patients: A study of attrition patterns in a clinical trial. *Comparative Psychiatry, 20,* 315–325.

Herz, M. I., Lamberti, J. S., & Mintz, J. (2000). A program for relapse prevention in schizophrenia: A controlled study. *Archives of General Psychiatry, 57(3),* 277–283.

Higgins, S. T., Wong, C. J., Badger, G. J., Haug Ogden, D. E., & Dantona, R. L. (2000). Contingent reinforcement increases cocaine abstinence during outpatient treatment and 1 year of follow-up. *Journal of Consulting and Clinical Psychology, 68(1),* 64–72.

Hobson, J. A. (2004). Rejoinder. *Scientific American, May,* 89.

Hogarty, G. E., Greenwald, D., Ulrich, R. F., Kornblith, S. J., DiBarry, A. L., Cooley, S., Carter, M., et al. (1997). Three-year trials of personal therapy among schizophrenic patients living with or independent of family, II: Effects of adjustment of patients. *American Journal of Psychiatry, 154(11),* 1514–1524.

Hogarty, G. E., Kornblith, S. J., & Greenwald, D. (1997). Three-year trials of personal therapy among schizophrenic patients living with or independent of family: I. Description of study and effects of relapse rates. *American Journal of Psychiatry, 154(11),* 1504–1513.

Hollon, S. D., & Kendall, P. C. (1980). Cognitive self-statements in depression: Development of an automatic thoughts questionnaire. *Cognitive Therapy and Research,* *4(4),* 383–395.

Horvath, A. O., & Greenberg, L. S. (1989). Development and validation of the Working Alliance Inventory. *Journal of Counseling Psychology, 36(2),* 223–233.

Hunt, M. M. (1999). *The new know-nothings: The political foes of the scientific study of human nature.* New Brunswick, NJ: Transaction Publishers.

Huppert, J. D., Bufka, L. F., Barlow, D. H., Gorman, J. M., Shear, M. K., & Woods, S. W. (2001). Therapist, therapist variables, and cognitive-behavioral therapy outcome in a multicenter trial for pain disorder. *Journal of Consulting and Clinical Psychology, 69(5),* 747–755.

Iguchi, M. Y., Belding, M. A., Morral, A. R., Lamb, R. J., & Husband, S. D. (1997). Reinforcing operants other than abstinence in drug abuse treatment: An effective alternative for reducing drug use. *Journal of Consulting and Clinical Psychology, 65 (3),* 421–428.

Imber, S. D., Pilkonis, P. A., Sotsky, S. M., Elkin, I., Watkins, J. T., Collins, J. F., Shea, M. T., et al. Mode-specific effects among three treatments for depression. *Journal of Consulting and Clinical Psychology, 58(3),* 352–359.

Insel, R. R., & Charney, D. S. (2003). Research on major depression. *Journal of the American Medical Association, 289(23),* 3167–3168.

Jackson, S. W. (1999). *Care of the psyche: A history of psychological healing.* New Haven, CT: Yale University Press.

Jacobson, N. S., Dobson, K. S., Truax, P. A., Addis, M. E., Koerner, K., Gollan, J. K., Gortner, E., et al. (1996). A component analysis of cognitive-behavioral treatment for depression. *Journal of Consulting and Clinical Psychology, 64(2),* 295–304.

Jacobson, N. S., Fruizzetti, A. E., Dobson, K., Whisman, M., & Hops, H. (1993). Couple therapy as a treatment for depression: The effects of relationship quality and therapy on depressive relapse. *Journal of Consulting and Clinical Psychology, 61(3),* 516–519.

James, R. K., & Gilliland, B. E. (2003). *Theories and strategies in counseling and psychotherapy.* Boston, MA: Allyn and Bacon.

Jarrett, R. B., Kraft, D., Doyle, J., Foster, B. M., Eaves, G. G., & Silver, P. C. (2001). Preventing recurrent depression using cognitive therapy with and without a continuation phase. *Archives of General Psychiatry, 58,* 381–388.

Jarrett, R. B., Schaffer, M., McIntire, D., Witt-Browder, A., Kraft, D., & Risser, R. C. (1999). Treatment of atypical depression with cognitive therapy or phenelzine: A double-blind, placebo-controlled trial. *Archives of General Psychiatry, 56,* 431–437.

Jeffrey, R. W., Wing, R. R., & Mayer, R. R. (1998). Are smaller weight losses or more achievable weight loss goals better in the long term for obese patients? *Journal of Consulting and Clinical Psychology, 66(4),* 641–645.

Jeffrey, R. W., Wing, R. R., Thorson, C., & Burton, L. R. (1998). Use of personal trainers and financial incentives to increase exercise in a behavioral weight-loss program. *Journal of Consulting and Clinical Psychology, 66(5),* 777–783.

Jouriles, E. N., McDonald, R., Spiller, L., Norwood, W. D., Swank, P. R., Stephens,

N., Ware, H., et al. (2001). Reducing conduct problems among children of battered women. *Journal of Consulting and Clinical Psychology, 69(5),* 774–785.

Jurjevich, R. M. (1974). *The hoax of Freudism: A study of brainwashing the American professionals and laymen.* Philadelphia: Dorrance.

Kaiser, A., Hahlweg, K., Fehm-Wolfsdorf, G., & Groth, T. (1998). The efficacy of a compact psychoeducational group training program for married couples. *Journal of Consulting and Clinical Psychology, 66(5),* 753–760.

Kantrowitz, J. L. (1986). The role of the patient-analyst "match" in the outcome of psychoanalysis. *Annals of Psychoanalysis, 14,* 273–297.

Kazdin, A. E., Siegel, T. C., & Bass, D. (1992). Cognitive problem-solving skills training and parent management training in the treatment of antisocial behavior in children. *Journal of Consulting and Clinical Psychology, 60(5),* 733–747.

Kelley, M. L., & Fals-Stewart, W. (2002). Couples- versus individual-based therapy for alcohol and drug abuse: Effects on children's psychosocial functioning. *Journal of Consulting and Clinical Psychology, 70(2),* 417–427.

Kelly, A. E. (2000). Helping construct desirable identities: A self-presentational view of psychotherapy. *Psychological Bulletin, 126(4),* 475–494.

Kendall, P. C., Flannery-Schroeder, E., Panichelli-Mindel, S. M., Southam-Gerow, M., Henin, A., & Warman, M. (1997). Therapy for youths with anxiety disorders: A second randomized clinical trial. *Journal of Consulting and Clinical Psychology, 65(3),* 366–380.

Kessler, R. C., Berglund, P., & Demler, O. (2003). The epidemiology of major depressive disorder: Results from the National Comorbidity Survey Replication (NCS.R). *JAMA: Journal of the American Medical Association, 289(23),* 3095–3105.

Killen, J. D., Fortmann, S. P., & Kraemer, H. C. (1996). Interactive effects of depression symptoms, nicotine dependence, and weight change on late smoking relapse. *Journal of Consulting and Clinical Psychology, 64(5),* 1060–1067.

Killen, J. D., Robinson, T. N., & Haydel, K. F. ((1997). Prospective study of risk factors for the initiation of cigarette smoking. *Journal of Consulting and Clinical Psychology, 65(6),* 1011–1016.

Kintz, B. L., Delprato, D. J. & Mettee, D. R. (1965). The experimenter effect. *Psychological Bulletin, 63(4),* 223–232.

Kirby, K. C., Marlowe, D. B., & Festinger, D. S. (1998). Schedule of voucher delivery influences initiation of cocaine abstinence. *Journal and Consulting and Clinical Psychology, 66(5),* 761–767.

Kirk, S. A., & Kutchins, H. (1992). *The selling of DSM: The rhetoric of science in psychiatry.* New York: A. de Gruyter.

Klesges, R. C., Haddock, C. K., & Lando, H. (1999). Efficacy of forced smoking cessation and an adjunctive behavioral treatment on long-term smoking rates. *Journal of Consulting and Clinical Psychology, 67(6),* 952–958.

Kolko, D. J., Brent, D. A., & Baugher, M. (2000). Cognitive and family therapies for adolescent depression: treatment specificity, mediation, and moderation. *Journal of Consulting and Clinical Psychology, 68(4),* 603–614.

Krijn, M., Emmelkamp, P. M. G., & Olafsson, R. P. (2004). Virtual reality exposure therapy of anxiety disorders: A review. *Clinical Psychology Review, 24(3)*, 259–281.

Kutchins, H., & Kirk, S. A. (1997). *Making us crazy: DSM, The psychiatric bible and the creation of mental disorders.* New York: Free Press.

Lambert, M., Weber, F. D., & Sykes, J. D. (1993). Psychotherapy versus placebo therapies: A review of the metaanalytic literature. Poster presented at the annual meeting of the Western Psychological Association, Phoenix, AZ.

Landman, J. T., & Dawes, R. M. (1982). Psychotherapy outcome: Smith and Glass's conclusions stand up under scrutiny. *American Psychologist, 37*, 504–516.

Latimer, W. W., Newcomb, M., & Winters, K. C. (2000). Adolescent substance abuse treatment outcome: The role of substance abuse problem severity, psychosocial, and treatment factors. *Journal of Consulting and Clinical Psychology, 68(4)*, 684–696.

Lazarus, A. A. (1989). *The practice of multimodal therapy: Systematic, comprehensive, and effective psychotherapy.* Baltimore, MD: Johns Hopkins University Press.

Leahy, R. L. (1996). *Cognitive therapy: Basic principles and applications.* Northvale, NJ: Jason Aronson.

Lehman, A. F., Dixon, L. B., & Kernan, E. (1997). A randomized trial of assertive community treatment for homeless persons with seere mental illness. *Archives of General Psychiatry, 54(11)*, 1038–1043.

Leigh, I. W., & Anthony-Tolbert, S. (2001). Reliability of the BDI-II with deaf persons. *Rehabilitation Psychology, 46(2)*, 195–202.

Lenze, E. J., Dew, M. A., & Mazumdar, S. (2002). Combined pharmacotherapy and psychotherapy as maintenance treatment for late-life depression: Effects on social adjustment. *American Journal of Psychiatry, 159(3)*, 466–468.

Lerman, P. (1975). *Community treatment and social control: A critical analysis of juvenile correctional policy.* Chicago: University of Chicago Press.

Levenson, H. (1995). *Time-limited dynamic psychotherapy: A guide to clinical practice.* New York: Basic Books.

Liebowitz, M. R., Heimberg, R. G., Schneier, F. R., Hope, D. A., Davies, S., Holt, C. S., Goetz, D., et al. (1999). Cognitive-behavioral group therapy versus phenelzine in social phobia: Long term outcome. *Depression and Anxiety, 10(3)*, 89–98.

Lilienfeld, S. O., Lynn, S. J., & Lohr, J. M. (Eds.). (2003). *Science and pseudoscience in clinical psychology.* New York: Guilford Press.

Lipke, H. (2001). Response to Devilly's (2001) claims on distraction and exposure. *Behavior Therapist, 24(9)*, 195.

Loftus, E., & Ketcham, K. (1994). *The myth of repressed memory: False memories and allegations of sexual abuse.* New York: St. Martin's Press.

Longabaugh, R., Wirtz, P. W., & Beattie, M. C. (1995). Matching treatment focus to patient social investment and support: 18-month follow-up results. *Journal of Consulting and Clinical Psychology, 63(2)*, 296–307.

Lowi, T. J. (1995). *The end of the republican era.* Norman, OK: University of Oklahoma Press.

Luborsky, L., Singer, B., & Luborsky, L. (1975). Comparative studies of psychother-apies: Is it true that "Everybody has won and all must have prizes"? *Archives of General Psychiatry, 32 (August),* 995–1008.

Luborsky, L., Woody, G. E., & Hole, A. V. (1995). Supportive-expressive dynamic psychotherapy for treatment of opiate drug dependence. In J. P. Barber & P. Crits-Christoph (Eds.), *Dynamic therapies for psychiatric disorders (Axis I)* (pp. 131–160). New York: Basic Books.

MacIntyre, A. (1967). Sigmund Freud. In P. Edwards (Ed.), *Encyclopedia of philoso-phy* (Vol. 3, pp. 249–252). New York: Macmillan.

Macmillan, M. (1997). *Freud evaluated: The completed arc.* Cambridge, MA: The MIT Press.

Madanes, C. (1995). *The violence of men: New techniques for working with abusive families, a therapy of social action.* San Francisco: Jossey-Bass.

Malcolm, J. (1982). *Psychoanalysis—The impossible profession.* New York: Vintage Books.

Mandino, O. *The greatest secret in the world.* New York: Bantam.

Marder, S. R., Wirshing, W. C., & Mintz, J. (1996). Two-year outcome of social skills training and group psychotherapy for outpatients with schizophrenia. *American Journal of Psychiatry, 153(12),* 1585–1592.

Markowitz, J. C., Klerman, G. L., Clougherty, K. F., Spielman, L. A., Jacobsber, L. B., Fishman, B., Frances, A. J., et al. (1995). Individual psychotherapies for depressed HIV-positive patients. *American Journal of Psychiatry, 152(10),* 1504–1509.

Marks, I., Lovell, K., Noshirvani, H., Livanou, M., & Thraher, S. (1998). Treatment of posttraumatic stress disorder by exposure and/or cognitive restructuring. *Archives of General Psychiatry, 55,* 317–325.

Martin, J. E., Calfas, K. J., Patten, C. A., Polarek, M., Hofstetter, C. R., Noto, J., & Beach, D. (1997). Prospective evaluation of three smoking interventions in 205 recovering alcoholics: One-year results of project scrap-tobacco. *Journal of Con-sulting and Clinical Psychology, 65(1),* 190–194.

Masson, J. M. (1988). *Against therapy: Emotional tyranny and the myth of psychologi-cal healing.* New York: Atheneum.

Maude-Griffin, P. M., Hohenstein, J. M., Humfleet, G. L., Reilly, P. M., Tusel, D. J., & Hall, S. M. (1998). Superior efficacy of cognitive-behavioral therapy for urban crack cocaine abusers: Main and matching effects. *Journal of Consulting and Clin-ical Psychology, 66(5),* 832–837.

McFarlane, W. R., Lukens, E., Link, B., Dushay, R., Deakins, S. A., Newmark, M., Dunne, E. J., et al. (1995). Multiple-family groups and psycho-education in the treatment of schizophrenia. *Archives of General Psychiatry, 52,* 679–687.

McGrath, P. J., Nunes, E. V., Stewart, J. W., Goldman, D., Agosti, V., Ocepek-Welik-son, K., & Quitkin, F. M. (1996). Imipramine treatment of alcoholics with pri-mary depression. *Archives of General Psychiatry, 54,* 232–240.

McKay, J. R., Alterman, A. I., Cacciola, J. S., Rutherford, M. J., O'Brien, C. P., & Koppenhaver, J. (1997). Group counseling versus individualized relapse prevention aftercare following intensive outpatient treatment for cocaine dependence: Initial results. *Journal of Consulting and Clinical Psychology, 65(5),* 778–788.

McKay, J. R., Alterman, A. I., McLellan, A. T., Boardman, C. R., Mulvaney, F. D., & O'Brien, C. P. (1998). Random versus nonrandom assignment in the evaluation of treatment for cocaine abusers. *Journal of Consulting and Clinical Psychology, 66(4),* 697–701.

McLean, P. D., & Taylor, S. (1992). Severity of unipolar depression and choice of treatment. *Behavioral Research and Therapy, 30(5),* 443–451.

McLean, P. D., Whittla, M. L., Thordarson, D. S., Taylor, S., Söchting, I., Kock, W. J., Paterson, R., et al. (2001). Cognitive versus behavior therapy in the group treatment of obsessive-compulsive disorder. *Journal of Consulting and Clinical Psychology, 69(2),* 205–214.

McLellan, A. T., Grisson, G. R., Zanis, D., Randall, M., Brill, P., & O'Brien, C. P. (1997). Problem-service "matching" in addiction treatment. *Archives of General Psychiatry, 54,* 730–735.

McMullin, C. M. (1986). Subjective body experience in adolescent females with varying degrees of weight preoccupation, body dissatisfaction and psychological features of anorexia nervosa and bulimia. *Dissertation Abstracts International, 46(12-B,pt.1).*

McMullin, R. E., & Giles, T. R. (1981). *Cognitive-behavior therapy.* New York: Grune and Stratton.

Meichenbaum, D. H. (1977). *Cognitive-behavior modification: An integrative approach.* New York: Plenum Press.

Meyers, A. W., Graves, T. J., & Whelan, J. P. (1996). An evaluation of a television-delivered behavioral weight loss program: Are the ratings acceptable? *Journal of Consulting and Clinical Psychology, 64(1),* 172–178.

Miller, W. R., Benefield, R. G., & Tonigan, J. S. (1993). Enhancing motivation for change in problem drinking: A controlled comparison of two therapist styles. *Journal of Consulting and Clinical Psychology, 61(3),* 455–461.

Moody, R. A. (1975). *Life after life: The investigation of a phenomenon—Survival of bodily death.* New York: HarperSanFrancisco.

———. (1999). *The last laugh: A new philosophy of near-death expereinces, apparitions, and the paranormal.* Charlottesville, VA: Hampton Roads.

———. (2001). *Life after loss: Conquering grief and finding hope.* New York: HarperSanFrancisco.

Morin, C. M., Kowatch, R. A., Barry, T., & Walton, E. (1993). Cognitive-behavior therapy for late-life insomnia. *Journal of Consulting and Clinical Psychology, 61(1),* 137–146.

MTA Cooperative Group. (1999). A 14-month randomized clinical trial of treatment strategies for attention-deficit/hyperactivity disorder. *Archives of General Psychiatry, 56,* 1073–1086.

Mufson, L., Weissman, M. M., Moreau, D., & Garfinkel, R. (1999). Efficacy of interpersonal psychotherapy for depressed adolescents. *Archives of General Psychiatry, 56,* 573–579.

Mynor-Wallis, L. M., Gath, D. H., Lloyd-Thomas, A. R., & Thomlison, D. (1995). Randomised controlled trial comparing problem solving treatment with amitriptyline and placebo for major depression in primary care. *British Medical Journal, 310,* 441–445.

Nickerson, R. S. (1998). Confirmation bias: A ubiquitous phenomenon in many guises. *Review of General Psychology, 2(2),* 175–220.

Norcross, J. C., Karg, R. S., & Prochaska, J. O. (1997). Clinical psychologists in the 1990s: II. *Clinical Psychologist, 50,* 4–11.

Norcross, J. C., Karpiak, C. P., & Lister, K. M. *What's an integrationist?* Unpublished manuscript.

Norcross, J. C., Karpiak, C. P., & Santoro, S. O. *Clinical psychologists across the years: The division of clinical psychology from 1960 to 2003.* Unpublished manuscript.

O'Hara, M. W., Stuart, S., Gorman, L. L., & Wenzel, A. (2000). Efficacy of interpersonal psychotherapy for postpartum depression. *Archives of General Psychiatry, 57,* 1039–1045.

O'Malley, S. S., Jaffe, A. J., Chang, G., Rode, S., Schottenfeld, R., Meyer, R. E., & Rounsaville, B. (1996). Six-month follow-up of naltrexone and psychotherapy for alcohol dependence. *Archives of General Psychiatry, 53,* 217–224.

Orne, M. T. (1959). The nature of hypnosis: Artifact and essence. *Journal of Abnormal and Social Psychology, 58,* 277–299.

———. (1962). The social psychology of the psychological experiment: With particular reference to demand characteristics and their implications. *American Psychologist, 17,* 776–783.

Öst, L.-G., Svensson, L., Hellström, K., & Lindwall, R. (2001). One-session treatment of specific phobias in youths: A randomized clinical trial. *Journal of Consulting and Clinical Psychology, 69(5),* 814–824.

Paivio, S. C., & Greenberg, L. S. (1995). Resolving "unfinished business": Efficacy of experimental therapy using empty-chair dialogue. *Journal of Consulting and Clinical Psychology, 63(3),* 419–425.

Palmer, T. (1974). The Youth Authority's Community Treatment Program. *Federal Probation, 38,* 3–14.

Park, R. L. (2000). *Science: The road from foolishness to fraud.* New York: Oxford University Press.

Paul, G. L., & Lentz, R. J. (1977). *Psychosocial treatment for chronic mental patients.* Cambridge, MA: Harvard University Press.

Paykel, E. S., Scott, J., & Teasdale, J. D. (1999). Prevention of relapse in residual depression by cognitive therapy: A controlled trial. *Archives of General Psychiatry, 56(9),* 829–835.

Payne, A., & Blanchard, E. B. (1995). A controlled comparison of cognitive therapy and self-help support groups in the treatment of irritable bowel syndrome. *Journal of Consulting and Clinical Psychology, 63(5),* 779–786.

Perkins, K. A., Marcus, M. D., Levine, M. D., D'Amico, D., Miller, A., Broge, M., Aschcom, J., et al. (2001). Cognitive-behavioral therapy to reduce weight concerns improves smoking cessation outcome in weight-concerned women. *Journal of Consulting and Clinical Psychology, 69(4)*, 601–613.

Perri, M. G., Martin, D., Leermakers, E. A., & Notelovitz, M. (1997). Effects of group- versus home-based exercise in the treatment of obesity. *Journal of Consulting and Clinical Psychology, 65(2)*, 278–285.

Perri, M. G., Nezu, A. M., Patti, E. T., & McCann, K. L. (1989). Effect of length of treatment on weight loss. *Journal of Consulting and Clinical Psychology, 57(3)*, 450–452.

Persons, J. B., Davidson, J., Tompkins, M. A. (2001). *Essential components of cognitive-behavior therapy for depression.* Washington, DC: American Psychological Association.

Petry, N. M., & Martin, B. (2002). Low-cost contingency management for treatment cocaine- and opioid-abusing methadone patients. *Journal of Consulting and Clinical Psychology, 70(2)*, 398–405.

Pfeffer, A. Z. (1959). A procedure for evaluating the results of psychoanalysis: A preliminary report. *Journal of the American Psychoanalytic Association, 7*, 418–444.

Pfiffner, L. J., & McBurnett, K. (1997). Social skills training with parent generalization: Treatment effects for children with attention deficit disorder. *Journal of Consulting and Clinical Psychology, 65(4)*, 749–757.

Pianta, R. C., Egeland, B., & Adam, E. K. (1996). Adult attachment classification and self-reported psychiatric symptomalogy as assessed by the Minnesota Multiphasic Personality Inventory-2. *American Psychological Association, 64(2)*, 273–281.

Piper, W. E., Joyce, A. S., McCallum, M., & Azim, H. F. (1998). Interpretive and supportive forms of psychotherapy and patient personality variables. *Journal of Consulting and Clinical Psychology, 66*, 558–567.

Piper, W. E., McCallum, M., Joyce, A. S., Azim, H. F., & Ogrodniczuk, J. S. (1999). Follow-up findings for interpretive and supportive forms of psychotherapy and patient personality variables. *Journal of Consulting and Clinical Psychology, 67*, 267–273.

Pope, H. G. (1997). *Psychology astray.* Boca Raton, FL: Upton Books.

Popper, K. R. (1962). *Conjectures and refutations.* New York: Basic Books.

Prioleau, L., Murdock, M., & Brody, N. (1983). An analysis of psychotherapy versus placebo studies. *Behavioral and Brain Sciences, 6*, 275–310.

Propst, L. R. (1980). The comparative efficacy of religious and nonreligious imagery for treatment of mild depression in religious individuals. *Cognitive Therapy and Research, 4*, 167–178.

Propst, L. R., Ostrom, R., Watkins, P., Dean, T., & Mashburn, D. (1992). Comparative efficacy of religious and nonreligious cognitive-behavioral therapy for the treatment of clinical depression in religious individuals. *Journal of Consulting and Clinical Psychology, 60(1)*, 94–103.

Raag, T., Pickens, J., Bendell, D., & Yando, R. (1997). Moderately dysphoric mothers behave more positively with their infants after completing the BDI. *Infant Mental Health Journal, 18(4),* 394–405.

Rachman, S. (1971). *The effects of psychological treatment.* Oxford: Perragon Press.

Randi, J. (1997) *Encyclopedia of claims, frauds, and hoaxes.* New York: St. Martin's Press.

Raue, P. J., Goldfried, M. R., & Barkham, M. (1997). The therapeutic alliance in psychodynamic-interpersonal and cognitive-behavioral therapy. *Journal of Consulting and Clinical Psychology, 65(4),* 582–587.

Reynolds, C. F., Miller, M. D., Pasternak, R. E., Frank, E., Perel, J. M., Cornes, C., Houck, P. R., et al. (1999). Treatment of bereavement-related major depressive episodes in later life: A controlled study of acute and continuation treatment with nortriptyline and interpersonal psychotherapy. *American Journal of Psychiatry, 156,* 202–208.

Reynolds, S., Barkham, M., Stiles, W. B., Shapiro, D. A., Hardy, G. E., & Rees, A. (1996). Acceleration of changes in session impact during contrasting time-limited psychotherapies. *Journal of Consulting and Clinical Psychology, 64,* 577–586.

Rieff, P. (1966). *Triumph of the therapeutic: Uses of faith after Freud.* New York: Harper and Row.

Rizvi, S. L., Peterson, C. B., Crow, S. J., & Agras, W. S. (2000). Test-retest reliability of the eating disorder examination. *International Journal of Eating Disorders, 28(3),* 311–316.

Robinson, L. A., Berman, J. S., & Neimeyer, R. A. (1990). Psychotherapy for the treatment of depression: A comprehensive review of controlled outcome research. *Psychological Bulletin, 108,* 30–49.

Rosen, J. C., Vara, L., & Wendt, S. (1990). Validity studies of the eating disorder examination. *International Journal of Eating Disorders, 9(5),* 519–528.

Rosenthal, R. (2003). Covert communication in laboratories, classrooms, and the truly real world. *Current Directions in Psychological Science, 12(5),* 151–154.

Rosenthal, R., & Rubin, D. B. (1978). Interpersonal expectancy effects: The first 345 studies. *Behavioral and Brain Sciences, 3,* 377–386.

Rossi, P. H. (1994). Review of the book *Families in crisis. Children and Youth Services Review, 16(5/6),* 461–465.

Rubovits-Seitz, P. F. D. (1998). *Depth-psychological understanding: Methodologic grounding of clinical interpretations.* Hillsdale, NJ: Analytic Press.

Rudd, D. M., Rajab, M. H., Orman, D. T., Joiner, T., Stulman, D. A., & Dixon, W. (1996). Effectiveness of an outpatient intervention targeting suicidal young adults: Preliminary results. *Journal of Consulting and Clinical Psychology, 64(1),* 179–190.

Sacco, W. P. (1981). Invalid use of the Beck Depression Inventory to identify depressed college-student subjects: A methodological comment. *Cognitive Therapy and Research, 5(2),* 143–147.

Salkovskis, P. M. (1996). *Frontiers of cognitive therapy.* New York: Guilford Press.

Sanders, M. R., Markie-Dadds, C., Tully, L. A., & Bor, W. (2000). The triple p-positive program: A comparison of enhanced, standard, and self-directed behavioral family intervention for parents of children with early onset conduct problems. *Journal of Consulting and Clinical Psychology, 68(4)*, 624–640.

Sanders, M. R., Shepherd, R. W., Cleghorn, G., & Woolford, H. (1994). The treatment of recurrent abdominal pain in children: A controlled comparison of cognitive-behavioral family intervention and standard pediatric care. *Journal of Consulting and Clinical Psychology, 62(2)*, 306–314.

Schmidt, N. B., & Woolaway-Bickel, K. (2000). The effects of treatment compliance on outcome in cognitive-behavioral therapy for panic disorder: Quality versus quantity. *Journal of Consulting and Clinical Psychology, 68(1)*, 13–18.

Schmitter-Edgecombe, M., Fahy, J. F., Whelan, J. P., & Long, C. J. (1995). Memory remediation after severe closed head injury: Notebook training versus supportive therapy. *Journal of Consulting and Clinical Psychology, 63(3)*, 484–489.

Schooler, N. R., Keith, S. J., Severe, J. B., Matthews, S. M., Bellack, A. S., Glick, I. D., Hargreaves, W. A., et al. (1997). Relapse and rehospitalization during maintenance treatment of schizophrenia. *Archives of General Psychiatry, 54*, 453–463.

Shulberg, H. C., Block, M. R., Madonna, M. J., Scott, C. P., Rodriguez, E., Imber, S. D., Perel, J., et al. (1996). Treating major depression in primary care practice: Eight-month clinical outcomes. *Archives of General Psychiatry, 53*, 913–919.

Scott, A. I., & Freeman, C. P. (1992). Edinburgh primary care depression study: Treatment outcome, patient satisfaction, and cost after 16 weeks. *British Medical Journal, 304*, 883–887.

Scott, J., Williams, J. M. G., & Beck, A. T. (1989). *Cognitive therapy in clinical practice.* New York: Routledge.

Sensky, T., Turkington, D., Kingdom, D., Scott, J. L., Scott, J., Siddle, R., et al. (2000). A randomized controlled trial of cognitive-behavioral therapy for persistent symptoms in schizophrenia resistant to medication. *Archives of General Psychiatry, 57*, 165–172.

Sexton, Harold. (1993). Exploring psychotherapeutic change sequence: Relating process to intersessional and posttreatment outcome. *Journal of Consulting and Clinical Psychology, 61(1)*, 128–136.

Shapiro, D. A., Barkham, M., Rees, A., Hardy, G. E., Reynolds, S., & Startup, M. (1994). Effects of treatment duration and severity of depression on the effectiveness of cognitive-behavioral and psychodynamic-interpersonal psychotherapy. *Journal of Consulting and Clinical Psychology, 62(3)*, 522–534.

Shear, K. M., Brown, T. A., Barlow, D. H., Money, R., Sholomskas, D. E., Woods, S. W., Gorman, J. M., et al. (1997). Multicenter collaborative panic disorder severity scale. *American Journal of Psychiatry, 154(11)*, 1571–1575.

Shear, K. M., Houck, P., Greeno, C., & Masters, S. (2001). Emotion-focused psychotherapy for patients with panic disorder. *American Journal of Psychiatry, 158(12)*, 1993–1998.

Shefler, G., Dasberg, H., & Ben-Shakhar, G. (1995). A randomized controlled outcome and follow-up study of Mann's time-limited psychotherapy. *Journal of Consulting and Clinical Psychology, 63(4), 585–593.*

Shier, D. A. (1969). Applying systematic exclusion to a case of bizarre behavior. In John D. Krumboltz & Carl E. Thoresen (Eds.), *Behavioral counseling: Cases and techniques* (pp. 114–123). New York: Holt, Rinehart and Winston.

Shulberg, H. C., Block, M. R., Madonia, M. J., Scott, C. P., Rodriguez, E., Imber, S. D., Perel, J., et al. (1996). Treating major depression in primary care practice: Eight-month clinical outcomes. *Archives of General Psychiatry, 53, 913–919.*

Sidman, M. (1960). *Tactics of scientific research: Evaluating experimental data in psychology.* New York: Basic Books.

Skinner, B. F. (1938). *The behavior of organisms.* Cambridge, MA: Harvard University Press.

Skutle, A., & Berg, G. (1987). Training in controlled drinking for early-stage problem drinking. *British Journal of Addiction, 82, 493–502.*

Smith, M. L., & Glass, G. V. (1977). Meta-analysis of psychotherapy outcome studies. *American Psychologist, 32(9), 752–760.*

Smith, M. L., & Glass, G. V., & Miller, T. I. (1980). *The benefits of psychotherapy.* Baltimore, MD: Johns Hopkins University Press.

Sobell, L. C., Sobell, M. B., & Riley, D. M. (1988). The reliability of alcohol abusers' self-reports of drinking and life events that occurred in the distant past. *Journal of Studies on Alcohol, 49(3), 225–232.*

Solms, M. (2004). Freud returns. *Scientific American, May, 82–88.*

Sotsky, S. M., Glass, D. R., Shea, T., Pilkonis, P. A., Collins, J. F., Elkin, I., Watkins, J. T., et al. (1991). Patient predictors of response to psychotherapy and pharmacotherapy: Findings in the NIMH Treatment of Depression Collaborative Research Program. *American Journal of Psychiatry 148(8), 997–1008.*

Spitzer, R. L., Forman, J. B., & Nee, J. (1979). DSM-III field trials: I. Initial interrater diagnostic reliability. *American Journal of Psychiatry, 136, 815–817.*

Spoth, R. L., Redmond, C., & Shin, C. (2001). Randomized trial of brief family interventions for general populations: Adolescent substance use outcomes 4 years following baseline. *Journal of Consulting and Clinical Psychology, 69(4), 627–642.*

Steer, R. A., Brown, G. K., & Beck, A. T. (2001). Mean Beck Depression Inventory-II scores by severity of major depressive disorder. *Psychological Reports, 88(3,pt.2), 1075–1076.*

Stein, L. I., & Test, M. A. (1980). Alternatives to mental hospital treatment. *Archives of General Psychiatry, 37, 392–412.*

Stephens, R. S., Roffman, R. A., & Simpson, E. E. (1994). Treating adult marijuana dependence: A test of the relapse prevention model. *Journal of Consulting and Clinical Psychology, (62)1, 92–99.*

Stern, R. S., Drummond, L. M., & Assin, M. (1991). *The practice of behavioral and cognitive psychotherapy.* New York: Cambridge University Press.

Stiles, W. B., Agnew-Dayles, R., Hardy, G. E., Barkham, M., & Shapiro, D. A. (1998). Relations of the alliance with psychotherapy outcome: Findings in the second Sheffield Psychotherapy Project. *Journal of Consulting and Clinical Psychology, 66(5),* 791–802.

Stiles, W. B., Shankland, M. C., Wright, J., & Field, S. D. (1997). Aptitude-treatment interactions based on clients' assimilation of their presenting problems. *Journal of Consulting and Clinical Psychology, 65(5),* 889–893.

Stiles, W. B., & Shapiro, D. A. (1994). Disabuse of the drug metaphor: Psychotherapy process-outcome correlations. *Journal of Consulting and Clinical Psychology, 62(5),* 942–948.

St. Lawrence, J. S., Brasfield, T. L., Jefferson, K. W., Alleyne, E., O'Bannon, III, R. E., & Shirley, A. (1995). Cognitive-behavioral intervention to reduce African American adolescents' risk for HIV infection. *Journal of Consulting and Clinical Psychology, 63(2),* 221–237.

Stone, M. H. (1997). *Healing the mind: A history of psychiatry from antiquity to the present.* New York: W. W. Norton.

Strupp, H. H., & Hadley, S. W. (1979). Specific vs. nonspecific factors in psychotherapy. *Archives of General Psychiatry, 36,* 1125–1136.

Stuart, R. B. (1973). *Trick or treatment.* Champaign, IL: Research Press.

Sylvain, C., Ladouceur, R., & Boisvert, J-M. (1997). Cognitive and behavioral treatment of pathological gambling: A controlled study. *Journal of Consulting and Clinical Psychology, 65(4),* 727–732.

Szasz, T. S. (1974). *The myth of mental illness.* New York: Harper and Row.

———. (1978). *The myth of psychotherapy.* Garden City, NY: Anchor Press.

Tanaka-Matsumi, J. & Kameoka, V. A. (1986). Reliabilities and concurrent validities of popular self-report measures of depression, anxiety, and social desirability. *Journal of Consulting and Clinical Psychology, 54(3),* 328–333.

Tarrier, N., Pilgrim, H., Sommerfield, C., Faragher, B., Reynolds, M., Graham, E., & Barrowclough, C. (1999). A randomized trial of cognitive therapy and imaginal exposure in the treatment of chronic posttraumatic stress disorder. *Journal of Consulting and Clinical Psychology, 67,* 13–18.

Teasdale, J. D., & Barnard, P. J. (1993). *Affect, cognition, and change: Re-modelling depressive thought.* Hillsdale, NJ: Lawrence Erlbaum Associates.

Teitelbaum, S. T. (1999). *Illusion and disillusionment: Core issues in psychotherapy.* Northvale, NJ: Transaction Publishers.

Telch, M. J., Schmidt, N. B., Jaimez, T. L., Jacquin, K. M., & Harrington, P. J. (1995). Impact of cognitive-behavioral treatment on quality of life in panic disorder patients. *Journal of Consulting and Clinical Psychology, 63(5),* 823–830.

Thase, M. E., Greenhouse, J. B., Frank, E., Reynolds, C. F., III, Pilkonis, P. A., Hurley, K., Grochocinski, V., et al. (1997). Treatment of major depression with psychotherapy or psychotherapy-pharmacotherapy combinations. *Archives of General Psychiatry, 54,* 1009–1015.

Tichenor, V., Marmar, C. R., Weiss, D. S., Metzler, T. J., & Ronfeldi, H. M. (1996). The relationship of peritraumatic dissociation and posttraumatic stress: Findings in female Vietnam theater veterans. *Journal of Consulting and Clinical Psychology,* 64(5), 1054–1059.

Toro, P. A., Passero Rabideau, J. M., Bellavia, C. W., Daeschler, C. V., Wall, D. D., Thomas, D. M., & Smith, S. J. (1997). Evaluating an intervention for homeless persons: Results of a field experiment. *Journal of Consulting and Clinical Psychology,* 65(3), 476–484.

Turk, D. C., Rudy, T. E., Kubinski, J. A., Zaki, H. S., & Greco, C. M. (1996). Dysfunctional patients with temporomandibular disorders: Evaluating the efficacy of a tailored treatment protocol. *Journal of Consulting and Clinical Psychology,* 64(1), 139–146.

Wadden, T. A., Foster, G. D., & Letizia, K. A. (1994). One-year behavioral treatment of obesity: Comparison of moderate and severe caloric restriction and the effects of weight management therapy. *Journal of Consulting and Clinical Psychology,* 62(1), 165–171.

Wadden, T. A., Vogt, R. A., Andersen, R. E., Bartlett, S. J., Foster, G. D., Kuehnel, R. H., Wilk, J., et. al. (1997). Exercise in the treatment of obesity: Effects of four interventions on body composition, resting energy expenditure, appetite, and mood. *Journal of Consulting and Clinical Psychology,* 65(2), 269–277.

Wagle, A. C., Ho, L. W., & Wagle, S. A. (2000). Psychometric behaviour of BDI in Alzheimer's disease patients with depression. *International Journal of Geriatric Psychiatry,* 15(1), 63–69.

Waldron, H. B., Slesnick, N., Brody, J. L., Turner, C., & Peterson, T. R. (2001). Treatment outcomes for adolescent substance abuse at 4- and 7-month assessments. *Journal of Consulting and Clinical Psychology,* 69(5), 802–813.

Walker, J. G., Johnson, S., & Manion, I. (1996). Emotionally focused marital intervention for couples with chronically ill children. *Journal of Consulting and Clinical Psychology,* 64(5), 1029–1036.

Wallerstein, R. S. (1986). *Forty-two lives in treatment: A study of psychoanalysis and psychotherapy.* New York: Guilford Press.

———. (1995). *The talking cures.* New Haven, CT: Yale University Press.

Walsh, B. T., Wilson, T., Loeb, K. L., Devlin, M. J., Pike, K. M., Roose, S. P., Fleiss, J., et al. (1997). Medication and psychotherapy in the treatment of bulimia nervosa. *American Journal of Psychiatry,* 154(4), 523–531.

Ward, S. C. (2002). *Modernizing the mind: Psychological knowledge and the remaking of society.* Westport, CT: Praeger.

Weber, J. J., Solomon, M., & Bachrach, H. M. (1985). Factors associated with the outcome of psychoanalysis: Report of the Columbia Psychoanalytic Center Research Project (I). *International Review of Psychoanalysis,* 12, 13–26.

Weber, J. J., Bachrach, H. M., & Solomon, M. (1985a). Factors associated with the outcome of psychoanalysis: Report of the Columbia Psychoanalytic Center Research Project (II). *International Review of Psychoanalysis,* 12, 127–141.

———. (1985b). Factors associated with the outcome of psychoanalysis: Report of the Columbia Psychoanalytic Center Research Project (III). *International Review of Psychoanalysis, 12,* 251–262.

Webster-Stratton, C. (1998). Preventing conduct problems in Head Start children: Strengthening parenting competencies. *Journal of Consulting and Clinical Psychology, 66(5),* 715–730.

Webster-Stratton, C., & Hammond, M. (1997). Treating children with early-onset conduct problems: A comparison of child and parent training interventions. *Journal of Consulting and Clinical Psychology, 65(1),* 93–109.

Wechsler, H., Nelson, T. F., Lee, J. E., Seibring, M., Lewis, C., & Keeling, R. P. (2003). Perception and reality: A national evaluation of social norms marketing interventions to reduce college students' heavy alcohol use. *Journal of Studies on Alcohol, 64(4),* 484–494.

Weersing, V. R., & Weisz, J. R. (2002). Community clinic treatment of depressed youth: Benchmarking usual care against CBT clinical trials. *Journal of Consulting and Clinical Psychology, 70(2),* 299–310.

Weissman, M. M., Prusoff, B. A., DiMascio, A., Neu, C., Goklaney, M., & Klerman, G. L. (1979). The efficacy of drugs and psychotherapy in the treatment of acute depressive episodes. *American Journal of Psychiatry, 136,* 555–558.

Weisz, J. R., Thurber, C. A., Sweeney, L., Proffitt, V. D., & LeGagnoux, G. L. (1997). Brief treatment of mild-to-moderate child depression using primary and secondary control enhancement training. *Journal of Consulting and Clinical Psychology, 65(4),* 703–707.

Whisman, M. A., Miller, I. W., Norman, W. H., & Keitner, G. I. (1991). Cognitive therapy with depressed inpatients: Specific effects on dysfunctional cognitions. *Journal of Consulting and Clinical Psychology, 59(2),* 282–288.

Wiborg, I. M., & Dahl, A. A. (1996). Does brief dynamic psychotherapy reduce the relapse rate of panic disorder? *Archives of General Psychiatry, 53,* 689–694.

Wilfley, D. E., Agras, W. S., Telch, C. F., Rossiter, E. M., Schneider, J. A., Golomb, A., Cole, A. G., et al. (1993). Group cognitive-behavioral therapy and group interpersonal psychotherapy for the nonpurging bulimic individual: A controlled comparison. *Journal of Consulting and Clinical Psychology, 61(2),* 296–305.

Willemsen-Swinkels, S. H. N., Buitelaar, J. K., Nijhof, G. J., & Van England, H. (1995). Failure of naltrexone hydrochloride to reduce self-injurious and autistic behavior in mentally retarded adults. *Archives of General Psychiatry, 52,* 766–773.

Williams, G. M. (1946). *Priestess of the occult.* New York: Alfred Knopf.

Williams, J. B., Gibbon, M., First, M. B., Spitzer, R. L., Davies, M., Borus, J., Howes, M. J., et al. (1992). The structured clinical interview for DSM-III-R (SCID) II. Multisite test reliability. *Archives of General Psychiatry, 49(8),* 630–636.

Wilson, G. T., Fairburn, C. C., Agras, W. S., Walsh, B. T., & Kraemer, H. (2002). Cognitive-behavioral therapy for bulimia nervosa: Time course and mechanisms of change. *Journal of Consulting and Clinical Psychology, 70(2),* 267–274.

Wilson, S. A., Becker, L. A., & Tinker, R. H. (1995). Eye movement desensitization and reprocessing (EMDR) treatment for psychologically traumatized individuals. *Journal of Consulting and Clinical Psychology, 63(6),* 928–937.

Wing, R. R., & Marcus, M. D. (1992). A "family-based" approach to the treatment of obese type II diabetic patients. *Journal of Consulting and Clinical Psychology, 59(1),* 156–162.

Wing, R. R., & Marcus, M. D., & Epstein, L. H. (1991). A "family-based" approach to the treatment of obese Type II dialbetic patients. *Journal of Consulting and Clinical Psychology, 59(1),* 156–162.

Winter, L. B., Steer, R. A., & Jones-Hicks, L. (1999). Screening for major depression disorders in adolescent medical outpatients with the Beck Depression Inventory for primary care. *Journal of Adolescent Health, 24(6),* 389–394.

Winters, J., Fals-Stewart, W., O'Farrell, T. J., Birchler, G. R., & Kelley, M. L. (2002). Behavioral couples therapy for female substance-abusing patients: Effects on substance use and relationship adjustment. *Journal of Consulting and Clinical Psychology, 70(2),* 344–355.

Wittgenstein, L. (1980). *Remarks on the philosophy of psychology, volume II.* Chicago: University of Chicago Press.

Wolpe, J. (1958). *Psychotherapy by reciprocal inhibition.* Stanford, CA: Stanford University Press.

———. (1973). *The practice of behavior therapy.* New York: Pergamon Press.

Woody, G. E., Luborsky, L., McLellan, A. T., O'Brien, C. P., Beck, A. T., Blaine, J., Herman, I., et al. (1983). Psychotherapy for opiate addicts: Does it help? *Archives of General Psychiatry, 40,* 639–645.

Woody, G. E., McLellan, A. T., Luborsky, L., & O'Brien, C. P. (1995). Psychotherapy in community methadone programs: A validation study. *American Journal of Psychiatry, 152(9),* 1302–1308.

Writing Committee for the ENRICHED Investigators. (2003). Effects of treating depression and low perceived social support on clinical events after myocardial infarction. *Journal of the American Medical Association 289(23),* 3106–3116.

Zeig, J. K. (1997). *Evolution of psychotherapy: The third conference.* New York: Brunner/Mazel.

Zhu, S., Stretch, V., Balabanis, M., Rosbrook, B., Sadler, G., & Pierce, J. (1996). Telephone counseling for smoking cessation: Effects of single-session and multiple-session interventions. *Journal of Consulting and Clinical Psychology, 64(1),* 202–211.

Zilbergeld, B. (1983). *The shrinking of America: Myths of psychological change.* Boston: Little, Brown.

Zuroff, D. C., Blatt, S. J., Sotsky, S. M., Krupnick, J. L., Martin, D. J., Sanislow, III, C. A., & Simmens, S. (2000). Relation of therapeutic alliance and perfectionism to outcome in brief outpatient treatment of depression. *Journal of Consulting and Clinical Psychology, 68(1),* 114–124.

Moreau, D. 32–33
Morin, C. M., 99
Morral, A. R., 67–68
motivational enhancement therapy, 75–76
MTA Cooperative Group, 97–98
Mufson, L., 32–33
Multimodal Treatment Study of Children
    with Attention-Deficit-Hyperactivity
    Disorder Cooperative Group. See
    MTA Cooperative Group
Muñoz, R. F., 77–78
Murdock, M. 10
Murdock, T. B., 59–60
Mynor-Wallis, L. M., 22–23

Nation, Carrie, 84
National Institute of Mental Health, 57,
    97, 20–21, 24, 102. See also Treatment
    of Depression Collaborative Research
    Program
National Institute on Alcohol Abuse and
    Alcoholism, 82
National Institute on Drug Abuse, 102
Newcomb, M., 70–71
Nezu, A. M., 87, 177–78
Nickerson, R. S., 123
Norcross, J. C., 234n3
norms: in cognitive-behavioral therapy,
    206; cultural, in psychotherapy,
    220–21; social, programs, 80–84, 85
Noshirvani, H., 60
Novaco, R. W., 98
Nunn, L. B., 175–76

obesity. See eating disorders
objectivity in cognitive-behavioral therapy,
    207, 208, 209
O'Brien, C. P., 65–67
obsessions without overt compulsions, 96
obsessive-compulsive disorder, 96–97
Oedipal conflict, 143, 150
O'Farrell, T. J., 63–65
O'Hara, M. W., 43

Olafsson, R. P., 178–80
O'Malley, S. S., 75
operant conditioning. See conditioning
Orne, M. T., 41, 121–22
orphanages. See under children
Öst, L.-G., 58
Ostrom, R. 29–30

panic disorder, 53–54, 116–17; Severity
    Scale, 116–17
paranoid delusions, 147–48
parental skills training, 90–93, 177
Park, R. L., 4
Pastor, D. A., 110
pastoral counseling, 29–30
patient self-assessment: in cognitive-
    behavioral therapy, 200–201; in ther-
    apeutic relationships, 127–28
Patti, E. T., 87, 177–78
Paul, G. L., 189–90
Paykel, E. S., 40
Perri, M. G., 87, 177–78
personal responsibility: in psychodynamic
    psychotherapy, 155–58; and Work
    Opportunity Reconciliation Act
    (1996), 62–63
Peterson, C. B., 115
Peterson, T. R., 71–72
Petry, N. M., 68
Pfeffer, A. Z., 153
phobias: adolescent, 58; behavioral
    therapy, 172–73, 179, 181–83; social,
    48–52. See also panic disorder
Pilgrim, H., 176
placebo. See under controls
Pope, H. G., 11
Popper, K. R., 9, 147–48, 233n1
post-traumatic stress disorder (PTSD),
    58–60, 176
PP. See psychodynamic psychotherapy
Preparing for the Drug Free Years, 99–102
preschoolers at risk, 93–94. See also
    children